Women's Me~~~~~~~ ŋ

Editors

SUSAN G. KORNSTEIN
ANITA H. CLAYTON

PSYCHIATRIC CLINICS
OF NORTH AMERICA

www.psych.theclinics.com

Consulting Editor
HARSH K. TRIVEDI

September 2023 • Volume 46 • Number 3

ELSEVIER

1600 John F. Kennedy Boulevard • Suite 1800 • Philadelphia, Pennsylvania, 19103-2899

http://www.theclinics.com

PSYCHIATRIC CLINICS OF NORTH AMERICA Volume 46, Number 3
September 2023 ISSN 0193-953X, ISBN-13: 978-0-443-18332-4

Editor: Megan Ashdown
Developmental Editor: Malvika Shah

© **2023 Elsevier Inc. All rights reserved.**

This periodical and the individual contributions contained in it are protected under copyright by Elsevier, and the following terms and conditions apply to their use:

Photocopying

Single photocopies of single articles may be made for personal use as allowed by national copyright laws. Permission of the Publisher and payment of a fee is required for all other photocopying, including multiple or systematic copying, copying for advertising or promotional purposes, resale, and all forms of document delivery. Special rates are available for educational institutions that wish to make photocopies for non-profit educational classroom use. For information on how to seek permission visit www.elsevier.com/permissions or call: (+44) 1865 843830 (UK)/(+1) 215 239 3804 (USA).

Derivative Works

Subscribers may reproduce tables of contents or prepare lists of articles including abstracts for internal circulation within their institutions. Permission of the Publisher is required for resale or distribution outside the institution. Permission of the Publisher is required for all other derivative works, including compilations and translations (please consult www.elsevier.com/permissions).

Electronic Storage or Usage

Permission of the Publisher is required to store or use electronically any material contained in this periodical, including any article or part of an article (please consult www.elsevier.com/permissions). Except as outlined above, no part of this publication may be reproduced, stored in a retrieval system or transmitted in any form or by any means, electronic, mechanical, photocopying, recording or otherwise, without prior written permission of the Publisher.

Notice

No responsibility is assumed by the Publisher for any injury and/or damage to persons or property as a matter of products liability, negligence or otherwise, or from any use or operation of any methods, products, instructions or ideas contained in the material herein. Because of rapid advances in the medical sciences, in particular, independent verification of diagnoses and drug dosages should be made.

Although all advertising material is expected to conform to ethical (medical) standards, inclusion in this publication does not constitute a guarantee or endorsement of the quality or value of such product or of the claims made of it by its manufacturer.

Psychiatric Clinics of North America (ISSN 0193-953X) is published quarterly by Elsevier Inc., 360 Park Avenue South, New York, NY 10010-1710. Months of issue are March, June, September, and December. Business and Editorial Offices: 1600 John F. Kennedy Blvd., Suite 1800, Philadelphia, PA 19103-2899. Periodicals postage paid at New York, NY and additional mailing offices. Subscription prices are $352.00 per year (US individuals), $781.00 per year (US institutions), $100.00 per year (US students/residents), $422.00 per year (Canadian individuals), $519.00 per year (international individuals), $983.00 per year (Canadian & international institutions), and $220.00 per year (international students/residents), $100.00 per year (Canadian & students/residents). Foreign air speed delivery is included in all *Clinics'* subscription prices. All prices are subject to change without notice. **POSTMASTER:** Send address changes to *Psychiatric Clinics of North America*, Elsevier Health Sciences Division, Subscription Customer Service, 3251 Riverport Lane, Maryland Heights, MO 63043. **Customer Service: 1-800-654-2452 (US). From outside the United States, call 1-314-447-8871. Fax: 1-314-447-8029. E-mail: journalscustomerservice-usa@elsevier.com (for print support)** and **journalsonlinesupport-usa@elsevier.com (for online support)**.

Reprints. For copies of 100 or more, of articles in this publication, please contact the Commercial Reprints Department, Elsevier Inc., 360 Park Avenue South, New York, New York 10010-1710. Tel.: 212-633-3874, Fax: 212-633-3820, E-mail: reprints@elsevier.com.

Psychiatric Clinics of North America is covered in *MEDLINE/PubMed (Index Medicus)*, *Current Contents/Social and Behavioral Sciences*, *Social Science Citation Index*, *Embase/Excerpta Medica,* and PsycINFO.

Contributors

CONSULTING EDITOR

HARSH K. TRIVEDI, MD, MBA
President and Chief Executive Officer, Sheppard Pratt, Clinical Professor of Psychiatry, University of Maryland School of Medicine, Baltimore, Maryland, USA

EDITORS

SUSAN G. KORNSTEIN, MD
Professor of Psychiatry and Obstetrics/Gynecology, Executive Director, Institute for Women's Health, Virginia Commonwealth University School of Medicine, Richmond, Virginia, USA

ANITA H. CLAYTON, MD
Wilford W. Spradlin Professor and Chair, Department of Psychiatry & Neurobehavioral Sciences, Professor of Clinical Obstetrics & Gynecology, University of Virginia School of Medicine, Charlottesville, Virginia, USA

AUTHORS

ELIZABETH ALPERT, PhD
National Center for PTSD Women's Health Sciences Division at VA Boston Healthcare System, Boston University Chobanian and Avedisian School of Medicine, Boston, Massachusetts, USA

ALLISON L. BAIER, PhD
National Center for PTSD Women's Health Sciences Division at VA Boston Healthcare System, Boston University Chobanian and Avedisian School of Medicine, Boston, Massachusetts, USA

NINA BALLONE, MD
Assistant Professor, Department of Psychiatry and Behavioral Science, Johns Hopkins University, Baltimore, Maryland, USA

RUTH M. BENCA, MD, PhD
Professor, Department of Psychiatry and Behavioral Medicine, Wake Forest School of Medicine, Winston-Salem, North Carolina, USA

KELLIE E. CARLYLE, PhD, MPH
Professor, Department of Social and Behavioral Health, Virginia Commonwealth University, Richmond, Virginia, USA

JULIA A.C. CASE, PhD
Postdoctoral Fellow, Gender Identity Program, Department of Psychiatry, Columbia University Irving Medical Center, New York, New York, USA

CAROLINE F. CENTENO, BS
Department of Psychiatry and Neurobehavioral Sciences, UVA Cancer Center, University of Virginia School of Medicine and Health System, Charlottesville, Virginia, USA

ABIGAIL H. CONLEY, PhD
Associate Professor, Department of Counseling and Special Education, Virginia Commonwealth University, Richmond, Virginia, USA

GARY CUDDEBACK, PhD, MSW, MPH
Associate Dean for Research and Professor, School of Social Work, Virginia Commonwealth University, Richmond, Virginia, USA

PAMELA DILLON, PharmD
Wright Center for Clinical and Translational Research, Virginia Commonwealth University, Richmond, Virginia, USA

GIHAN ELNAHAS, MD
Professor of Psychiatry, Head of Women Mental Health Program, NeuroPsychiatry, Department Faculty of Medicine, Ain Shams University, Egypt; Secretary of International Association for Women Mental Health

TARA E. GALOVSKI, PhD
National Center for PTSD Women's Health Sciences Division at VA Boston Healthcare System, Boston University Chobanian and Avedisian School of Medicine, Boston, Massachusetts, USA

GABRIELLE HASHMAN, MSc
Medical Student, Medical School for International Health, Faculty of Health Sciences, Ben-Gurion University of the Negev, Beer Sheva, Israel; Mathison Centre for Mental Health Research and Education, University of Calgary, Calgary, Alberta, Canada

NANCY A. HAUG, PhD
Department of Psychology, Palo Alto University, Palo Alto, California, USA

MASHAEL HUSSAIN, MBBS
Clinical Research Assistant, Department of Psychiatry, University of Calgary, Calgary, Alberta, Canada

JENNIFER V.A. KEMP, MSc
Clinical Research Assistant, Department of Psychiatry, University of Calgary, Calgary, Alberta, Canada

SUSAN G. KORNSTEIN, MD
Professor of Psychiatry and Obstetrics/Gynecology, Executive Director, Institute for Women's Health, Virginia Commonwealth University School of Medicine, Richmond, Virginia

VIVEK KUMAR, MBBS, MPH
Clinical Research Coordinator, Department of Psychiatry, University of Calgary, Calgary, Alberta, Canada

KAREEN M. MATOUK, PhD
Assistant Professor in Medical Psychology (in Psychiatry), Assistant Program Director, Gender Identity Program, Clinical Psychologist, Department of Psychiatry, Columbia University Irving Medical Center, New York, New York, USA

GRETCHEN N. NEIGH, PhD
Associate Professor, Department of Anatomy and Neurobiology, Virginia Commonwealth University, Richmond, Virginia, USA

PAUL OKOYEH, MD
Post-Doctoral Fellow, Department of Psychiatry and Behavioral Medicine, Wake Forest School of Medicine, Winston-Salem, North Carolina, USA

JENNIFER L. PAYNE, MD
Professor and Vice Chair of Research, Department of Psychiatry and Neurobehavioral Sciences, University of Virginia, Charlottesville, Virginia, USA

DAVID R. PENBERTHY, MD, MBA
Associate Professor of Radiation Oncology, Medical Director of Radiation Oncology, Department of Radiation Oncology, Penn State Cancer Institute, Penn State Health Milton S. Hershey College of Medicine, Hershey, Pennsylvania, USA

JENNIFER KIM PENBERTHY, PhD
Chester F. Carlson Professor of Psychiatry and Neurobehavioral Sciences, Department of Psychiatry and Neurobehavioral Sciences, UVA Cancer Center, University of Virginia School of Medicine and Health System, Charlottesville, Virginia, USA

KATHARINE A. PHILLIPS, MD
Professor of Psychiatry, DeWitt Wallace Senior Scholar, NewYork-Presbyterian/Weill Cornell Medical Center, Weill Cornell Medical College, Weill Cornell Psychiatry Specialty Center, New York, New York, USA

KATHRYN POLAK, PhD
Postdoctoral Fellow, Department of Psychiatry, Virginia Commonwealth University, Richmond, Virginia, USA

ERICA RICHARDS, MD, PhD
Assistant Professor, Department of Psychiatry and Behavioral Science, Johns Hopkins University Baltimore, Maryland, USA

MEREDITH E. RUMBLE, PhD
Associate Professor, Department of Psychiatry, University of Wisconsin-Madison, Madison, Wisconsin, USA

APRIL SALEEM, BSc
Graduate Student, Department of Pathology and Molecular Medicine, Gastrointestinal Disease Research Unit (GIDRU), Queen's University, Kingston, Ontario, Canada

JULIE K. SCHULMAN, MD
Assistant Professor of Psychiatry, CUIMC/Columbia University Vagelos College of Physicians and Surgeons, Attending, Consultation-Liaison Psychiatry, NewYork-Presbyterian/Columbia University Irving Medical Center, New York, New York, USA

MARY V. SEEMAN, OC, MDCM, DSc
Professor Emerita, Department of Psychiatry, University of Toronto, Toronto, Ontario
Canada

CLAUDIO N. SOARES, MD, PhD, FRCPC, MBA
Professor and Head, Department of Psychiatry, Queen's University School of Medicine,
Kingston, Ontario, Canada

HANNAH STADTLER, BS
Graduate Student, Department of Anatomy and Neurobiology, Virginia Commonwealth
University, Richmond, Virginia, USA

ANNE LOUISE STEWART, MD
Assistant Professor, Department of Psychiatry and Neurobehavioral Sciences, UVA
Cancer Center, University of Virginia School of Medicine and Health System, University of
Virginia, Charlottesville, Virginia, USA

NADA LOGAN STOTLAND, MD, MPH
Formerly, Professor of Psychiatry, Rush University, Chicago, Illinois, USA

LEAH C. SUSSER, MD
Assistant Professor of Clinical Psychiatry, NewYork-Presbyterian/Weill Cornell Medical
Center, Weill Cornell Medical College, Outpatient Department, White Plains, New York,
USA

DACE S. SVIKIS, PhD
Professor, Department of Psychology, Deputy Director, Institute for Women's Health,
Virginia Commonwealth University, Richmond, Virginia, USA

VALERIE H. TAYLOR, MD, PhD
Professor and Head, Department of Psychiatry, University of Calgary, Calgary, Alberta,
Canada

FLORENCE THIBAUT, MD, PhD
Professor of Psychiatry, University Paris Cité, INSERM U1266 Institute of Psychiatry and
Neurosciences, Department of Psychiatry and Addiction, University Hospital Cochin (Site
Tarnier), AP-HP, Paris, France

Contents

> Women are at the highest risk of pandemic adversities as they represent the majority of health and frontline workers in addition to their essential roles at home. We review gender differences during the COVID-19 pandemic by demonstrating risk-exposure during specific situations such as pregnancy, women's mental health fallouts, COVID-19 disease itself and exposure to different forms of violence. We discuss the particularities that women face in developing countries with depicted examples from some countries in Africa and the Middle East. Women mental health care service stands out as an essential component of the national response to pandemics. Women's integration and leadership in the national pandemic response planning is crucial.

> This review highlights the existing knowledge and data that explain the physiologic impacts of stress, especially pertaining to neurobiology, and how these impacts differ by sex. Furthermore, this review explains the benefits of interventions aimed at preventing or mitigating the adverse effects of stress, because of both the significant toll of stress on the body and the disproportionate impact of these changes experienced by women.

> Perinatal depression is a common psychiatric condition that has negative effects on pregnancy and infant outcomes. Screening for the condition is relatively easy and should be done routinely in all medical care of the pregnant and postpartum woman and her infant. The risk–benefit analysis favors the use of antidepressant medications during pregnancy and lactation compared with the risk of untreated maternal depression. Other, non-pharmacological treatments will be discussed as well as new treatments, including a new class of medications that act on the inhibitory GABAergic neurotransmitter system.

> Depression is a disabling condition that often leads to significant burden. Women are more vulnerable to depression during reproductive-related "windows of vulnerability" such as the menopause transition and early postmenopausal years. This heightened vulnerability can be attributed, at least in

part, to the neuromodulatory effects of estrogen on mood and cognition and the exposure to rapid fluctuations of estradiol levels during midlife years. The management of midlife depression can be challenging due to the presence and severity of other complaints such as vasomotor symptoms and sleep disturbances. Psychopharmacologic, behavioral, and hormonal interventions should be part of the treatment armamentarium.

Men and women, for biologic and sociocultural reasons, differ in the nature of their risks for schizophrenia and also in their care needs. Women with schizophrenia have several reproduction-associated risks and care needs that require special clinical consideration. They also have several specific risks related to antipsychotics and gender-associated needs not necessarily related to biology. These require clinicians' diagnostic acumen, treatment skills, cultural sensitivity, and advocacy know-how. Although this does not pertain to everyone, awareness on the part of clinicians is essential. This article addresses the current evidence for difference.

Substance use disorder (SUD) is among the leading causes of premature morbidity and mortality and imposes significant health, economic, and social burdens. Gender differences have been found in the development, course, and treatment of SUD, with women at increased risk for physiologic and psychosocial consequences compared with men. Reasons for these differences are multifold and include biological, genetic, environmental, and behavioral factors. This article discusses SUD among women, emphasizing clinical considerations for care. Specific topics include epidemiology, sex and gender differences, common comorbidities, screening, diagnosis, treatment, pregnancy, and sociocultural factors.

Body dysmorphic disorder (BDD) consists of distressing or impairing preoccupation with perceived defects in physical appearance that are actually nonexistent or only slight. This common and often-severe disorder, which affects more women than men, frequently goes unrecognized. BDD is associated with marked impairment in functioning, poor quality of life, and high rates of suicidality. Most patients seek cosmetic treatment, which virtually never improves BDD symptoms. In contrast, serotonin-reuptake inhibitors, often at high doses, and cognitive behavioral therapy that is tailored to BDD's unique clinical features are often effective. This article provides a clinical overview of BDD, including BDD in women.

Women have increased risks for both sleep disturbances and disorders and for mental health issues throughout their lives, starting in adolescence.

Women have a higher prevalence of insomnia disorder and restless legs syndrome (RLS) versus men, and obstructive sleep apnea (OSA) is more likely as women age. Hormonal transitions are important to consider in women's sleep. For women, insomnia, OSA, and RLS are predictive of depression, and insomnia and sleep-disordered breathing are predictive of Alzheimer disease. These findings underscore the importance of assessment, treatment, and future research examining sleep and mental health in women, given their unique and increased vulnerability.

Obesity is a common comorbidity associated with mental illness. It is important to understand the many ways weight gain and obesity can impact the cause and course of mental illness in women, with a special focus on vulnerable life stages. Women seem disproportionally impacted by the weight gain side effects of medications, and issues such as weight gain are more likely to impact symptoms of mental illness, impacting self-esteem. This article summarizes the existing literature on the associations between women's mental health and obesity. Understanding this association will lead to better health outcomes.

Breast cancer is the most commonly diagnosed cancer in women. Associated psychological symptoms include stress, adjustment difficulties, anxiety, depression, impaired cognitive function, sleep disturbances, altered body image, sexual dysfunction, and diminished overall well-being. Distress screening and assessment identifies women who will benefit from therapeutic interventions. Addressing these symptoms improves compliance with treatment and outcomes including disease-related outcomes, psychological symptoms, and quality of life. The most effective treatments include teaching coping skills such as expressing emotion, along with other structured cognitive behavioral, interpersonal, and mindfulness approaches. Patients should be provided these psychosocial supports throughout their cancer journey.

Racial and ethnic disparities are apparent in many areas of health care. Within mental health, women experience increased rates of some mental health disorders particularly noted within the reproductive life cycle starting at puberty and ending with the menopause transition. Hormone and endocrine processes along with individual vulnerability and various stressors all likely play a major role. Among these women, a disproportionate number are racial and ethnic minorities in the United States. Cultural influences and systemic barriers are explored to provide competent and necessary mental health care for women.

PSYCHIATRIC CLINICS OF NORTH AMERICA

SERIES OF RELATED INTEREST

Child and Adolescent Psychiatric Clinics of North America
https://www.childpsych.theclinics.com/

Neurologic Clinics
https://www.neurologic.theclinics.com/

Advances in Psychiatry and Behavioral Health
https://www.advancesinpsychiatryandbehavioralhealth.com/

THE CLINICS ARE AVAILABLE ONLINE!
Access your subscription at:
www.theclinics.com

Preface

Women's Mental Health

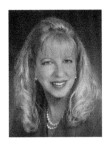
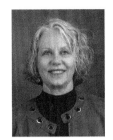

Susan G. Kornstein, MD   Anita H. Clayton, MD
Editors

This issue of *Psychiatric Clinics of North America* on Women's Mental Health represents our fourth issue on this topic in the past 20 years. Women's mental health has broadened in its scope beyond reproductive psychiatry, and research has revealed a greater understanding of sex differences in neuroendocrine systems and the multiple contributions of various factors to the onset of psychiatric illness. In addition, there have been exciting advances to improve the care of women, including the availability of the first medication approved by the FDA for postpartum depression. Progress has been made in addressing unmet needs, although other concerns have emerged, including the threat to women's reproductive rights, awareness of the significant impact of military service on women veterans, the collective trauma of the COVID-19 pandemic, disparities in the care of racial, ethnic, and sexual minorities, and the dramatic rise in substance use disorders (SUD) in women. Sex and gender differences have become increasingly evident in the onset, diagnosis, and course of mental health conditions, response to treatment, and long-term outcomes.

The issue begins with a focus on COVID-19 by Thibaut and El Nahas. The authors address the significant impact that COVID-19 has had on women's mental health, with increased rates of depression, anxiety, and posttraumatic stress disorder. Although men are at higher risk of severe COVID-19 symptoms and death, the risk of long-COVID is higher in women. Next, Stadtler and Neigh provide an overview of sex differences in the neurobiology of stress. They note that differences in neural plasticity related to hormonal differences between women and men may contribute to increased susceptibility of women to stress. Chronic stress can increase hypothalamic-pituitary-adrenal axis dysregulation and disrupt glucocorticoid balance in women, which negatively impacts neurobiology and cognition. Interventions aimed at mitigating chronic stress are warranted especially in women, considering the long-term physical effects of stress.

Psychiatr Clin N Am 46 (2023) xiii–xv
https://doi.org/10.1016/j.psc.2023.04.016
0193-953X/23/© 2023 Published by Elsevier Inc.

psych.theclinics.com

The next two articles present updates on reproductive mood disorders. Stewart and Payne review perinatal depression, which is common, is serious, and has negative effects on pregnancy and infant outcomes. Screening should be done routinely during pregnancy and the postpartum period. The risk-benefit analysis favors treatment with antidepressants during pregnancy and lactation over the risks of untreated maternal depression. Soares discusses menopause and mood, noting that women are more vulnerable to depression during the menopause transition and early post-menopausal years. The management of midlife depression includes psychopharmacologic, behavioral, and hormonal interventions, which can be especially challenging due to the presence of vasomotor symptoms and sleep disturbances.

The next several articles provide overviews of several different psychiatric disorders in women. Clinical considerations in the treatment of schizophrenia are summarized by Seeman. Women may experience delays in diagnosis and treatment due to atypical symptom presentation with preserved social skills and a broad range of affect. Women with schizophrenia have a number of risks and care needs related to reproductive function, as well as sex-specific side effects and sequelae related to the use of antipsychotics. Polak, Haug, Dillon, and Svikis discuss sex/gender differences in presentation and adverse consequences of SUD, as well as the need for gender-specific treatments to address the lower rates of treatment engagement and retention among women. They also emphasize the importance of universal screening to identify women with SUD. Phillips and Susser present an overview of body dysmorphic disorder, which is more common in women and is associated with marked functional impairment, poor quality of life, and high rates of suicidality. Most women with body dysmorphic disorder seek cosmetic surgery, which is ineffective and can make them worse, whereas serotonin reuptake inhibitors (SRIs) and cognitive behavioral therapy are often effective.

The next set of articles focuses on sleep, obesity, and breast cancer. The association between sleep and women's mental health is examined by Rumble, Okoyeh, and Benca. Women are more likely than men to experience insomnia disorder and restless legs syndrome, and obstructive sleep apnea is more likely as women age. Hormonal transitions are important to consider when evaluating sleep disturbances and disorders in women. The topic of obesity and women's mental health is reviewed by Kemp, Kumar, Saleem, Hashman, Hussain, and Taylor. Weight gain symptoms are common in depression and binge eating disorder, both of which are more prevalent in women than in men. Reproductive life stages can also impact weight gain in women. In addition, women are more likely to experience weight gain as a side effect of psychotropic medications. Penberthy, Stewart, Centeno, and Penberthy discuss psychological aspects of breast cancer. The most common psychological symptoms and disorders in women with breast cancer include anxiety, depression, cognitive impairment, adjustment disorders, sleep disturbance and associated fatigue, posttraumatic stress, body image issues, and sexual dysfunction. Addressing these disturbances can improve compliance with treatment, disease-related outcomes, and quality of life.

The final set of articles concentrates on the needs of specific populations, including racial and ethnic underrepresented minority women, sexual minority and transgender women, survivors of sex trafficking, women seeking abortion, and women veterans. Ballone and Richards discuss racial and ethnic disparities and women's mental health. They note that racial and ethnic minority women are more likely to experience psychiatric disorders but are less likely to receive treatment, and that mental health providers have a duty to educate themselves on how to provide culturally sensitive care to all women. Mental health disparities in sexual minority and transgender women and considerations for treatment are reviewed by Matouk, Schulman, and Case. Sexual minority and transgender women are at high risk of discrimination, marginalization, harassment, violence, and a wide range of mental health issues. They often avoid mental health treatment due to previous negative experiences or fears of discrimination. It is important for clinicians to seek out education to develop cultural competence in treating sexual minority and transgender patients. Conley, Carlyle, Cuddeback, and Kornstein discuss working with survivors of sex trafficking and the mental health implications. Sex trafficking is the most common form of human trafficking, and survivors experience significant physical, emotional, and sexual trauma that places them at increased risk of poor health outcomes. Clinicians should become familiar with screening protocols for trafficking and evidence-based, trauma-informed mental health treatment interventions. Stotland discusses reproductive rights and women's mental health. Barriers, misinformation, intrusion, and coercion affecting sex education, contraception, abortion, and perinatal care are an ongoing danger to women's mental and physical health. A solid body of evidence demonstrates that abortion does not cause mental illness. Mental health professionals should know the facts and laws affecting reproductive health care and be able to communicate them clearly to patients and help them to make informed decisions about their care. Psychiatric issues in women veterans are summarized by Alpert, Baier, and Galovski. Women veterans have unique life experiences and mental health needs, likely related to their high rates of exposure to traumatic events, including military sexual trauma, combat trauma, and intimate partner violence. It is important for providers to ask women patients about military history and to develop military cultural competence in order to maximize clinical outcomes.

We are grateful to the authors for their excellent contributions and to the publisher for granting us this opportunity. We hope that the readers will find this issue useful in their evaluation and treatment of women patients.

Susan G. Kornstein, MD
Department of Psychiatry and Institute for Women's Health
Virginia Commonwealth University School of Medicine
PO Box 980319
Richmond, VA 23298, USA

Anita H. Clayton, MD
Department of Psychiatry and Neurobehavioral Sciences and Obstetrics & Gynecology
University of Virginia School of Medicine
2955 Ivy Road, Suite 210
Charlottesville, VA 22903, USA

E-mail addresses:
susan.kornstein@vcuhealth.org (S.G. Kornstein)
ahc8v@uvahealth.org (A.H. Clayton)

Women's Mental Health and Lessons Learnt from the COVID-19 Pandemic

Florence Thibaut, MD, PhD[a,b,*], Gihan ELNahas, MD[c]

KEYWORDS

- COVID-19 • SARS-CoV-2 • Women • Mental health • Perinatal health • Africa
- Middle east • Violence

KEY POINTS

- Most pregnant women have asymptomatic or midly symptomatic COVID-19 disease but about 10% of them may present with severe disease. Preterm delivery, low birth weight may be observed in COVID + women. All these uncertainties have increased the risk of anxiety and/or depression or even PTSD in pregnant women. Prescription of contraception and medical abortions should be maintained during pandemics.
- Even if men were at higher risk of death and severe COVID-19 disease, the risk of long COVID is two times higher in women as compared to men.
- Anxiety, depression, and PTSD are more prevalent in women (especially in health care professionals), however, longitudinal studies will be necessary to conclude if there was only a transient increase of psychological symptoms due to a particularly stressful situation or if this will last in the long term.
- Females, young aged, and low- and middle-income countries have been the most affected by COVID 19-related mental health fallouts and economic crisis.

INTRODUCTION

The COVID-19 pandemic is an unprecedented health crisis that rapidly impacted every country around the globe in a matter of few weeks. Initially, the United Nations (UN) Director General drew attention to certain populations who will be the most impacted by the pandemic adversities namely, those living in poverty and in conflict zones, the elderly, children, and importantly frontline health workforce. The former UN Women Executive Director emphasized that women are at the highest risk as they represent the majority of health workers, in addition to being already burdened

a University Paris Cité, Paris, France; b INSERM U1266 Institute of Psychiatry and Neurosciences, Department of Psychiatry and Addiction, University Hospital Cochin (Site Tarnier), AP-HP; c NeuroPsychiatry Department Faculty of Medicine, Ain Shams University, Egypt
* Corresponding author. Hôpital Tarnier, 89 rue d'assas, Paris 75006, France.
E-mail address: florence.thibaut@aphp.fr

Psychiatr Clin N Am 46 (2023) 415–426
https://doi.org/10.1016/j.psc.2023.04.001
0193-953X/23/© 2023 Elsevier Inc. All rights reserved.

by their essential roles as parents and caregivers to other family members.[1] Developing countries were hit the hardest with the pandemic and its related fallouts, which extended to impact every sphere of lives. Importantly, the pandemic is not just a health crisis; it also brings drastic social and economic costs. The pandemic and its adverse impact continue to hit hard, and it is projected to drive up to 40 million people into extreme poverty across sub-Saharan Africa, with African women and girls being hit the hardest.[2] Our article will review the specific impact of COVID-19 pandemic on women and also the consequences of COVID-19 pandemic on women in different parts of the world capturing experiences from developed and developing countries.

THE SPECIFIC SITUATION OF PREGNANCY

The pandemic has been particularly distressing to pregnant women. Most pregnant women with SARS-CoV-2 infection are asymptomatic or mildly symptomatic. They often present with fever and cough and less often with myalgia and chill. Ma and colleagues[3] have conducted a metaanalysis in 19,884 individuals with confirmed COVID-19. The pooled percentage of asymptomatic infections was 54.1% in pregnant women as compared to 40.5% in the general population. Yet, Vouga and colleagues[4] reported 9.9% of severe COVID-19 disease in a cohort of 926 pregnant women positive for SARS-CoV-2. In these pregnant women, risk factors for severe COVID-19 were pulmonary comorbidities, hypertension, and diabetes. Symptomatic COVID-19 pregnant women were also more likely to experience hospitalization (RR 5.4), intensive care unit admission (RR 1.5), intubation and mechanical ventilation (RR 1.7), and even death.[5] Maternal death due to all causes was 11.3% in pregnant women as compared with 6.4% in non-pregnant hospitalized women.[6]

The adverse outcomes most often reported in pregnant women with SARS-CoV-2 infection were preterm delivery and low birth weight.[7] Other obstetric complications include stillbirth, miscarriage, preeclampsia-like syndrome, fetal growth restriction, coagulopathy, premature rupture of membranes and postpartum hemorrhage, all of which remained rare.[7,8] The severity of maternal disease was associated with a higher risk of cesarean section, preterm delivery and requirement of neonatal intensive care unit.

Maternal–fetal transmission was considered low during SARS-CoV-2 maternal infection; rate of SARS-CoV2 positive test in neonates born to mothers with COVID-19 was 8% in[6]; 2.9% in[4] and 6% in[9] respectively and two neonates died. Respiratory symptoms were observed in these COVID-positive neonates. Vivanti and colleagues[10] described a case of congenital COVID-19 infection associated with neurological symptoms following neonatal viremia and transplacental transmission. Magnetic resonance imaging showed bilateral lesions of the neonate brain white matter. The risk of bipolar disorders or schizophrenia during adolescence remains unknown after exposure to SARS-CoV2 during pregnancy.

The transmission of SARS-CoV-2 through breast milk remains unclear. The World Health Organization (WHO) considers that the benefit of breastfeeding is higher than the potential risk of maternal transmission whereas the Centers for Disease Control and Prevention recommends temporary separation of the newborn from a mother with confirmed or suspected COVID-19.[7]

All these uncertainties may have contributed to increased levels of stress which may in turn increase the risk of mental health problems in pregnant women and, of pregnancy terminations. Indeed, high levels of posttraumatic stress (43%), anxiety and depression (31%), were reported in 6894 pregnant women from 64 countries,[11] while 86% were somewhat or very worried about medical care and their future babies. A pooled prevalence of 25% to 30% for depression and 34% to 42% for anxiety was reported in pregnant women during the pandemic[12] (prevalence two times higher in pregnant vs nonpregnant women).[13,14]; Berthelot and colleagues[15] have compared 1258 women recruited online during the pandemic with 496 pre–COVID-19 pregnant women and reported higher levels of depressive and anxiety symptoms (OR:1.94). Previous psychiatric diagnosis or low income were risk factors for elevated distress and psychiatric symptoms during the COVID-19 pandemic.[15,16] In contrast, several studies have reported a lower prevalence of anxiety, depression, insomnia, or PTSD in pregnant woman during the first lockdown compared to nonpregnant women or prepandemic rates.[17,18]

It is also of upmost importance to note that the COVID-19 pandemic was associated with major disruptions in access to essential health services including family planning, mental health services, and perinatal health services.[19] Furthermore, the notable limited access to women-specific critical services may have resulted in riskier home births and an increase in maternal mortality.[20] In addition, it is reported that institutional deliveries dropped below prepandemic levels in 6 out of 10 sub-Saharan African countries.[21]

Even before the COVID-19 pandemic, several countries had limited access to sexual and reproductive health services, and social stigma on sexuality was observed in certain communities. During the pandemic, the United Nations Population Fund estimated that 12 million women in 115 countries have lost access to birth control and 1.4 million unplanned pregnancies might have occurred during the pandemic. Moreover, abortion was considered as non-essential in many countries during the lockdown periods.[22] These social factors have increased the risk of psychiatric symptoms in women.

Women at Increased Risk of Psychiatric Symptoms During the COVID-19 Pandemic?

COVID-19 disease was associated with a significant increase in the prevalence of both anxiety and depressive symptoms in the general population. Most studies have reported a gender effect in the increased prevalence of psychological distress, anxiety, and depressive symptoms or loneliness during the lockdowns but most studies were conducted in Europe, China, and North America, were cross-sectional and based on self reports[23](female gender was a risk factor)[24]; (OR 1.48 for women and anxiety).[25–27]; Finally, in a review of 2020 Western European and North American studies, females were more affected than males for major depressive and anxiety disorders respectively (29.8% vs 24% and 27.9% vs 21.7%).[28] In contrast several studies did not report any gender effect.[29]

In developing countries, mental ill-being has been, and continues to be a major fallout of the pandemic. This comes as a result of the direct pandemic-related adversities, which challenges human coping and adaptation, and heightens the sense of threat, uncertainty, and negative expectations. The World Health Organization (WHO) provided evidence that females, young aged and low- and middle-income countries (LMICs) were the most affected by COVID 19-related mental health fallouts.[30] A study of the mental health impact of COVID-19 in 7 Arab countries reveals that COVID-19 traumatic stress significantly contributes to increased mental distress. This effect correlates with population density and economic status.[31] Ethiopia's Amhara reported high levels of anxiety and depression with a three-fold increase compared to prepandemic levels.[32] Similarly, there are heightened levels of depression and anxiety among women when comparing pre to postpandemic studies in Pakistan.[32,33]

A significantly higher prevalence of posttraumatic stress disorder was observed in women (7%–53.8%).[23]

Suicide rate in Japan increased by 16% especially in females and younger individuals after the first lockdown.[34] Dubé and colleagues[35] have reported increased rates for suicide ideation (10.8%), suicide attempts (4.7%), and self-harm (9.6%) during the COVID-19 pandemic as compared to prepandemic studies. Women and ethnic minorities were at higher risk of suicide ideation during the pandemic.

Women at Increased Risk of Addictive Disorders During the COVID-19 Pandemic?

Historically, women have used tobacco, alcohol, or illicit drugs less often than men. The gradual change of societal role of women over time and lessening of social taboos have led to a gradual increase in the frequency and amount of psychoactive substance use in women, particularly in Europe and North America.[36] Even if 50% of adults did not report any change in alcohol and/or tobacco consumption during the COVID-19 pandemic, women and past-year harmful alcohol users had a higher risk of change in alcohol and/or tobacco use.[37] In most studies, women reported more emotional distress[38–40] and a higher risk of drinking prevalence was observed in women in some studies.[38,39,41,42] In contrast several studies did not report any gender effect or even higher risk in men.[40,43,44] Currie[45] reported a slight increase in illicit substance use (13.4%) while Malandain and colleagues[43] reported a decrease in 27.8% of cases without any gender effect.

Malandain and colleagues[43] reported an increase in internet use (gambling, cybersex (4%–24%), creation of new social networks) in 14.4% of cases without any gender effect as well as an increased risk of behavioral addictions. In contrast, Huang and colleagues[46] have reported a higher increase in internet use in women as compared to men. Grubbs and colleagues[47] reported a trend downwards for problematic pornography use in men without any change in women (already low users). Furthermore, women were 1.6 times more likely than men to lose control on diet and 2.3 times more likely to increase smartphone use. No gender effect was reported for videogaming.[48]

Gender Inequalities

The pandemic has increased the inequality between men and women. The constraints, lockdowns, and other measures enforced in order to contain the spread of the disease have drastically impacted all aspects of human lives and livelihoods, education, domestic life, economic wellbeing, traditional gender roles and overall health, interlocking life spheres which are inevitably affecting mental wellbeing directly and indirectly as discussed in **Fig. 1**.[49] Women were more likely to take care of children because of closed schools and adapt their job with reduced working hours and lower

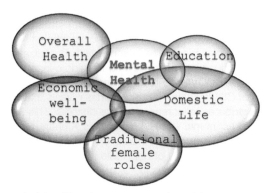

Fig. 1. Impact of Interlocking life spheres on Mental Health.

income. They have more often insecure jobs and jobs with lower social security coverage. They were also more affected by lockdown-related closures, reduced work and job losses in the hotels, restaurants, services, and retail. According to the U.S. Bureau of Labor Statistics,[50] women accounted for 55% of the 20.5 million jobs lost and at a faster rate than men in April 2020. Notably, the limited access to health services and increased partner violence were also contributing factors.[51,52]

It is noteworthy that 85% of women in Africa (58% of self-employed population in Africa) are employed informally with no employment security or benefits, which makes women the most vulnerable sector to be laid off by employers.[53] Lessons learnt from previous epidemics, such as the Ebola outbreak in West Africa in 2014 showed that women suffered more income losses as a result of such crisis. The direct effect of the crisis, in addition to the preventive measures (which included travel restrictions), severely impacted women's livelihoods and economic security. In Yemen 1:5 people live in conflict zones and express high need for mental health and psychosocial support.[54,55] On the other hand, in South Sudan, it was estimated that around 5 million people were affected by the ongoing prepandemic humanitarian emergency in the country representing one of the largest mental health gaps in the world, which got even worse with the COVID outbreak.[56] The UN urged for mental health care to be incorporated into all Governments' COVID- 19 national response.

COVID-19 Disease and Gender Differences

Interestingly, a study based on health records from US hospitals reported that a recent diagnosis of mental disorder increased the risk for COVID-19 infection. The strongest effects were observed for depression (OR 7.6) and schizophrenia (OR 7.34), especially in women and African-Americans.[57]

In Western Europe and North America, men represented a slight majority of coronavirus deaths (52%–58%). The largest proportion of deaths (male-to-female ratio) in confirmed cases was observed in Taiwan, Denmark, Thailand, Tunisia, and Albania (ratio>2).[58] For every 10 female intensive care admissions (ICU) there were 17 male ICU admissions and 15 male confirmed deaths. The highest death ratio observed in men could be partly explained by pre-existing cardio-vascular or metabolic diseases, a higher prevalence of alcohol abuse, or tobacco smoking. Women are also more likely to follow hand hygiene practices, which may decrease infection risk.[59] Finally, sex chromosomes, sex hormones may contribute to the differences in the immune responses observed between males and females.[60]

Long COVID occurred in individuals with a history of probable or confirmed SARS-CoV-2 infection, usually 3 months from the onset of COVID-19 (symptoms may appear following initial recovery from an acute infection or persist from the initial infection). Symptoms last for at least 2 months and cannot be explained by another diagnosis. The most common symptoms are fatigue, shortness of breath, and cognitive dysfunction. Being a female is a risk factor for long COVID. Approximately 10% to 20% of patients with COVID-19 experience persistent symptoms following an acute SARS-CoV-2 infection.[61] Long COVID was more frequently observed in women (10.6%) as compared to men (5.4%).[62] An estimated 15.1% continued to experience symptoms at 12 months. Huang and colleagues[63] reported that 3/4 of patients with SARS-CoV-2 positive had at least one symptom at 6 months of follow-up, the percentage was higher in women (fatigue, muscle weakness, and sleep difficulties, OR 1.33; anxiety and/or depression, OR 1.80).

Health Care Professionals

Worldwide, more than 70% of front-line health workers and essential service staff are women (including nurses, midwives, social workers, employees in pharmacies, cleaning, canteens, child or elderly care, grocery retail, laundry, and so forth). Women were, therefore, more exposed to SARS-CoV-2 infection, sustained distress, and higher workload levels as compared to the general population.[64,65] In Italy and Spain, 66% and 72% of health workers SARS-CoV-2 positive were women vs. 34% and 28% men respectively.[32] Many women required smaller-sized N95 masks than those made available to them, which was a matter of safety and put them at higher risk of SARS CoV-2 infection.[66] Shortages of personal protective equipment was also observed in many sectors and increased the infectious risk in women.

Health care professionals were at higher risk of psychological distress compared to the general population. Higher risk of insomnia, PTSD, depression, anxiety and burn out were observed during and after the pandemic peak[64,67]; especially in female front-line workers (47.1% for insomnia, 33% for depression, and 16.3% for PTSD respectively).[68] Risk factors were lack of rest (for insomnia), death of friends or relatives (for depression) and personal COVID-19 status (for PTSD). In a survey conducted in Pakistan among healthcare workers, more than 35% and around 50% showed substantial symptoms of depression and anxiety respectively, notably young women.[69]

The societal norms and structures stating that women assume caregiving roles are increased during pandemics.[70] This resulted in a high workload level in female health care professionals. Health care professionals had also encountered higher social isolation and discrimination.[71] In addition there were insufficient specialized services to detect and manage anxiety, depression, suicidal ideation and to give advice to health workers without stigmatization. Yet, longitudinal studies will be necessary to conclude if there was only a transient increase of psychological symptoms due to a particularly stressful situation or if this will last in the long term.

Increased Violence Against Women

An increase of 25% to 30% in intimate partner violence was observed during the COVID-19 pandemic.[72,73] Like many parts of the world, the Arab States and Sub Saharian Africa witnessed a staggering surge of domestic violence in different parts of both regions including Tunisia, South Africa, Jordan, Egypt, Kenya, Uganda, Nigeria and many more as compared to pre-pandemic figures. Kenya, Yemen, Morocco, Egypt, and Tunisia have reported an increase in domestic violence (**Fig. 2**).[74]

All male psychiatric diagnoses were associated with an increased risk of domestic violence against women (alcohol and mostly substance use disorders were associated with the highest risk).[75,76]

Likewise, increased verbal and physical aggression was reported toward caregivers in China, Italy, France, and Singapore.[77] Violence during pandemics is even more complex including prevent women from accessing health or social services, inability for women to escape or call social services, increased risk of being put on the streets without shelters.[78]

COVID-19 impact on Domestic Violence

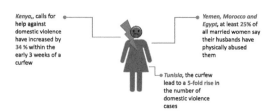

Fig. 2. The surge in domestic violence in different developing countries.

According to estimates by the UNFPA,[22] the COVID-19 pandemic may result in two million cases of female genital mutilation.

Gendered adversities extended to become a witnessed gender-based violence with reported incidences of online violence faced by many women when they used smartphones, the Internet, social media platforms, and emails. This type of gendered violence took several forms as for instance: cyberbullying, sexual harassment, zoom bombing, social media harassment, threats, and so forth. The negative consequences of this escalating form of gendered violence are expected to impact women and girls negatively in several ways limiting their access to online services, use of helplines and other information systems, hindering their education and employment opportunities, and minimizing women's participation as active digital citizens.[79] Sixty percent of women across nine Arab states reported experiencing online violence during the pandemic. Moreover, two-thirds of 100 East African women journalists reported that online harassment had increased during the pandemic.[53] Importantly, health services provided to survivors of gender-based violence continued to be disrupted, with health facilities repurposed into quarantine centers.

Impact on Education

Over a 100 million girls in developing countries struggle to access proper education. In the wake of COVID-19, the closure of thousands of schools was part of confinement measures taken to limit the spread of the coronavirus, there are deep concerns that this will exacerbate gender gaps in education and lead to increased risk of sexual exploitation, early and unintended pregnancy, child abuse, child labor, and forced early marriage in some societies. In Kenya, the dropout of girls has tripled (3.2% to 9.4%).[21] This will result in a rollback on previous preemptive measures taken during the previous years to narrow the gender disparity in education.

SUMMARY

It is quite obvious that women and girls are facing multiple challenges as a result of the pandemic, a situation which requires a multipronged response. In order to achieve this, women's participation and leadership in pandemic response planning is critical. Unfortunately, data compiled by[53] monitoring women's representation and leadership in COVID-19 taskforces, showed that women are significantly underrepresented or notably excluded from the assemblies assigned to this purpose, even at the national levels. The adversity of the COVID-19 pandemic is not a thing of the past, it continues to teach us lessons as we witness the red flags of long-haul COVID; with a long list of somatic, cognitive, and neuropsychiatric manifestations. The pandemic remains a public health emergency of international concern and it is yet too early to cease efforts on combating it as declared by the COVID-19 Emergency Committee of the WHO. Telehealth services, insurance coverage should be increased. Prescription of contraception and medical abortions should be maintained during pandemics. The development of novel vaccines and therapies must include pregnant and breastfeeding women. Emergency aid should be gender-based as proposed by the World Health Organization to take into account existing economic gender disparities.[19] Countries national preparedness and response to this pandemic is now stemming from an enhanced understanding of the impact of a global crisis on mental health, and how this impact is gender-specific. We need to turn our lens to mental health. It is quite obvious that women mental health care service stands out as an essential component of the national preparedness and response to disease outbreaks. Mental wellbeing and effective coping with crisis now being recognized as an integral part of the immediate, short-term and long-term of national public health strategy, which yet need to be gender-responsive.

We learnt a lesson: Women Mental Health matters-this is what we learnt. Putting women first in mental health support should be part of the holistic approach aiming to curb the post-pandemic adversities. As front-liners and key mobilizers in the community, fostering women mental well-being is a way to empower them to pursue their roles and improve their lives.

DISCLOSURE

The authors have nothing to disclose.

REFERENCES

1. UN 2020. United Nations leads call to protect most vulnerable from mental health crisis during and after COVID-19, May 2020. Available at: https://news.un.org/en/story/2020/05/1063882. Accessed 1 December, 2022.
2. Semo BW, Frissa SM. The Mental Health Impact of the COVID-19 Pandemic: implications for Sub-Saharan Africa. Psychol Res Behav Manag 2020;13:713–20.
3. Ma Q, Liu J, Liu Q, et al. Global Percentage of Asymptomatic SARS-CoV-2 Infections Among the Tested Population and Individuals With Confirmed COVID-19 Diagnosis: A Systematic Review and Meta-analysis. JAMA Netw Open 2021;4(12):e2137257.
4. Vouga M, Favre G, Martinez-Perez O, et al. Maternal outcomes and risk factors for COVID-19 severity among pregnant women. Sci Rep 2021;11:13898.
5. Zambrano LD, Ellington S, Strid P, et al. Update: characteristics of symptomatic women of reproductive age with laboratory-confirmed SARS-CoV-2 infection by pregnancy status-United States, January 22-October 3, 2020. MMWR (Morb Mortal Wkly Rep) 2020. Available at: https://www.cdc.gov/mmwr/volumes/69/wr/mm6944e3.htm. Accessed 1 December, 2022.
6. Jafari M, Pormohammad A, Aghayari S, et al. Clinical characteristics and outcomes of pregnant women with COVID-19 and comparison with control patients: a systematic review and meta-analysis. Rev Med Virol 2021;31:e2208.
7. Kotlar B, Gerson E, Petrillo S, et al. The impact of the COVID-19 pandemic on maternal and perinatal health: a scoping review. Reprod Health 2021;18:10.
8. Mirbeyk M, Saghazadeh A, Rezaei N. A systematic review of pregnant women with COVID-19 and their neonates. Arch Gynecol Obstetrics 2021;304:5–38.
9. Capobianco G, Saderib L, Alibertic S, et al. COVID-19 in pregnant women: a systematic review and meta-analysis. Eur J Obstetr Gynecol Reprod Biol 2020;252:543–58.
10. Vivanti AJ, Vauloup-Fellous C, Prevot S, et al. Transplacental transmission of SARS-CoV-2 infection. Nat Commun 2020;11:3572.
11. Basu A, Kim HH, Koenen KC. A cross-national study of factors associated with women's perinatal mental health and wellbeing during the COVID-19 pandemic. PLoS One 2021;16(4):e0249780.
12. Sun F, Zhu J, Tao H, et al. A systematic review involving 11,187 participants evaluating the impact of COVID-19 on anxiety and depression in pregnant women. J Psychosom Obstet Gynaecol 2020;42(2):91–9.
13. Fan S, Guan J, Cao L, et al. Psychological effects caused by COVID-19 pandemic on pregnant women: a systematic review with meta-analysis. Asian J Psychiatr 2020;56:102533.

14. Davenport MH, Meyer S, Meah VL, et al. Moms Are Not OK: COVID-19 and Maternal Mental Health. Front Glob Womens Health 2020;1:1.
15. Berthelot N, Lemieux R, Garon-Bissonnette J, et al. Uptrend in distress and psychiatric symptomatology in pregnant women during the coronavirus disease 2019 pandemic. Acta Obstet Gynecol Scand 2020;99:848–55.
16. Liu CH, Erdei C, Mittal L. Risk factors for depression, anxiety, and PTSD symptoms in perinatal women during the COVID-19 Pandemic. Psychiatry Res 2021; 295(11):35–52.
17. Zhou Y, Shi H, Liu Z, et al. The prevalence of psychiatric symptoms of pregnant and non-pregnant women during the COVID-19 epidemic. Transl Psychiatry 2020;10:319.
18. Sade S, Sheiner E, Wainstock T, et al. Risk for depressive symptoms among hospitalized women in high-risk pregnancy units during the COVID-19 pandemic. J Clin Med 2020;9(8):2449.
19. Connor J, Madhavan S, Mokashi M, et al. Health risks and outcomes that disproportionately affect women during the Covid-19 pandemic: a review. Soc Sci Med 2020;266:113364.
20. Chmielewska B, Barratt I, Townsend R, et al. Effects of the COVID-19 pandemic on maternal and perinatal outcomes: a systematic review and meta-analysis [published correction appears in Lancet Glob Health. 2021 Jun;9(6):e758]. Lancet Glob Health 2021;9(6):e759–72.
21. World Bank Infograph, 2022: Assessing the Damage: Early Evidence on Impacts of the COVID-19 Crisis on Girls and Women in Africa. Available at: https://www.worldbank.org/en/news/infographic/2022/05/25/assessing-the-damage-early-evidence-on-impacts-of-the-covid-19-crisis-on-girls-and-women-in-africa. Accessed 1 December, 2022.
22. UNFPA 2020. Impact of the COVID-19 pandemic on family planning and ending gender-based violence, female genital mutilation and child marriage. UNFPA; 2020. Available at: https://www.unfpa.org/resources/impact-covid-19-pandemic-family-planning-and-ending-gender-based-violence-female-genital. Accessed 1 December, 2022..
23. Xiong J, Lipsitz O, Nasri F, et al. Impact of COVID-19 pandemic on mental health in the general population: A systematic review. J Affect Disord 2020;277:55–64.
24. Wang Y, Kala MP, Jafar TH. Factors associated with psychological distress during the coronavirus disease 2019 (COVID-19) pandemic on the predominantly general population: a systematic review and meta-analysis. PLoS One 2020;15: e0244630.
25. Smirnova D, Syunyakov T, Pavlichenko A, et al. Interactions between Anxiety Levels and Life Habits Changes in General Population during the Pandemic Lockdown: Decreased Physical Activity, Falling Asleep Late and Internet Browsing about COVID-19 Are Risk Factors for Anxiety, whereas Social Media Use Is not. Psychiatr Danub 2021;33(S9):119–29.
26. Li LZ, Wang S. Prevalence and predictors of general psychiatric disorders and loneliness during COVID-19 in the United Kingdom. Psychiatry Res 2020;291: 113267.
27. Wathelet M, Duhem S, Vaiva G, et al. Factors associated with mental health disorders among university students in France confined during the COVID-19 pandemic. JAMA Netw Open 2020;3:e2025591.
28. COVID-19 Mental Disorders Collaborators. Global prevalence and burden of depressive and anxiety disorders in 204 countries and territories in 2020 due to the COVID-19 pandemic. Lancet 2021;398(10312):1700–12.

29. Thibaut F, van Wijngaarden-Cremers P. Women's mental health in the time of Covid-19 pandemic. Front Glob Womens Health 2020;1:588372.
30. WHO EURO 2022. Mental health impacts of Covid-19 across the European region and associated opportunities for action. Available at: https://apps.who.int/iris/bitstream/handle/10665/362637/WHO-EURO-2022-6108-45873-66068-eng.pdf?sequence=1. Accessed 1 December, 2022.
31. Shuwiekh HAM, Kira IA, Sous MSF, et al. The differential mental health impact of COVID-19 in Arab countries. Curr Psychol 2022;41(8):5678–92.
32. UN Policy Brief 2020. COVID-19 and the Need for Action on Mental Health. Available at: https://unsdg.un.org/resources/policy-brief-covid-19-and-need-action-mental-health. Accessed 1 December, 2022.
33. Asim SS, Ghani S, Ahmed M, et al. Assessing Mental Health of Women Living in Karachi During the COVID-19 Pandemic. Front Glob Women's Health 2021;1:594970.
34. Tanaka T, Okamoto S. Increase in suicide following an initial decline during the COVID-19 pandemic in Japan. Nat Hum Behav 2021;5:229–38.
35. Dubé JP, Smith MM, Sherry SB, et al. Suicide behaviors during the COVID-19 pandemic: a meta-analysis of 54 studies. Psychiatry Res 2021;301:113998.
36. Thibaut F. Overview of Women and Addiction. In: Chandra P, Herrman H, Fisher J, et al, editors. Mental health and illness of women. Mental health and illness worldwide. Singapore: Springer; 2019.
37. Kilian C, Neufeld M, Manthey J, et al. Self-reported changes in alcohol and tobacco use during COVID-19: Findings from the eastern part of WHO European Region. Eur J Public Health 2022;32:474–80.
38. Rodriguez LM, Litt DM, Stewart SH. Drinking to cope with the pandemic: the unique associations of COVID-19-related perceived threat and psychological distress to drinking behaviors in American men and women. Addict Behav 2020;110:106532.
39. Mougharbel F, Sampasa-Kanyinga H, Heidinger B, et al. Psychological and demographic determinants of substance use and mental health during the COVID-19 pandemic. Front Public Health 2021;9:680028.
40. Thompson K, Dutton DJ, McNabb K, et al. Changes in alcohol consumption during the COVID-19 pandemic: exploring gender frontiers in differences and the role of emotional distress. Health Promot Chronic Dis Prev Can 2021;41:254–63.
41. Jackson SE, Beard E, Angus C, et al. Moderators of changes in smoking, drinking and quitting behaviour associated with the first COVID-19 lockdown in England. Addiction 2022;117:772–83.
42. Barbosa C, Cowell AJ, Dowd WN. Alcohol consumption in response to the COVID-19 pandemic in the United States. J Addict Med 2021;15:341–4.
43. Malandain L, Fountoulakis KN, Syunyakov T, et al. Psychoactive substance use, internet use and mental health changes during the COVID-19 lockdown in a French population: a study of gender effect. Front Psychiatry 2022;13:958988.
44. Fountoulakis KN, Karakatsoulis G, Abraham S, et al. The effect of different degrees of lockdown and self-identified gender on anxiety, depression and suicidality during the COVID-19 pandemic: data from the international COMET-G study. Psychiatry Res 2022;315:114702.
45. Currie CL. Adult PTSD symptoms and substance use during Wave 1 of the COVID-19 pandemic. Addict Behav Rep 2021;13:100341. Erratum in: Addict Behav Rep. 2021 Jun 12;14:100361.
46. Huang Q, Chen X, Huang S, et al. Substance and Internet use during the COVID-19 pandemic in China. Transl Psychiatry 2021;11(1):491.

47. Grubbs JB, Perry SL, Grant, et al. Porndemic? A longitudinal study of pornography use before and during the COVID-19 pandemic in a nationally representative sample of Americans. Arch Sex Behav 2022;51:123–37.
48. Attanasi G, Maffioletti A, Shalukhina T, et al. Gender Differences in the Impact of COVID-19 Lockdown on Potentially Addictive Behaviors: an Emotion-Mediated Analysis. Front Psychol 2021;12:703897.
49. Chuku C, Mukasa A, Yenice Y. Putting women and girls' safety first in Africa's response to COVID19. Brookings 2020. Available at: https://www.brookings.edu/blog/africa-in-focus/2020/05/08/putting-women-and-girls-safety-first-in-africas-response-to-covid-19/. Accessed 1 December, 2022.
50. U.S. Bureau of Labor Statistics, 2020. Staff of the National Estimates Branch. Current Employment Statistics Highlights. Available at: https://www.bls.gov/web/empsi t/ceshi ghlig hts.pdf. Accessed 1 December, 2022.
51. Seedat S, Rondon M. Women's wellbeing and the burden of unpaid work. BMJ 2021;374:n1972.
52. Xue B, McMunn A. Gender differences in unpaid care work and psychological distress in the UK Covid-19 lockdown. PLoS One 2021;16:e0247959.
53. UN Women and United Nations Development Program (UNDP): Government Responses to COVID-19: Lessons on gender equality for a world in turmoil. 2022;eISBN: 9789210019194. Available at: https://www.unwomen.org/sites/default/files/2022-06/Government-responses-to-COVID-19-Lessons-on-gender-equality-for-a-world-in-turmoil-en_0.pdf. Accessed 1 December, 2022.
54. UN 2020. Seven Possible Actions-Women's Rights and COVID-19. African Union Commission Women, Gender & Development. April 2020. Available at: https://www.ohchr.org/en/documents/tools-and-resources/7-possible-actions-womens-rights-and-covid-19-africa. Accessed 1 December, 2022.
55. Charlson F, van Ommeren M, Flaxman A, et al. New WHO prevalence estimates of mental disorders in conflict settings: a systematic review and meta-analysis. Lancet 2019;394(10194):240–8.
56. Shoib S, Osman Elmahi OK, Siddiqui MF, et al. Sudan's unmet mental health needs: a call for action. Ann Med Surg (Lond) 2022;78:103773.
57. Wang Q, Xu R, Volkow ND. Increased risk of COVID-19 infection and mortality in people with mental disorders: analysis from electronic health records in the United States. World Psychiatr 2021;20(1):124–30.
58. UNDP-UN Women COVID-19 Gender Response Tracker. Available at: https://data.undp.org/gendertracker/. Accessed 1 December, 2022.
59. Johnson HD, Sholcosky D, Gabello K, et al. Sex differences in public restroom handwashing behavior associated with visual behavior prompts. Percept Mot Skills 2003;97:805–10.
60. Klein SL, Flanagan KL. Sex differences in immune responses. Nat Rev Immunol 2016;16:626–38.
61. WHO 2022. Post COVID-19 condition (Long Covid). Available at https://www.who.int/europe/news-room/fact-sheets/item/post-covid-19-condition. Accessed 1 December, 2022.
62. Global Burden of Disease Long COVID Collaborators. Estimated Global Proportions of Individuals With Persistent Fatigue, Cognitive, and Respiratory Symptom Clusters Following Symptomatic COVID-19 in 2020 and 2021. JAMA 2022;328(16):1604–5.
63. Huang C, Huang L, Wang Y, et al. 6-month consequences of COVID-19 in patients discharged from hospital: a cohort study. Lancet 2021;397(10270):220–32. Epub 2021 Jan 8.

64. Boniol M, McIsaac M, Xu L, et al. Gender equity in the health workforce: analysis of 104 countries. World Health Organization; 2019. Available at: https://apps.who.int/iris/handle/10665/311314. License: CC BY-NC-SA 3.0 IGO. Accessed 1 December, 2022.
65. Abu-Jaber M. Recognizing women's important role in Jordan's COVID-19 response. April 29th 2020. Available at: https://www.brookings.edu/blog/education-plus-development/2020/04/29/recognizing-womens-important-role-in-jordans-covid-19-response/ . Accessed December 1 2022.
66. Rabinowitz LG, Rabinowitz DG. Women on the Frontline: a Changed Workforce and the Fight Against COVID-19. Acad Med 2021;96(6):808–12.
67. Lai J, Ma S, Wang Y, et al. Factors Associated With Mental Health Outcomes Among Health Care Workers Exposed to Coronavirus Disease 2019. JAMA Netw Open 2020;3(3):e203976.
68. Robles R, Rodríguez E, Vega-Ramírez H, et al. Mental health problems among healthcare workers involved with the COVID-19 outbreak. Braz J Psychiatry 2021;43(5):494–503.
69. Ullah I, Khan KS, Ali I, et al. Depression and anxiety among Pakistani healthcare workers amid COVID-19 pandemic: a qualitative study. Ann Med Surg 2022;78: 103863.
70. Smith J. Overcoming the 'tyranny of the urgent': integrating gender into disease outbreak preparedness and response. Gend Dev 2019;27(2):355–69.
71. Goyal K, Chauhan P, Chhikara K, et al. Fear of COVID 2019. Asian J Psychiatr 2020;49:101989.
72. UN Women. COVID-19 and Ending Violence Against Women and Girls. 2020. Available online at: https://www.unwomen.org//media/headquarters/attachments/sections/library/publications/2020/issue-briefcovid-19-and-ending-violence-against-women-and-girls-en.pdf?la=en&vs=5006. Accessed 1 December, 2022.
73. Mengin A, Allé MC, Rolling J, et al. Conséquences psychopathologiques du confinement. Encephale 2020;46:S43–52.
74. UN Women 2021. Measuring the shadow pandemic: Violence against Women during COVID-19. November 2021. Available at: https://data.unwomen.org/sites/default/files/documents/Publications/Measuring-shadow-pandemic.pdf. Accessed 1 December, 2022.
75. Gulati G, Kelly BD. Domestic violence against women and the COVID-19 pandemic: what is the role of psychiatry? Int J Law Psychiatry 2020;71:101594.
76. Yu R, Nevado-Holgado AJ, Molero Y, et al. Mental disorders and intimate partner violence perpetrated by men towards women: a Swedish population-based longitudinal study. PLoS Med 2019;16:e1002995.
77. Ajayi T. Violence Against Women and Girls in the Shadow of Covid-19. 2020. Available online at: http://www.sddirect.org.uk/media/1881/vawg-helpdesk-284-covid-19-and-vawg.pdf. Accessed 1 December, 2022.
78. Roesch E, Amin A, Gupta J, et al. Violence against women during covid-19 pandemic restrictions. BMJ 2020;369:m1712.
79. UN Women 2020. Online and ICT facilitated violence against women and girls during COVID-19. 2020. Available at: https://www.unwomen.org/sites/default/files/Headquarters/Attachments/Sections/Library/Publications/2020/Brief-Online-and-ICT-facilitated-violence-against-women-and-girls-during-COVID-19-en.pdf. Accessed 1 December, 2022.

Sex Differences in the Neurobiology of Stress

Hannah Stadtler, BS, Gretchen N. Neigh, PhD*

KEYWORDS

- Stress • Sex differences • Neurobiology • Estrogen • Stress-mitigating interventions

KEY POINTS

- Women disproportionally experience lasting physical effects of stress when compared with their male counterparts.
- Chronic stress can increase HPA axis dysregulation and disrupt glucocorticoid balance in women, which negatively impact neurobiology and cognition.
- Differences in neural plasticity fueled by hormonal differences between women and men could contribute to increased susceptibility of women to stress.

INTRODUCTION

When a person perceives a stressor, their body undergoes distinct physical reactions to respond to the stressor. Allostasis refers to the body's coordinated response to a stressor to respond to the challenge and bring organ systems back to homeostatic conditions after the stressor has dissipated. The cumulative cost of experiencing many stressors and having to undergo allostasis frequently is referred to as "allostatic load," which manifest as the primarily negative health effects of stress.[1–3] Allostatic load has been associated with chronic diseases including cardiovascular disease, reproductive difficulties, and overall worse health outcomes.[2,4–6] In addition to diseases and disorders of somatic systems, allostatic load is associated with neuropsychiatric disorders including depression, anxiety, and post-traumatic stress disorder (PTSD). Women are disproportionately affected by the neuropsychiatric repercussions of allostatic load. Women are twice as likely to experience depression in their lifetime compared with their male counterparts.[7–11] Similarly, the incidence of anxiety and the development of PTSD is higher in women than men.[12–14] The susceptibility to disease is further increased in women who identify with a minority group and women who have a low socioeconomic status.[15–19] These epidemiological differences can be attributed to both increased societal pressures on women and sex-specific neurobiological

Department of Anatomy and Neurobiology, 1101 East Marshall Street Box 980709, Virginia Commonwealth University, Richmond, VA, USA
* Corresponding author. 1101 East Marshall Street Box 980709, Richmond, VA 23298.
E-mail address: gretchen.mccandless@vcuhealth.org

Psychiatr Clin N Am 46 (2023) 427–446
https://doi.org/10.1016/j.psc.2023.04.002
0193-953X/23/© 2023 Elsevier Inc. All rights reserved.

responses to experiencing stress.[6,20] Although societal experiences and pressures can vary between communities, there are established biological differences between men and women that contribute to the differing physical effects of stress on the body, which could contribute to the higher incidence of neuropsychiatric disease in women. This review highlights the existing knowledge and data that explain the physiologic impacts of stress, especially pertaining to neurobiology, and how these impacts differ from sex.

THE HYPOTHALAMIC-PITUITARY-ADRENAL AXIS, STRESS, AND NEUROBIOLOGY
The Hypothalamic-Pituitary-Adrenal Axis

When an organism experiences a psychological stressor, the brain sends signals to prepare the body to respond to a host of potential exposures and experiences, including escape and injury. The mechanism for initiating, sending, and stopping the physical response to stress is achieved through communication between the hypothalamus, pituitary gland, and adrenal gland, often referred to as the hypothalamic-pituitary-adrenal (HPA) axis. When a stressor is perceived, the paraventricular nucleus of the hypothalamus releases corticotrophin-releasing hormone (CRH), which stimulates the anterior pituitary gland in the brain. The anterior pituitary gland then releases adrenocorticotropic hormone (ACTH), which travels through the bloodstream to stimulate the zona fasciculata layer of the adrenal gland; on stimulation, the adrenal gland increases release of cortisol, which creates physiologic changes throughout the body to effectively respond to the stressor (**Fig. 1**). Cortisol is a steroid hormone that under homeostatic conditions is secreted in a diurnal pattern; thus physiologically, there are higher levels of cortisol in the morning that slowly decrease throughout the day.[21] Cortisol acts on both mineralocorticoid and glucocorticoid receptors, which are found throughout the body; mineralocorticoid receptors are more involved within homeostasis, whereas glucocorticoid receptors are most involved in stress response activity. Following a stressor, cortisol secretion increases via HPA axis activation, and glucocorticoid receptors serve as the primary effector of stress-induced functions of cortisol. Glucocorticoid receptors are found within the nervous system, immune system, heart, lungs, reproductive and gastrointestinal tracts, muscles, and skin, which allows for a body-wide response to the perceived stressor. On binding to cortisol, the cortisol/glucocorticoid complex acts as a transcription factor to regulate transcriptional changes depending on the particular cell type and previous experiences of the individual. These changes are evolutionarily favored to provide the brain as many nutrients as possible for fuel during stressful events to facilitate the physical ability to generate energy in the form of adenosine triphosphate (ATP) to appropriately respond to a stressor.[22] For example, cortisol acts on the liver, muscles, adipose tissues, and pancreas to promote the availability of blood glucose. Readily available blood glucose is critical, as it contributes to the generation of ATP, and thus gives the body more energy for the cardiovascular or muscular system to respond to an imminent threat, such as running away from a fear. The HPA axis is activated when any stressor is perceived whether that be a fear that necessitates escape or a psychological stressor that does not require the same degree of energy mobilization. Thus, psychological stressors can lead to an energy mismatch, as HPA axis-mediated energy mobilization is prioritized without the corresponding physical need for that energy.

Sex Differences in Glucocorticoid Receptors

There are established sex differences associated with the glucocorticoid receptor, which influence the response to a stressor from sex.[23] Glucocorticoid receptors

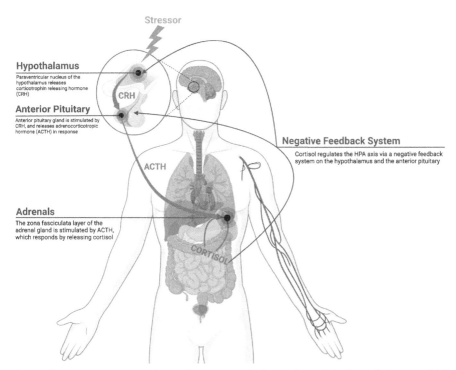

Fig. 1. The HPA axis. Stress activates the paraventricular nucleus of the hypothalamus, which releases corticotropin-releasing hormone (CRH). CRH stimulates the anterior pituitary gland, which releases adrenocorticotropic hormone (ACTH). ACTH activates the zona fasciculata layer of the adrenal glands to release cortisol, which travels all throughout the body to coordinate the physical stress response. The HPA axis is turned off via a negative feedback system, when cortisol levels reach threshold, the hypothalamus and anterior pituitary are signaled to turn off, which ceases the physical response to stress. This system becomes faulty during chronic stress, however, as chronic stress impairs this negative feedback loop. (Figure created with biorender.com.)

require many steps for activation, which is part of how they are regulated; for activation, cortisol must bind to two glucocorticoid receptors intracellularly, which then form a homodimer and are transported to the nucleus via heat shock proteins and co-chaperone proteins that facilitate translocation, including the proteins PPID and FKBP52, which are both influenced by sex.[23–25] PPID has been shown to have interactions with estrogen receptors and is transcriptionally upregulated by estradiol.[26] FKBP52 has been observed in several breast cancer cell lines, supporting a role of estradiol in its regulation.[27] Another protein implicated in the glucocorticoid receptor activation is SRC1, a nuclear coactivator of glucocorticoid receptors, which is also influenced by sex.[23] Testosterone or estradiol supplementation has been shown to increase SCR1 expression, and accordingly SCR1 expression varies during the estrous cycle, illustrating mechanisms by which sex differences and differing hormone levels influence glucocorticoid receptors and thus the HPA axis.[28–30]

Chronic stress further influences the interaction between sex and glucocorticoid chaperones and associated proteins. For example, chronic stress has been shown to alter glucocorticoid receptor translocation in the form of increased transcription of the glucocorticoid receptor and co-chaperones such as PPID, FKBP5, and SCR1, which results in attenuation of glucocorticoid receptor translocation and a delayed resolution of plasma corticosterone levels in response to acute stress.[31] Furthermore, childhood maltreatment is associated with a decrease in methylation of the FKBP5 gene, implicating early-life stress as a mechanism for potentiation of glucocorticoid translocation and alterations in the stress response (p 5).[32–34] Gene variants in FKBP5 chaperone have also been associated with increased incidence of depression.[35–37] Thus, stress augments already existing sex differences in the glucocorticoid receptor and corresponding proteins.

HPA Axis and the Brain

The response initiated by HPA axis activation and subsequent engagement of glucocorticoid receptors is also critical for the brain during a stressor, as the brain needs a constant supply of glucose under normal conditions but has an increased demand during times of stress. Facilitative glucose transporters (GLUT), which allow the uptake of glucose into cells, are modified in the brain during perceived stress.[38,39] At homeostatic conditions, GLUT isoform 3 (GLUT3) is present within the brain, which allows a constant flow of glucose to be supplied to the brain; GLUT3 is specific to the brain and the placenta, because it requires the lowest concentration of glucose to be activated, which prioritizes these structures to receive glucose over other organs in periods of low glucose concentrations.[40] During times of stress, however, GLUT4, another isoform of these transporters, is upregulated and inserted into neuronal axonal membranes to ensure glucose delivery to the brain in addition to typical delivery via GLUT3.[38,41,42] GLUT1 is also upregulated in times of cellular stress.[39] These changes in GLUT expression in response to stress are location-dependent and chiefly occur in neuroanatomical structures associated with the stress response: the prefrontal cortex (PFC), the amygdala, and the hippocampus.[43] The PFC mediates higher order cognition and is activated by HPA axis activation; studies have shown that distinct PFC metabolic glucose patterns are linked to endocrine stress measures as well as subjective perception of stress, indicating the significant role that the PFC has within the stress response.[44] The amygdala plays a role in HPA axis activation, as it regulates emotional responses and interprets whether something is a stressor warranting HPA axis activation.[45] The hippocampus is involved in learning and memory and aids in turning off HPA axis activation.[46,47] The function of each of these areas makes them especially relevant to responding to a stressor, and thus, upregulating GLUT expression in these areas during times of stress is evolutionarily favored. HPA axis activation relies on the brain for perception of a stressor and supports brain function during a stressor in the form of increased energy supply for heightened short-term neurologic functioning.

Chronic Stress, the HPA Axis, and Cortisol

Activation of the HPA axis during stressful events is beneficial, as it is a short-term way to allow efficient physical and neurologic function during stress. However, with chronic stress, the HPA axis becomes dysfunctional. Dysfunction could manifest in an inability to properly turn off or HPA axis activation in response to events that are not actually stressors, such as initiating a response to a perceived stressor that is not proportional to the actual stressor. The HPA axis is regulated via a negative feedback system, when cortisol binds to glucocorticoid receptors in the hypothalamus and pituitary glands, CRH and ACTH secretion is suppressed, which stops the propulsion of the HPA axis response. The hypothalamus is also impacted by neuronal projections from the hippocampus, which when activated further suppress the release of CRH and thus contributes to halting the stress response.[46] Under chronic stress or when HPA axis function is compromised, this negative feedback system is impaired, becomes inefficient, and release of cortisol is not regulated appropriately.

The prolonged glucocorticoid exposure that can result from HPA axis dysfunction and exposure to repeated or extreme stressors is associated with an increased risk of developing neuropsychiatric disorders including depression, anxiety, and PTSD.[6,20] Glucocorticoids are well established as being neurotoxic, especially to areas such as the hippocampus, and thus, maintaining homeostatic levels of cortisol is key.[48] Acutely, cortisol improves cognition by acting on mineralocorticoid receptors in brain regions specific to the task at hand; for example, learning and memory are improved via stimulation of mineralocorticoid receptors in the limbic system of the brain as that system is highly associated with consolidation and retrieval of memories.[49,50] A transient increase in cortisol levels can further highlight those pathways associated with learning and memory, hence the benefit of acute HPA axis stimulation. However, when cortisol levels significantly increase, or stay elevated for prolonged periods of time, a disproportionate number of glucocorticoid receptors are stimulated, which conversely decreases cognitive function.[21,49] Too little cortisol makes completing tasks difficult, but too much cortisol also negatively impacts tasks.[21,22] For example, study participants who were give exogenous cortisol performed significantly worse in a simple sequence learning task, indicating the neurobiological ramifications of abnormally high levels of cortisol.[51] There is also a correlation between neuropsychiatric diseases such as depression, a disease characterized by cortisol and other neurotransmitter imbalances, and cognition, as patients with major depression performed significantly worse than healthy controls in a battery of tests assessing verbal memory, attention, working memory, and executive function, suggesting imbalanced cortisol as a contributor to these outcomes.[52] Although just correlative, it is reasonable that imbalanced cortisol could be mediating negative cognitive outcomes considering that the addition of exogenous cortisol resulted in similar findings. This is further supported by findings from patients who require long-term corticosteroid medication to manage a particular disease, for example, patients on steroids to prevent multiple sclerosis flare ups; long-term corticosteroid use has been found to increase neuropsychiatric disorders such as depression, increase mood fluctuations, and decrease cognitive function.[53–59] Glucocorticoids have a negative impact on memory, attention, mood, and cognition, suggesting a connection between chronic stress and increased incidence of neuropsychiatric diseases.

Furthermore, there are sex-specific effects of cortisol imbalances on neurocognition. For example, low-dose hydrocortisone administration transiently enhances cognition in women, a finding that was not consistent in men; this effect is present up to 4 hours of dosing but fades and becomes detrimental beyond 4 hours of hydrocortisone exposure.[60] This further indicates how HPA axis activation can be initially beneficial but can quickly become damaging with over-activation from chronic stress. In addition, women who were treated with low-dose hydrocortisone in order to explore cortisol as a mechanism for neurologic changes had a heightened ability to recognize fearful faces when compared with men; this heightened efficacy in threat detection was only present in women, and especially women who had lower psychological burdens and who had experienced minimal trauma. This enhanced threat detection was lost in women who had experienced a significant amount of trauma, indicating that cortisol can be beneficial for responding to stressful situations, but this system becomes dysfunctional in women who experience settings of prolonged stress exposure and long-term increases in glucocorticoids.[61] In another study, high cortisol was again associated with worse memory and visual perception in both women and men, but in individuals with high cortisol, a variety of microstructural brain changes were seen in women only.[62] Similarly, cortisol levels that are too low also negatively impact cognition, as there are not high enough amounts to active mineralocorticoid receptors.[50] The impact of cortisol on learning is also influenced by past experiences specific to individuals, indicating how life experiences and dispositional traits can influence these pathways.[49,63–65] Potential mechanisms of these individualistic influences have been hypothesized to be of an epigenetic origin of the glucocorticoid receptor and its expression, but more research is warranted to fully understand how individual experiences play a role on resulting stress responses.[66]

The impact of chronic stress on the brain can endure long after the stressor exposure has concluded, and these effects are particularly pronounced in women as compared with men. For example, imbalanced cortisol, indicative of HPA axis dysregulation following chronic stress, can persist in some female patients who have experienced a depressive episode in the past, regardless of whether that depression is in remission or active; this indicates the possibility of lasting effects of chronic stress on physiologic processes for women, as this pattern is not present for men.[67] Furthermore, patients with remitted major depressive disorder demonstrated a decrease in learning and memory, suggesting that there are lasting impacts of neuropsychiatric diseases.[67] However, more research is warranted to understand those dynamics and different mechanisms contributing to the effects of stress, as that is not the case for all women who have experienced a depressive episode. Lasting effects of stress on structural and functional neurologic differences between men and women are heightened by imbalanced cortisol levels, and women seem to be especially susceptible to potential changes.

The negative impacts of stress and neuropsychiatric disease on cognitive function co-occur with neuroanatomical modifications. Childhood trauma has been shown to correlate negatively with brain volume, indicating the physical effect stress can have on neuroanatomy.[68] Patients who have experienced chronic stress and depression have also been found to have decreased amounts of gray matter; patients' hippocampus, amygdala, and PFCs were all affected. Depression has been associated with structural and functional alterations in the hippocampus and medial PFC.[69] Specifically, structural imaging of the hippocampus in patients diagnosed with major depressive disorder showed that these patients consistently had reduced hippocampal volumes when compared with healthy controls. Patients who had other neuropsychiatric conditions beyond depression had even more significant reductions in hippocampal and PFC volumes, indicating a more significant effect with additional neuropsychiatric conditions.[70–74] Neuroanatomical changes resulting from stress are also influenced by sex. In a study, the association between early morning serum cortisol, cognitive performance and brain structural integrity, and higher cortisol was inversely associated with cerebral brain volume in women; high cortisol levels resulted in decreased regional fractional anisotropy, a measure of connectivity within the brain, especially in the splenium of corpus callosum and the posterior corona radiata, two areas critical to coordination between brain hemispheres and neural traffic.[62] The experience of trauma as a form of chronic stress has also been shown to alter the neuroanatomy of women. In a study of mothers who had experienced childhood maltreatment and those who had not, maltreatment was associated with greater gray matter volume in brain regions associated with emotional empathy and less maternal sensitivity when interacting with their children.[75,76] Although these studies and the effects of stress and sex on neuroanatomical changes are still being investigated, assessing neuroanatomical changes as a basis of stress exposure and sex is an important consideration.[77–80] These studies all demonstrate that dysfunctional

HPA axis activation by chronic stress has physical ramifications and that women experience different neurobiological changes than men as a result of stress (**Fig. 2**).

THE HYPOTHALAMIC–PITUITARY–GONADAL AXIS
Hypothalamic–Pituitary–Gonadal Axis

One explanation for sex-specific differences in neurobiological responses to stress is differing hormone profiles between men and women, the system of which is referred to as the hypothalamic–pituitary–gonadal (HPG) axis. Similar to the HPA axis, where the brain perceives a stressor, the hypothalamus secretes CRH to stimulate the pituitary to secrete ACTH to stimulate the adrenals to secrete glucocorticoids, the HPG axis is characterized by hypothalamus and pituitary influence over the gonads and reproductive tract.[81] The parvocellular neurosecretory cells within the hypothalamus secrete gonadotropin-releasing hormone, which stimulates the anterior pituitary.[81] On stimulation, the anterior pituitary releases luteinizing hormone (LH) and follicle-stimulating hormone (FSH) into the general circulation, which act on the gonads of both men and women. In response to LH and FSH, the testes primarily release testosterone, an androgen, and the ovaries release estradiol, an estrogen. The HPG axis becomes activated around 10 weeks of gestational development and, in conjunction with sex chromosomes, drives organizational, or permanent, sex differences in males in females.[82] It continues throughout the lifespan to influence activational or transient sex differences via these different hormone profiles.[82]

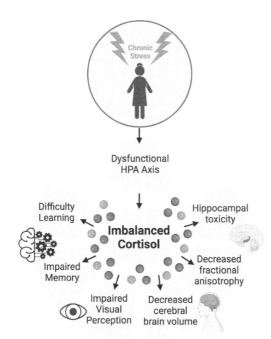

Fig. 2. Lasting neurobiological effects in women with a history of chronic stress. Chronic stress is associated with a variety of lasting physical effects in women. It results in a dysfunctional HPA axis, which leads to imbalanced cortisol levels even after the stress is no longer present. Imbalanced cortisol mediates neurobiological changes in women, such as cognitive dysfunction and neuroanatomical modifications. (Figure created with biorender.com.)

Estrogen

One of the significant hormones that potentiate sex-differences via the HPG axis is estrogen. There are three predominant estrogens—estrone (E1) is a weak estrogen with higher levels present after menopause.[83] Estradiol (E2) is predominant throughout the lifespan and the most common form of estrogen, and estriol (E3) is a weak estrogen that increases during pregnancy, as it is important for maintaining the fetus.[84,85] Both males and females are physically affected by estrogen, but the degree of which and the location of these effects are part of what distinguishes sex. During development, when the HPG axis is first initiated, estrogen receptors and estrogen signaling in the brain have a significant impact on brain development; in males, the testes briefly activate at birth, give a surge of testosterone, which is converted to estrogen via neural aromatase.[86] This estrogen works via estrogen receptor alpha to establish sex-specific differences in cell number and connectivity, an organizational effect of estrogen, which lays the groundwork for neurobiological differences between sexes in conjunction with sex chromosomes.[84,87,88] Following development, estrogen continues to have physical influences specific to sex by influencing protein expression and function via activational effects. First, the degree of which estrogen is produced varies between men and women and varies as a function of age. Men produce primarily testosterone from the testes in a consistent fashion and experience some peripheral conversion to estrogen and progesterone, whereas women produce primarily estrogen and progesterone from the ovaries in a cyclical pattern, dependent on age, with a small amount of testosterone produced peripherally.[89]

Estrogen has been implicated as a key regulator of neurotransmitters and correlative neurotransmitter circuitry. Estrogen influences transcriptional changes via nuclear receptors, specifically estrogen receptors alpha and beta, which on binding serve as a transcription factor complex and directly influence gene expression in neural cells.[90] For example, estrogen has been found to increase dopamine synthesis in the brain and regulate dopamine receptors in response to varying dopamine levels.[91–94] It also upregulates the expression of tryptophan hydroxylase, an enzyme involved in synthesizing serotonin, to increase serotonin biosynthesis in the brain.[91,92,95] In addition, estrogen regulates the serotonin receptors 5HT2 and 2C in response to varying serotonin levels.[96,97] The regulation of dopamine and serotonin allows estrogen to be a chief regulator of mood and behavioral responses and thus is further implicated in neuropsychiatric disorders that so frequently modulate mood and behavioral responses. Estrogen as a transcription factor also has benefits to cognitive function, especially learning and memory, as it has been shown to upregulate N-methyl-D-aspartate (NMDA) glutamate receptors, which are critical to learning and memory.[91,98–100] Considering the detrimental impact of neuropsychiatric diseases on learning and memory, it is noteworthy that estrogen has a role in both.

Beyond influencing genomic effects via transcription factors, there are also membrane-bound estrogen receptors alpha and beta as well as membrane bound G-protein-coupled estrogen receptors, which can facilitate non-genomic effects, further expanding estrogen's influence in the brain.[101] Membrane-bound estrogen receptors facilitate rapid responses resulting from estrogen, rather than pathways characterized by nuclear receptor activation which typically require time to facilitate transcriptional changes.[101] Rapid estrogen signaling via these receptors can lead to axospinous synapse formation in the hippocampus and increases structural plasticity of postsynaptic neuronal spines, which both enhance glutamatergic transmission and long-term potentiation and plasticity, further supporting estrogen's role in learning and memory.[101] These different receptors complement the transcriptional function of estrogen, and the combination of both makes estrogen a key modulator of neurotransmitter systems and learning and memory within the brain.

Because estrogen and other HPG axis sex hormones influence transcription and work via nuclear receptors, similar to the glucocorticoid receptor and proteins associated with the HPA axis, there are key interactions between the HPG and HPA axes, as there are overlapping proteins and chaperones involved within each. Thus, the HPG and HPA axes can transactivate and transrepress each other. For example, FKBP5, one of the co-chaperones that impact glucocorticoid translocation to the nucleus and thus the potentiation of the HPA axis-mediated stress response influences and is influenced by estrogen.[102] FKBP5 has been found to interact with nuclear receptors beyond the glucocorticoid receptor, including estrogen nuclear receptors.[102] Estrogen has been found to potentiate the increase in FKBP5 expression in conjunction with cortisol.[103] Conversely, estradiol treatment resulted in decreased expression of peptidylprolyl isomerase D (PPID), another key glucocorticoid receptor chaperone, an effect that was further exacerbated by the administration of progesterone.[103]

Estrogen specifically has been shown as a key regulator within the HPA axis in both men and women.[104] For example, estrogen influences CRH neurons which are key regulators within the limbic system of sensory inputs and play a significant role in identification of physiologic stressors and thus the HPA axis; these neurons contribute to regulation of behavior, perception, and autonomic and neuroendocrine responses.[104–106] Estrogen receptor alpha is expressed throughout CRH neuronal circuitry, and treatment with estrogen has been shown to increase CRH neuronal activity, thus increasing CRH levels, and furthering the HPA axis response.[107,108] In addition, in a preclinical study assessing the impact of chronic stress in offspring from mothers exposed to chronic prenatal stress, estrogen was found to mediate an increase in visceral hypersensitivity as a result of chronic stress in these offspring via an increase in brain-derived neurotropic factor expression, potentiating the HPA axis response to chronic stress.[109] Estrogen can also work against the HPA axis and mitigate the physical stress response. For example, high concentrations of estrogen receptor beta have been identified within neurons within the paraventricular hypothalamic nucleus, which are classically antagonistic to CRH-releasing neurons, and thus mitigate HPA axis activation.[110] Furthermore, estrogen can work in a synergistic manner to oxytocin, a hormone associated with maternal behaviors, parturition, lactation, and mitigating the physical stress response launched by the HPA axis. Estrogen enhances oxytocin's effect via modulation of oxytocin neuron function via estrogen receptor beta-driven reductions of cortisol and ACTH levels within these hypothalamic paraventricular nucleus (PVN) neurons.[104,111]

These differing effects of estrogen within HPA axis regulation are likely due to differences in estrogen receptor alpha and estrogen receptor beta. Estrogen receptor alpha has been found to facilitate estrogen-mediated impairment of the negative feedback loop on the HPA axis.[112,113] In a study assessing estradiol treatment on the effects of the synthetic glucocorticoid, dexamethasone, treatment with an estrogen receptor alpha agonist increased stress-induced cortisol via activation of gamma-aminobutyric acid (GABAergic) neurons; conversely, treatment with an estrogen receptor beta agonist resulted in the opposite effect, primarily via the reduction of glucocorticoid receptors.[112] In another study, peripheral treatment with an estrogen receptor beta agonist prevented HPA axis reactivity as well as decreased anxiety-like behaviors seen in female rats in response to a glucocorticoid receptor agonist.[114] Both of these findings suggest a strong role of estrogen within HPA axis regulation, either in upregulation of the stress response via estrogen receptor alpha or downregulation via estrogen receptor beta. The ability of estrogen to increase HPA axis hyperactivity via disruption of the negative feedback loop can potentiate increased cortisol in women who experience chronic stress. Furthermore, the neuroprotective aspect of estrogen via activation of estrogen receptor beta could explain why neurobiological effects of childhood trauma can be shielded until menopause, a time when estrogen levels are decreased significantly in women.[115]

More research is warranted to discern the balance between the neuroprotective effects of estrogen and the transcriptional changes that can increase stress susceptibility mediated by estrogen as well as estrogen's conflicting role in HPA axis hyperactivity. Regardless, estrogen and similar sex hormones provide a significant basis for neurobiological changes resulting from stress as a function of sex and contribute to the increased physical burden of stress on women. The increased concentrations of circulating estrogen within women, as well as the fluctuations women experience throughout their lifespan, heighten these effects for women, which is better understood by assessing the incidence and resulting impacts of stress and neuropsychiatric disease in women throughout the lifespan.

ESTROGEN THROUGH THE LIFESPAN, NEUROPSYCHIATRIC DISEASE, AND CLINICAL INTERVENTIONS
Estrogen and Stress Through the Lifespan

Estrogen and other sex hormones change throughout a woman's life with the core hormonal stages being prepubertal, puberty and reproductive years, perimenopause, and menopause.[116–118] Prepubertal males and females have similar hormone levels with the biggest differences developing during puberty. That being said, prepubertal children are still susceptible to neurobiological changes due to stress. For example, early abuse and neglect have been found to reduce resilience to stressful events and decreased ability to emotionally regulate responses.[119] Neuroimaging studies in individuals who experienced childhood trauma indicate hypoactivity in the frontal lobe and corresponding decreases in executive function.[119] Childhood trauma has been associated with hypersensitivity to threat and signs of anger and a corresponding increase in synapse formation and dendritic spines in the amygdala, where threats and emotions are processed.[119] Children who have experienced childhood trauma have been found to be more susceptible to having difficulty regulating their emotions.[119] Furthermore, there is an association between experiencing childhood trauma and the development of psychosis with the number of traumatic events increasing the likelihood of developing psychosis.[120,121] Early life stress has been associated with complex clinical profiles of both neurobiological changes and other diseases.[122–124] Although there is no known sex difference in the experience of early life stress in the prepubertal phase, experiencing early life stress correlates to neuropsychiatric diseases more significantly in women later in life.[125]

There are two stages of puberty: adrenarche, hallmarked by adrenal androgen production and gonadarche, hallmarked by the activation of the HPG axis.[126,127] During puberty, males have an increase in testosterone while females undergo menarche, the initiation of the menstrual cycle, which introduces another layer of hormonal fluctuations beyond what is seen within different life stages.[128] During each menstrual cycle, estradiol levels fluctuate to prepare the reproductive system for fertilization and shed the uterine lining that is created if fertilization does not occur. The average menstrual cycle is 28 days. From days 0 to 12 estradiol gradually increases, and it sharply decreases on ovulation, from days 13 to 17. After ovulation, estradiol increases again from day 18 to 24 and decreases again from day 24 to 28, which is when uterine shedding occurs.[129] Neurobiology is affected by these monthly fluctuations of estradiol.

Structural and functional neural plasticity increases throughout the menstrual cycle as estradiol levels vary, and mood changes are more likely to occur during the period of low estradiol that precedes ovulation.[130–132] With the onset of puberty, women enter their reproductive years, where they are twice as likely to develop depression when compared with their male counterparts.[10,20,133] Furthermore, the timing of trauma during puberty can influence the development of neuropsychiatric diseases: in a study of pubescent girls, trauma during puberty conferred significantly more risk of anxiety disorder diagnoses, whereas prepubertal trauma conferred significantly more risk of depressive disorder diagnoses, indicating that timing of trauma and stress can influence resulting neuropsychiatric outcomes.[134] Early life stress can also affect the timing of puberty. Experiencing early life stress is positively associated with the development of early puberty in girls and late puberty in boys when compared with their peers.[135] Early life puberty was predicative of the development of anxiety in girls but not boys, indicating further differences between early life stress and how stress impacts neuropsychiatric outcomes.[135]

The role of estrogen in neurobiological changes as a result of stress becomes even more apparent when considering incidence of neuropsychiatric diseases within women during perimenopause and after. Increased susceptibility to developing depression is further heightened when women enter perimenopause, the period before menopause when periods become irregular and estrogen levels begin to decrease.[136] On average, perimenopause begins in the late 40s and lasts 4 to 5 years until women stop having a menstrual period completely and they enter menopause.[136] The more significant hormone fluctuations introduced in the perimenopausal stage, and the subsequent decreases in estrogen could contribute to the higher incidence of neuropsychiatric diseases in this population. Furthermore, it has been well established that childhood trauma or experiencing chronic adolescent stress is associated with the development of neuropsychiatric disorders and physical ramifications in both males and females.[119,124] That being said, the increase in incidence of neuropsychiatric disorders in women during the perimenopausal phase has been associated with experiencing childhood trauma—a woman is more likely to develop depression during perimenopause if she experienced childhood trauma, a pattern that is not observed for men.[137] In addition, the effects of childhood trauma can be shielded until menopause, when neuroprotective estrogen is depleted.[137,138] Furthermore, estrogen treatment has shown to be effective as an antidepressant in women who experience depression during perimenopause, further implicating hormonal changes as a chief modulator for neurobiological changes and the potential development of psychiatric diseases.[136,139] Because of the increased susceptibility to developing depression in this population, women undergoing perimenopause and then menopause should be consistently screened for depression.[138]

These differences in neurobiological changes as a result of stress as a function of age and pubertal stage implicates estrogen as a key modulator. Understanding neuroprotective and deleterious effects of estrogen is essential to further elucidating these dynamics, especially considering the effect of cycling gonadal steroids on the HPA axis and neurotransmitter systems in women.[140]

Clinical Interventions

Considering the significant physical consequences that women especially experience as a result of chronic stress, it should be evident how beneficial interventions mitigating stress would be. The neurobiological changes that women especially experience as a result of stress have implications for disease; HPA axis dysregulation has been associated with not only depression but also cardiovascular disease, diabetes, hypertension, suppressed immune function, and impaired wound healing.[140,141] Accordingly, interventions aimed at mitigating stress should be taken as seriously as preventative interventions to mitigate diabetes, as the physical effects are similarly impactful. Although there are some interventions that seem efficacious in reducing stress and remission rates in people who experience neuropsychiatric diseases, more research should be done to investigate different interventional approaches. For example, eye movement desensitization and reprocessing and trauma-focused cognitive behavioral therapies have both been found to decrease remission rates and symptoms associated with PTSD.[142,143] Simple mindfulness interventions have also been found to decrease stress in a variety of populations.[144–149] Interventions have various levels of involvement and detail, and yet can still have similar preventative effects, which exemplifies how these interventions can be easily accessible while still having significant potential to decrease these significant physical changes that result from stress.

SUMMARY

This review provides an overview of neurobiological differences between men and women, and how men and women have alternate responses to stress as a result of these neurobiological changes. These conclusions should hopefully impact medical practitioners, policy makers, and researchers to understand the following:

Practice: Awareness that stress, regardless of if that is an established clinical disease such as depression, PTSD, anxiety, or if that is just a general stressful state, impacts women via direct physical ramifications rather than being a fleeting emotion.

Policy: Interventions aimed at mitigating the burden of chronic stress should be highly considered, especially in light of all of the physical processes associated with chronic stress.

Research: More research is warranted to further elucidate the mechanisms underlying the increased susceptibility to physical changes women experience when compared with men as a result of stress. Further investigation of the differing effects of stress on estrogen and correlative enzymes such as aromatase should especially be considered.

CLINICS CARE POINTS

- Women are significantly more likely to develop a neuropsychiatric disorder when compared with their male counterparts, a major risk factor of which is experiencing chronic stress.
- Chronic stress can lead to HPA axis dysfunction in women.
- Women experience long-term imbalanced cortisol and resulting impacts as a result of chronic stress, whereas men are not as longitudinally impacted.
- Estrogen levels are a key protein difference between women and men that could be contributing to the different neurobiological impacts of chronic stress.
- Interventions aimed at mitigating chronic stress are warranted especially in women, considering the long-term physical effects stress has on the body.

DISCLOSURE

Dr G.N. Neigh's effort was supported by the Emory SCORE (NIH U54 AG062334).

REFERENCES

1. McEwen B, Lasley EN. Allostatic load: When protection gives way to damage. Adv Mind Body Med 2003;19:28–33.
2. Guidi J, Lucente M, Sonino N, et al. Allostatic Load and Its Impact on Health: A Systematic Review. Psychother Psychosom 2021;90(1):11–27.
3. McEwen BS. Stress, adaptation, and disease. Allostasis and allostatic load. Ann N Y Acad Sci 1998;840:33–44.
4. Negris O, Lawson A, Brown D, et al. Emotional stress and reproduction: what do fertility patients believe? J Assist Reprod Genet 2021;38(4):877–87.
5. Cohen BE, Edmondson D, Kronish IM. State of the Art Review: Depression, Stress, Anxiety, and Cardiovascular Disease. Am J Hypertens 2015;28(11):1295–302.
6. Bekhbat M, Neigh GN. Sex differences in the neuro-immune consequences of stress: Focus on depression and anxiety. Brain Behav Immun 2018;67:1–12.
7. Dudek KA, Dion-Albert L, Kaufmann FN, et al. Neurobiology of resilience in depression: immune and vascular insights from human and animal studies. Eur J Neurosci 2021;53(1):183–221.
8. Pu D, Luo J, Wang Y, et al. Prevalence of depression and anxiety in rheumatoid arthritis patients and their associations with serum vitamin D level. Clin Rheumatol 2018;37(1):179–84.
9. Kessler RC, Berglund P, Demler O, et al. Lifetime Prevalence and Age-of-Onset Distributions of DSM-IV Disorders in the National Comorbidity Survey Replication. Arch Gen Psychiatry 2005;62(6):593–602.
10. Sassarini DJ. Depression in midlife women. Maturitas 2016;94:149–54.
11. Serpytis P, Navickas P, Lukaviciute L, et al. Gender-Based Differences in Anxiety and Depression Following Acute Myocardial Infarction. Arq Bras Cardiol 2018;111(5):676–83.
12. Welzel FD, Luppa M, Pabst A, et al. Incidence of Anxiety in Latest Life and Risk Factors. Results of the AgeCoDe/AgeQualiDe Study. Int J Environ Res Public Health 2021;18(23):12786.
13. Christiansen DM, Berke ET. Gender- and Sex-Based Contributors to Sex Differences in PTSD. Curr Psychiatry Rep 2020;22(4):19.
14. Faravelli C, Alessandra Scarpato M, Castellini G, et al. Gender differences in depression and anxiety: the role of age. Psychiatry Res 2013;210(3):1301–3.
15. Foubert L, Noël Y, Spahr CM, et al. Beyond WEIRD: Associations between socioeconomic status, gender, lifetime stress exposure, and depression in Madagascar. J Clin Psychol 2021;77(7):1644–65.
16. Sumner LA, Olmstead R, Azizoddin DR, et al. The contributions of socioeconomic status, perceived stress, and depression to disability in adults with systemic lupus erythematosus. Disabil Rehabil 2020;42(9):1264–9.
17. Han KM, Han C, Shin C, et al. Social capital, socioeconomic status, and depression in community-living elderly. J Psychiatr Res 2018;98:133–40.
18. Patel JS, Oh Y, Rand KL, et al. Measurement invariance of the patient health questionnaire-9 (PHQ-9) depression screener in U.S. adults across sex, race/ethnicity, and education level: NHANES 2005-2016. Depress Anxiety 2019;36(9):813–23.
19. Wyman MF, Jonaitis EM, Ward EC, et al. Depressive role impairment and subthreshold depression in older black and white women: race differences in the clinical significance criterion. Int Psychogeriatr 2020;32(3):393–405.

20. Young E, Korszun A. Sex, trauma, stress hormones and depression. Mol Psychiatry 2010;15(1):23–8.
21. Tortosa-Martínez J, Manchado C, Cortell-Tormo JM, et al. Exercise, the diurnal cycle of cortisol and cognitive impairment in older adults. Neurobiol Stress 2018;9:40–7.
22. Thau L, Gandhi J, Sharma S. Physiology, Cortisol. In: StatPearls. StatPearls Publishing; 2021. Available at: http://www.ncbi.nlm.nih.gov/books/NBK538239/. Accessed 23 July, 2021.
23. Bourke CH, Harrell CS, Neigh GN. Stress-Induced Sex Differences: Adaptations Mediated by the Glucocorticoid Receptor. Horm Behav 2012;62(3):210–8.
24. Binder EB. The role of FKBP5, a co-chaperone of the glucocorticoid receptor in the pathogenesis and therapy of affective and anxiety disorders. Psychoneuroendocrinology 2009;34(Suppl 1):S186–95.
25. Grad I, Picard D. The glucocorticoid responses are shaped by molecular chaperones. Mol Cell Endocrinol 2007;275(1–2):2–12.
26. Kumar P, Mark PJ, Ward BK, et al. Estradiol-regulated expression of the immunophilins cyclophilin 40 and FKBP52 in MCF-7 breast cancer cells. Biochem Biophys Res Commun 2001;284(1):219–25.
27. Ward BK, Mark PJ, Ingram DM, et al. Expression of the estrogen receptor-associated immunophilins, cyclophilin 40 and FKBP52, in breast cancer. Breast Cancer Res Treat 1999;58(3):267–80.
28. Meijer OC, Kalkhoven E, van der Laan S, et al. Steroid receptor coactivator-1 splice variants differentially affect corticosteroid receptor signaling. Endocrinology 2005;146(3):1438–48.
29. Charlier TD, Ball GF, Balthazart J. Plasticity in the expression of the steroid receptor coactivator 1 in the Japanese quail brain: effect of sex, testosterone, stress and time of the day. Neuroscience 2006;140(4):1381–94.
30. Camacho-Arroyo I, Neri-Gómez T, González-Arenas A, et al. Changes in the content of steroid receptor coactivator-1 and silencing mediator for retinoid and thyroid hormone receptors in the rat brain during the estrous cycle. J Steroid Biochem Mol Biol 2005;94(1–3):267–72.
31. Bourke CH, Raees MQ, Malviya S, et al. Glucocorticoid sensitizers Bag1 and Ppid are regulated by adolescent stress in a sex-dependent manner. Psychoneuroendocrinology 2013;38(1):84–93.
32. Parade SH, Parent J, Rabemananjara K, et al. Change in FK506 binding protein 5 (FKBP5) methylation over time among preschoolers with adversity. Dev Psychopathol 2017;29(5):1627–34.
33. Tyrka AR, Parade SH, Eslinger NM, et al. Methylation of exons 1D, 1F, and 1H of the glucocorticoid receptor gene promoter and exposure to adversity in preschool-aged children. Dev Psychopathol 2015;27(2):577–85.
34. Klengel T, Mehta D, Anacker C, et al. Allele-specific FKBP5 DNA demethylation mediates gene–childhood trauma interactions. Nat Neurosci 2013;16(1):33–41.
35. Menke A, Klengel T, Rubel J, et al. Genetic variation in FKBP5 associated with the extent of stress hormone dysregulation in major depression. Genes Brain Behav 2013;12(3):289–96.
36. Appel K, Schwahn C, Mahler J, et al. Moderation of Adult Depression by a Polymorphism in the FKBP5 Gene and Childhood Physical Abuse in the General Population. Neuropsychopharmacology 2011;36(10):1982–91.
37. Klinger-König J, Hertel J, Van der Auwera S, et al. Methylation of the FKBP5 gene in association with FKBP5 genotypes, childhood maltreatment and depression. Neuropsychopharmacology 2019;44(5):930–8.

38. Koepsell H. Glucose transporters in brain in health and disease. Pflüg Arch - Eur J Physiol 2020;472(9):1299–343.
39. McCall AL. Glucose transport. In: Fink G, editor. *Encyclopedia of stress*. 2nd edition. Academic Press; 2007. p. 217–22. https://www.elsevier.com/books/encyclopedia-of-stress/fink/978-0-12-373947-6.
40. Mora S. and Pessin J., Glucose/sugar transport in mammals, In: Lennarz W.J. and Lane M.D., *Encyclopedia of biological Chemistry*, 2nd edition, 2013, Academic Press, 391–394. Available at: https://www.sciencedirect.com/science/article/abs/pii/B9780123786302000414?via%3Dihub.
41. Ashrafi G, Wu Z, Farrell RJ, et al. GLUT4 Mobilization Supports Energetic Demands of Active Synapses. Neuron 2017;93(3):606–15.e3.
42. Rangaraju V, Calloway N, Ryan TA. Activity-Driven Local ATP Synthesis Is Required for Synaptic Function. Cell 2014;156(4):825–35.
43. Kelly SD, Harrell CS, Neigh GN. Chronic Stress Modulates Regional Cerebral Glucose Transporter Expression in an Age-Specific and Sexually-Dimorphic Manner. Physiol Behav 2014;126:39–49.
44. Kern S, Oakes TR, Stone CK, et al. Glucose metabolic changes in the prefrontal cortex are associated with HPA axis response to a psychosocial stressor. Psychoneuroendocrinology 2008;33(4):517–29.
45. Diano M, Celeghin A, Bagnis A, Tamietto M. Human Amygdala in Sensory and Attentional Unawareness: Neural Pathways and Behavioural Outcomes. InTech 2017. https://doi.org/10.5772/intechopen.69345.
46. Anand KS, Dhikav V. Hippocampus in health and disease: An overview. Ann Indian Acad Neurol 2012;15(4):239–46.
47. Wingenfeld K, Wolf OT. Stress, Memory, and the Hippocampus. Hippocampus Clin Neurosci 2014;34:109–20.
48. Sapolsky RM. The Physiological Relevance of Glucocorticoid Endangerment of the Hippocampusa. Ann N Y Acad Sci 1994;746(1):294–304.
49. van Ast VA, Cornelisse S, Marin MF, et al. Modulatory mechanisms of cortisol effects on emotional learning and memory: Novel perspectives. Psychoneuroendocrinology 2013;38(9):1874–82.
50. Otte C, Wingenfeld K, Kuehl LK, et al. Mineralocorticoid Receptor Stimulation Improves Cognitive Function and Decreases Cortisol Secretion in Depressed Patients and Healthy Individuals. Neuropsychopharmacology 2015;40(2):386–93.
51. Römer S, Schulz A, Richter S, et al. Oral cortisol impairs implicit sequence learning. Psychopharmacology (Berl) 2011;215(1):33–40.
52. Keller J, Gomez R, Williams G, et al. HPA axis in major depression: cortisol, clinical symptomatology and genetic variation predict cognition. Mol Psychiatry 2017;22(4):527–36.
53. Feinstein A, Freeman J, Lo AC. Treatment of progressive multiple sclerosis: what works, what does not, and what is needed. Lancet Neurol 2015;14(2):194–207.
54. Räikkönen K, Gissler M, Kajantie E. Associations Between Maternal Antenatal Corticosteroid Treatment and Mental and Behavioral Disorders in Children. JAMA 2020;323(19):1924–33.
55. Pullen RLJ. Mental status changes with corticosteroid therapy. Nurs Made Incred Easy 2021;19(1):55–6.
56. Ros LT. Symptomatic depression after long-term steroid treatment: a case report. Afr J Med Med Sci 2004;33(3):263–5.
57. Brown ES, Chandler PA. Mood and Cognitive Changes During Systemic Corticosteroid Therapy. Prim Care Companion J Clin Psychiatry 2001;3(1):17–21.

58. Kenna HA, Poon AW, de los Angeles CP, et al. Psychiatric complications of treatment with corticosteroids: Review with case report. Psychiatry Clin Neurosci 2011;65(6):549–60.

59. Thibaut F. Corticosteroid-induced psychiatric disorders: genetic studies are needed. Eur Arch Psychiatry Clin Neurosci 2019;269(6):623–5.

60. Rubin LH, Phan KL, Keating SM, et al. A single low dose of hydrocortisone enhances cognitive functioning in HIV-infected women. AIDS Lond Engl 2018; 32(14):1983–93.

61. Kamkwalala AR, Maki PM, Langenecker SA, et al. Sex-specific effects of low-dose hydrocortisone on threat detection in HIV. J Neurovirol 2021;27(5):716–26.

62. Echouffo-Tcheugui JB, Conner SC, Himali JJ, et al. Circulating cortisol and cognitive and structural brain measures: The Framingham Heart Study. Neurology 2018;91(21):e1961–70.

63. Abercrombie HC, Wirth MM, Hoks RM. Inter-individual differences in trait negative affect moderate cortisol's effects on memory formation: Preliminary findings from two studies. Psychoneuroendocrinology 2012;37(5):693–701.

64. Bagot RC, van Hasselt FN, Champagne DL, et al. Maternal care determines rapid effects of stress mediators on synaptic plasticity in adult rat hippocampal dentate gyrus. Neurobiol Learn Mem 2009;92:292–300.

65. Champagne DL, Bagot RC, van Hasselt F, et al. Maternal care and hippocampal plasticity: evidence for experience-dependent structural plasticity, altered synaptic functioning, and differential responsiveness to glucocorticoids and stress. J Neurosci Off J Soc Neurosci 2008;28(23):6037–45.

66. Weaver ICG, Cervoni N, Champagne FA, et al. Epigenetic programming by maternal behavior. Nat Neurosci 2004;7(8):847–54.

67. Rubin LH, Langenecker SA, Phan KL, et al. Remitted depression and cognition in HIV: The role of cortisol and inflammation. Psychoneuroendocrinology 2020; 114:104609.

68. Rosada C, Bauer M, Golde S, et al. Association between childhood trauma and brain anatomy in women with post-traumatic stress disorder, women with borderline personality disorder, and healthy women. Eur J Psychotraumatology 2021;12(1):1959706.

69. Sneider JT, Cohen-Gilbert JE, Hamilton DA, et al. Brain Activation during Memory Retrieval is Associated with Depression Severity in Women. Psychiatry Res Neuroimaging 2021;307:111204.

70. Belleau EL, Treadway MT, Pizzagalli DA. The Impact of Stress and Major Depressive Disorder on Hippocampal and Medial Prefrontal Cortex Morphology. Biol Psychiatry 2019;85(6):443–53.

71. McKinnon MC, Yucel K, Nazarov A, et al. A meta-analysis examining clinical predictors of hippocampal volume in patients with major depressive disorder. J Psychiatry Neurosci JPN 2009;34(1):41–54.

72. Bremner JD, Narayan M, Anderson ER, et al. Hippocampal volume reduction in major depression. Am J Psychiatry 2000;157(1):115–8.

73. Roddy DW, Farrell C, Doolin K, et al. The Hippocampus in Depression: More Than the Sum of Its Parts? Advanced Hippocampal Substructure Segmentation in Depression. Biol Psychiatry 2019;85(6):487–97.

74. Han KM, Won E, Sim Y, et al. Hippocampal subfield analysis in medication-naïve female patients with major depressive disorder. J Affect Disord 2016;194:21–9.

75. Mielke EL, Neukel C, Bertsch K, et al. Maternal sensitivity and the empathic brain: Influences of early life maltreatment. J Psychiatr Res 2016;77:59–66.

76. Kim P. How stress can influence brain adaptations to motherhood. Front Neuro-endocrinol 2021;60:100875.
77. Collins MA, Chung Y, Addington J, et al. Discriminatory experiences predict neuroanatomical changes and anxiety among healthy individuals and those at clinical high risk for psychosis. NeuroImage Clin 2021;31:102757.
78. Mychasiuk R, Gibb R, Kolb B. Prenatal bystander stress induces neuroanatomical changes in the prefrontal cortex and hippocampus of developing rat offspring. Brain Res 2011;1412:55–62.
79. Teimouri M, Heidari MH, Amini A, et al. Neuroanatomical changes of the medial prefrontal cortex of male pups of Wistar rat after prenatal and postnatal noise stress. Acta Histochem 2020;122(6):151589.
80. McEwen BS, McKittrick CR, Tamashiro KLK, et al. The brain on stress: Insight from studies using the Visible Burrow System. Physiol Behav 2015;146:47–56.
81. Henley C. HPG Axis. Published online January 1, 2021. Available at: https://openbooks.lib.msu.edu/neuroscience/chapter/hpg-axis/. Accessed 7 November, 2022.
82. Arnold AP, Breedlove SM. Organizational and activational effects of sex steroids on brain and behavior: a reanalysis. Horm Behav 1985;19(4):469–98.
83. Davis SR, Martinez-Garcia A, Robinson PJ, et al. Estrone Is a Strong Predictor of Circulating Estradiol in Women Age 70 Years and Older. J Clin Endocrinol Metab 2020;105(9):dgaa429.
84. McCARTHY MM. Estradiol and the Developing Brain. Physiol Rev 2008;88(1):91–134.
85. Ali Es, C Mangold, Peiris AN. Estriol: emerging clinical benefits. Menopause N Y N 2017;24(9). https://doi.org/10.1097/GME.0000000000000855.
86. Clarkson J, Herbison AE. Hypothalamic control of the male neonatal testosterone surge. Philos Trans R Soc B Biol Sci 2016;371(1688):20150115.
87. Gegenhuber B, Wu MV, Bronstein R, et al. Gene regulation by gonadal hormone receptors underlies brain sex differences. Nature 2022;606(7912):153–9.
88. Simerly RB. Wired for Reproduction: Organization and Development of Sexually Dimorphic Circuits in the Mammalian Forebrain. Annu Rev Neurosci 2002;25(1):507–36.
89. Lauretta R, Sansone M, Sansone A, et al. Gender in Endocrine Diseases: Role of Sex Gonadal Hormones. Int J Endocrinol 2018;2018:4847376.
90. Luine VN. Estradiol and cognitive function: Past, present and future. Horm Behav 2014;66(4):602–18.
91. Hwang WJ, Lee TY, Kim NS, et al. The Role of Estrogen Receptors and Their Signaling across Psychiatric Disorders. Int J Mol Sci 2020;22(1):E373.
92. Pecins-Thompson M, Brown NA, Kohama SG, et al. Ovarian Steroid Regulation of Tryptophan Hydroxylase mRNA Expression in Rhesus Macaques. J Neurosci 1996;16(21):7021–9.
93. Maharjan S, Serova LI, Sabban EL. Membrane-initiated estradiol signaling increases tyrosine hydroxylase promoter activity with ERα in PC12 cells. J Neurochem 2010;112(1):42–55.
94. Becker JB. Estrogen rapidly potentiates amphetamine-induced striatal dopamine release and rotational behavior during microdialysis. Neurosci Lett 1990;118(2):169–71.
95. Bethea CL, Mirkes SJ, Shively CA, et al. Steroid regulation of tryptophan hydroxylase protein in the dorsal raphe of macaques. Biol Psychiatry 2000;47(6):562–76.

96. Gundlah C, Pecins-Thompson M, Schutzer WE, et al. Ovarian steroid effects on serotonin 1A, 2A and 2C receptor mRNA in macaque hypothalamus. Brain Res Mol Brain Res 1999;63(2):325–39.

97. Rivera HM, Santollo J, Nikonova LV, et al. Estradiol increases the anorexia associated with increased 5-HT2C receptor activation in ovariectomized rats. Physiol Behav 2012;105(2):188–94.

98. Adams MM, Fink SE, Janssen WGM, et al. Estrogen modulates synaptic N-methyl-D-aspartate receptor subunit distribution in the aged hippocampus. J Comp Neurol 2004;474(3):419–26.

99. Woolley CS, Weiland NG, McEwen BS, et al. Estradiol increases the sensitivity of hippocampal CA1 pyramidal cells to NMDA receptor-mediated synaptic input: correlation with dendritic spine density. J Neurosci 1997;17(5):1848–59.

100. Kurata K, Takebayashi M, Kagaya A, et al. Effect of beta-estradiol on voltage-gated Ca(2+) channels in rat hippocampal neurons: a comparison with dehydroepiandrosterone. Eur J Pharmacol 2001;416(3):203–12.

101. Hara Y, Waters EM, McEwen BS, et al. Estrogen Effects on Cognitive and Synaptic Health Over the Lifecourse. Physiol Rev 2015;95(3):785–807.

102. Zannas AS, Wiechmann T, Gassen NC, et al. Gene–Stress–Epigenetic Regulation of FKBP5: Clinical and Translational Implications. Neuropsychopharmacology 2016;41(1):261–74.

103. Malviya SA, Kelly SD, Greenlee MM, et al. Estradiol stimulates an anti-translocation expression pattern of glucocorticoid co-regulators in a hippocampal cell model. Physiol Behav 2013;122:187–92.

104. Oyola MG, Handa RJ. Hypothalamic-pituitary-adrenal and hypothalamic-pituitary-gonadal axes: sex differences in regulation of stress responsivity. Stress Amst Neth 2017;20(5):476–94.

105. Bale TL, Vale WW. CRF and CRF receptors: role in stress responsivity and other behaviors. Annu Rev Pharmacol Toxicol 2004;44:525–57.

106. Füzesi T, Daviu N, Wamsteeker Cusulin JI, et al. Hypothalamic CRH neurons orchestrate complex behaviours after stress. Nat Commun 2016;7:11937.

107. Laflamme N, Nappi RE, Drolet G, et al. Expression and neuropeptidergic characterization of estrogen receptors (ERalpha and ERbeta) throughout the rat brain: anatomical evidence of distinct role of each subtype. J Neurobiol 1998; 36(3):357–78.

108. Zhou JN, Fang H. Transcriptional regulation of corticotropin-releasing hormone gene in stress response. IBRO Rep 2018;5:137–46.

109. Chen J, Li Q, Saliuk G, et al. Estrogen and serotonin enhance stress-induced visceral hypersensitivity in female rats by up-regulating brain-derived neurotrophic factor in spinal cord. Neuro Gastroenterol Motil 2021;33(10):e14117.

110. Handa RJ, Mani SK, Uht RM. Estrogen Receptors and the Regulation of Neural Stress Responses. Neuroendocrinology 2012;96(2):111–8.

111. Vamvakopoulos NC, Chrousos GP. Evidence of direct estrogenic regulation of human corticotropin-releasing hormone gene expression. Potential implications for the sexual dimophism of the stress response and immune/inflammatory reaction. J Clin Invest 1993;92(4):1896–902.

112. Weiser MJ, Handa RJ. Estrogen impairs glucocorticoid dependent negative feedback on the hypothalamic–pituitary–adrenal axis via estrogen receptor alpha within the hypothalamus. Neuroscience 2009;159(2):883–95.

113. Panagiotakopoulos L, Neigh GN. Development of the HPA axis: where and when do sex differences manifest? Front Neuroendocrinol 2014;35(3):285–302.

114. Weiser MJ, Foradori CD, Handa RJ. Estrogen receptor beta activation prevents glucocorticoid receptor-dependent effects of the central nucleus of the amygdala on behavior and neuroendocrine function. Brain Res 2010;1336:78–88.
115. Epperson CN, Sammel MD, Bale TL, et al. Adverse Childhood Experiences and Risk for First-Episode Major Depression During the Menopause Transition. J Clin Psychiatry 2017;78(3):e298–307.
116. Zacur HA. Hormonal changes throughout life in women. Headache 2006; 46(Suppl 2):S49–54.
117. Burger HG, Hale GE, Robertson DM, et al. A review of hormonal changes during the menopausal transition: focus on findings from the Melbourne Women's Midlife Health Project. Hum Reprod Update 2007;13(6):559–65.
118. Stevenson JC. A woman's journey through the reproductive, transitional and postmenopausal periods of life: impact on cardiovascular and musculo-skeletal risk and the role of estrogen replacement. Maturitas 2011;70(2): 197–205.
119. Giotakos O. Neurobiology of emotional trauma. Psychiatr Psychiatr 2020;31(2): 162–71.
120. Loewy RL, Corey S, Amirfathi F, et al. Childhood trauma and clinical high risk for psychosis. Schizophr Res 2019;205:10–4.
121. Quidé Y, Tonini E, Watkeys OJ, et al. Schizotypy, childhood trauma and brain morphometry. Schizophr Res 2021;238:73–81.
122. Herzog JI, Schmahl C. Adverse Childhood Experiences and the Consequences on Neurobiological, Psychosocial, and Somatic Conditions Across the Lifespan. Front Psychiatry 2018;9:420.
123. Anda RF, Felitti VJ, Bremner JD, et al. The enduring effects of abuse and related adverse experiences in childhood. A convergence of evidence from neurobiology and epidemiology. Eur Arch Psychiatry Clin Neurosci 2006;256(3):174–86.
124. van der Kolk BA. The neurobiology of childhood trauma and abuse. Child Adolesc Psychiatr Clin N Am 2003;12(2):293–317, ix.
125. An X, Guo W, Wu H, et al. Sex Differences in Depression Caused by Early Life Stress and Related Mechanisms. Front Neurosci 2022;16:797755.
126. Grumbach MM. The neuroendocrinology of human puberty revisited. Horm Res 2002;57(Suppl 2):2–14.
127. Hoyt LT, Falconi A. Puberty and Perimenopause: Reproductive Transitions and their Implications for Women's Health. Soc Sci Med 2015;132:103–12.
128. Patton GC, Viner R. Pubertal transitions in health. Lancet Lond Engl 2007; 369(9567):1130–9.
129. Zhang K, Pollack S, Ghods A, et al. Onset of Ovulation after Menarche in Girls: A Longitudinal Study. J Clin Endocrinol Metab 2008;93(4):1186–94.
130. Comasco E, Sundström-Poromaa I. Neuroimaging the Menstrual Cycle and Premenstrual Dysphoric Disorder. Curr Psychiatry Rep 2015;17(10):77.
131. Sundström-Poromaa I. The Menstrual Cycle Influences Emotion but Has Limited Effect on Cognitive Function. Vitam Horm 2018;107:349–76.
132. Gonda X, Telek T, Juhász G, et al. Patterns of mood changes throughout the reproductive cycle in healthy women without premenstrual dysphoric disorders. Prog Neuro-Psychopharmacol Biol Psychiatry 2008;32(8):1782–8.
133. Labaka A, Goñi-Balentziaga O, Lebeña A, et al. Biological Sex Differences in Depression: A Systematic Review. Biol Res Nurs 2018;20(4):383–92.
134. Marshall AD. Developmental Timing of Trauma Exposure Relative to Puberty and the Nature of Psychopathology Among Adolescent Girls. J Am Acad Child Adolesc Psychiatry 2016;55(1):25–32.e1.

135. Stenson AF, Michopoulos V, Stevens JS, et al. Sex-Specific Associations Between Trauma Exposure, Pubertal Timing, and Anxiety in Black Children. Front Hum Neurosci 2021;15. Available at: https://www.frontiersin.org/articles/10.3389/fnhum.2021.636199. Accessed 6 November, 2022.
136. Schmidt PJ, Rubinow DR. Sex hormones and mood in the perimenopause. Ann N Y Acad Sci 2009;1179:70–85.
137. Hodes GE, Epperson CN. Sex Differences in Vulnerability and Resilience to Stress Across the Life Span. Biol Psychiatry 2019;86(6):421–32.
138. Bromberger JT, Epperson CN. Depression During and After the Perimenopause: Impact of Hormones, Genetics, and Environmental Determinants of Disease. Obstet Gynecol Clin North Am 2018;45(4):663–78.
139. Voytko ML, Tinkler GP, Browne C, et al. Neuroprotective effects of estrogen therapy for cognitive and neurobiological profiles of monkey models of menopause. Am J Primatol 2009;71(9):794–801.
140. Albert KM, Newhouse PA. Estrogen, Stress, and Depression: Cognitive and Biological Interactions. Annu Rev Clin Psychol 2019;15:399–423.
141. Moulton CD, Pickup JC, Ismail K. The link between depression and diabetes: the search for shared mechanisms. Lancet Diabetes Endocrinol 2015;3(6):461–71.
142. Mavranezouli I, Megnin-Viggars O, Daly C, et al. Psychological treatments for post-traumatic stress disorder in adults: a network meta-analysis. Psychol Med 2020;50(4):542–55.
143. Fodor KE, Bitter I. [Psychological interventions following trauma to prevent post-traumatic stress disorder. A systematic review of the literature]. Orv Hetil 2015;156(33):1321–34.
144. Hathaisaard C, Wannarit K, Pattanaseri K. Mindfulness-based interventions reducing and preventing stress and burnout in medical students: A systematic review and meta-analysis. Asian J Psychiatry 2022;69:102997.
145. Huberty J, Green J, Glissmann C, et al. Efficacy of the Mindfulness Meditation Mobile App "Calm" to Reduce Stress Among College Students: Randomized Controlled Trial. JMIR MHealth UHealth 2019;7(6):e14273.
146. Boyd JE, Lanius RA, McKinnon MC. Mindfulness-based treatments for posttraumatic stress disorder: a review of the treatment literature and neurobiological evidence. J Psychiatry Neurosci JPN 2018;43(1):7–25.
147. Janssen M, Heerkens Y, Kuijer W, et al. Effects of Mindfulness-Based Stress Reduction on employees' mental health: A systematic review. PLoS One 2018;13(1):e0191332.
148. Yang J, Tang S, Zhou W. Effect of Mindfulness-Based Stress Reduction Therapy on Work Stress and Mental Health of Psychiatric Nurses. Psychiatr Danub 2018;30(2):189–96.
149. Hofmann SG, Gómez AF. Mindfulness-Based Interventions for Anxiety and Depression. Psychiatr Clin North Am 2017;40(4):739–49.

Perinatal Depression
A Review and an Update

Anne Louise Stewart, MD, Jennifer L. Payne, MD*

KEYWORDS

- Perinatal depression • Antenatal depression • Postpartum depression • Lactation
- Infant • Antidepressants • Allopregnanolone • GABAergic neurotransmission

KEY POINTS

- Perinatal depression is common, serious, and has negative effects on pregnancy and infant outcomes.
- Screening for and treatment of perinatal depression is imperative.
- Most antidepressants can be used during pregnancy and lactation with the risk–benefit ratio favoring treatment over the risks of untreated psychiatric illness.
- Other treatments for perinatal depression that can be considered include transcranial magnetic stimulation, electroconvulsive therapy, psychotherapy such as interpersonal therapy and light box therapy.
- New treatments with a unique mechanism of action, acting on the GABAergic neurotransmitter system, are available to treat postpartum depression.

INTRODUCTION

Perinatal depression is a serious psychiatric illness that can have severe and deleterious effects on the mother, the exposed infant, and the family unit. By definition, perinatal depression is depression occurring during pregnancy (antenatal depression) or during the immediate postpartum time period (postpartum depression [PPD]). It should be identified as quickly as possible and treated effectively and expediently in order to support a healthy perinatal period. Perinatal depression can also lead to devastating and preventable consequences such as suicide and infanticide and is associated with negative pregnancy outcomes as well as effects on infant development and cognition. With maternal depression only increasing during the coronavirus disease 2019 pandemic,[1,2] understanding screening, diagnosis, and treatment is more important than ever. This article will review why it is important to screen for,

Department of Psychiatry and Neurobehavioral Sciences, University of Virginia, PO Box 800548, Charlottesville, VA 22908, USA
* Corresponding author.
E-mail address: jlp4n@uvahealth.org

Psychiatr Clin N Am 46 (2023) 447–461
https://doi.org/10.1016/j.psc.2023.04.003
0193-953X/23/© 2023 Elsevier Inc. All rights reserved.

psych.theclinics.com

identify and treat perinatal depression, and discuss the treatment options, as well as the safety of the treatment options for perinatal depression.

EFFECTS OF PERINATAL DEPRESSION ON PREGNANCY AND INFANT OUTCOMES

Maternal depression both during and after pregnancy is associated with adverse pregnancy and infant outcomes. Antenatal depression is associated with multiple negative pregnancy outcomes including preterm birth,[3,4] and low birth weight,[5] as well as higher rates of gestational diabetes, preeclampsia, and C-section.[5] Mothers with antenatal depression can also experience low maternal weight gain, increased rates of substance use, ambivalence about pregnancy, and overall worse health status.[6,7] Infants that are exposed to antenatal depression have also been shown to have higher serum cortisol levels than infants who are not exposed to maternal depression, likely due to elevated maternal cortisol and inflammation associated with depression.[8] Although the long-term effects of elevated cortisol on the infant need further research, the elevated cortisol levels continue into adolescence and could partially explain a mechanism for the development of psychiatric illness in children.[8] Importantly, if antenatal depression is treated during pregnancy, cortisol levels seem to normalize, indicating a potential pathway to prevent long-term psychiatric illness in vulnerable children.[9] After pregnancy, PPD has repeatedly been shown to interfere with normal infant development. PPD is associated with impaired maternal infant bonding and increased infant colic.[10] Because it also interferes with flexible parenting behavior and maternal–infant bonding, PPD has been shown to subsequently have negative effects on infant development, including lower IQ, slower language development, and behavioral issues.[11]

If left untreated, PPD can have devastating consequences such as suicide and infanticide. In fact, suicides account for up to 20% of all postpartum deaths and are a leading cause of perinatal mortality in the year following childbirth.[12] Infanticide and its relationship with PPD is not well documented in the literature but there are almost 3000 infanticides in the United States per year,[13] and notably few mothers turning to this devastating action actually received any prenatal care including psychiatric care.[14]

SCREENING FOR PERINATAL DEPRESSION

The US Preventative Services Task Force (USPSTF) recommendations for screening for depression continue to change and have been encompassing more populations, including women and children. In 2016, the USPSTF recommended screening for depression in the perinatal population,[15] and recently recommended to screen children aged 12 years and older for depression,[16] indicating a growing problem for even the youngest of the population. With adolescent PPD occurring in up to 50% of mothers in some studies,[17] inclusive screening is necessary. In line with growing screening practices, The American College of Obstetricians and Gynecologists (ACOG) recommends screening for depression (and anxiety) symptoms at least once during the perinatal period with repeat screening being part of the comprehensive postpartum visit.[18] The American Psychiatric Association position statement published 2018, recommends depression screening with a validated screening tool twice during pregnancy and during pediatric visits throughout the first 6 months postpartum.[19] Validated screening tools include (but are not limited to): Edinburgh Postnatal Depression Scale (EPDS),[20] Patient Health Questionnaire 9,[21] and the Hospital Anxiety and Depression Scale.[22]

Although no official organization has made recommendations on how to screen for bipolar disorder in the perinatal period, bipolar depression is a common complication of childbirth. One study has demonstrated that the addition of the Mood Disorder Questionnaire[23] to the EPDS increased the identification of women with bipolar depression as opposed to unipolar depression in the perinatal period.[24]

RELAPSE RISK OF PREPREGNANCY MOOD DISORDERS

Treatment of perinatal depression should continue throughout pre-existing and throughout the postpartum period. Discontinuation of psychiatric medications is associated with high relapse rates of both major depressive disorder (MDD) and bipolar disorder. For mothers with a history of MDD, discontinuation of treatment is linked to another major depressive episode in 60% to 70% of women.[25] For mothers with bipolar disorder, 80% to 100% of women will have a recurrent mood episode after discontinuing mood stabilizers, whereas 29% to 37% of women will have a recurrent mood episode if continued on their mood stabilizer.[26,27] These rates show that although there is a lower risk of relapse on medications, a significant amount of women relapse despite ongoing medication use. Pregnancy is time of significant changes in pharmacokinetics and metabolism subsequent to variations in blood volume and distribution, body weight, and metabolic changes associated with pregnancy. The concentration of some medications has been shown to decrease, particularly in the third trimester[28] and may represent a possible underlying cause of psychiatric relapse during pregnancy despite ongoing medication use.

UNITED STATES FOOD AND DRUG ADMINISTRATION DRUG LABELING RULES

In 2014, the US Food and Drug Administration (FDA) published the "Pregnancy and Lactation Labeling Rule (PLLR),"[29] which replaces the previous pregnancy categories with a summary narrative describing the currently available information for a particular medication well. The pregnancy categories (A, B, C, D, and X) were thought to represent an over simplistic interpretation and created confusion about how to make a decision about medication use in pregnancy or breastfeeding. For example, some Category B drugs had not been studied in humans but clinicians often assumed that Category B drugs were safer than Category C or D drugs when, in fact, there was no human data.

The new system will attempt to summarize all currently available information to help the clinician and the patient weigh the risks and benefits of prescribing a drug during pregnancy or breastfeeding as well as in the new category of "females and males of reproductive potential." This new section gives valuable information and guidance on pregnancy testing, contraception, and infertility. A potentially impactful change will be that the PLLR will explicitly state when there is no data available and provide a risk summary based on known human data, animal data, and provide some clinical considerations. In addition, there is now a pregnancy exposure registry as well as sections discussing dose adjustment during pregnancy and the postpartum period as well as labor and delivery information.[29]

TREATMENT PRINCIPLES
Prepregnancy Planning

The most important time to identify and treat depressive illness is before pregnancy. Because as many as 50% of pregnancies are unplanned in the United States, [30,31] physicians should assume that every woman of reproductive age will get pregnant and discuss the safety of medications versus the risks of the untreated depressive illness during pregnancy—before pregnancy and preferably when medications are first prescribed. During these discussions, the physician should also support the woman's reproductive choices and discuss contraception options, especially in the case of medication use that is absolutely contraindicated in pregnancy. If a woman is taking a psychiatric medication contraindicated in pregnancy (such valproic acid or carbamazepine), a discussion should be held with the woman and, if possible, her partner, to plan what should be done if she were to become pregnant. It is important to understand whether that particular medication is crucial for the stability of the patient. This prepregnancy planning is an important collaboration between the obstetrician-gynecologist, psychiatrist, patient, and family so that critical medications are continued, and the risk of relapse is minimized in the case of unplanned pregnancy.

General principles that apply when planning for pregnancy include using medications for which we have data during pregnancy (meaning older medications usually have more than newer ones), and minimizing the number of medications to those necessary to maintain a woman's psychiatric wellness. Many psychiatric patients get on complicated regimens in the process of recovering and there is often a reluctance to changing the regimen once they get well. Careful trimming of medications in order to see what medication is actually helping should be done before pregnancy. Any medication changes should ideally be done 6 to 12 months before attempting pregnancy to ensure stability and to limit the number of medication and illness exposures. For example, if a patient and physician are planning before pregnancy, a newer, less-studied medication could be switched to a medication with more safety data before attempting pregnancy. Another important principle is to not undertreat. Undertreatment increases the number of exposures for the baby—the baby is exposed to both the psychiatric medication as well as maternal illness. Treat to wellness.

Importantly, if the patient or partner is against medication use during pregnancy, it is essential to discuss the risks of no treatment of the infant, the risks of no treatment of the mother, and the risk of relapse. If the patient and/or the partner insist on eliminating psychiatric medications for pregnancy, rather than insist on a specific treatment plan, the clinician should focus on keeping an open line of communication, outlining home symptom monitoring, and scheduling close follow-up. This approach can maintain a doctor–patient relationship that keeps patients safe and in treatment.

Unplanned Pregnancy

The rate of unplanned pregnancies in the United States remains at about 50% including both pregnancies resulting from failed contraception efforts and pregnancies from no contraception efforts.[30,31] Given the high rate of unplanned pregnancies, all physician will eventually care for a patient requesting medication guidance in the setting of an unplanned pregnancy. The same principles apply to an unplanned pregnancy as to a planned pregnancy with some additional considerations. Importantly, do not stop all psychiatric medications abruptly because this can cause stress for patient and family, can precipitate withdrawal or discontinuation symptoms, can trigger relapse of a depressive illness, and subsequently can expose the fetus to the risks of all of the above. Similarly, do not abruptly lower the dosages or alter the timing of medications—that is, transform a scheduled medication to an as needed medication. The patient may need more treatment, not less, in the setting of the pharmacokinetic changes of drugs in pregnancy.[28]

The best approach is to review the medication list with the patient and family in a systematic fashion as soon as possible. In an unplanned pregnancy, the fetus is already exposed to regularly scheduled medications, so while some changes might be necessary, such as stopping a teratogenic medication, it should be done in a calm and logical fashion, fostering trust and open discussion to keep the mother in treatment. Because the fetus has already been exposed to medications, it might *not* make sense to change a medication with no safety data to a medication with known safety data because this plan increases the number of medication exposures to the baby. In addition, there is the risk of precipitating a relapse when switching medications. If the treatment plan includes stopping a certain medication, it should be tapered to eliminate the risk of withdrawal and discontinuation symptoms to mother and fetus.

Breastfeeding

The American Academy of Pediatrics and the World Health Organization advocate for exclusively providing breastmilk for baby throughout the first 6 months of life. The benefits breastfeeding or providing breastmilk for baby and mother are well documented. Breastfeeding provides protection against gastrointestinal infections and decreases newborn mortality,[32] which in turn can lower the stress a mother can experience caring for a sick child. Breastfeeding is also associated with downstream benefits for baby including healthier weight, higher income in adult life, higher school attendance, and better intelligence tests.[32,33] Direct benefits for the mother include a lower risk of ovarian and breast cancer.[33] Although the association between depression and breastfeeding needs further prospective study, there is a signal in the current literature that depressive symptoms may be associated with early cessation of breastfeeding.[33,34] This underscores that for the baby and mother to gain the benefits of breastfeeding, depressive illnesses should be safely and effectively treated.

If medications do need to change during breastfeeding due to worsening of the mother's psychiatric illness or side effects for the infant, the discussion should include whether continued breastfeeding is worth the risks of increasing the number of exposures to medications and/or psychiatric illness for the infant. For example, a mother with a history of depression with psychotic features requiring previous psychiatric hospitalization, stable on an antidepressant and antipsychotic, might notice sedation in her baby, reducing its desire to feed and resulting in poor weight gain. Because the mother's depression has historically been severe, the risk of relapse by changing medications might outweigh the benefits of breastfeeding for that specific infant and mother pair. The pediatrician should be involved in this decision-making process because they help monitor side effects and can draw blood levels in the baby as needed. In general, common side effects in the baby can include sleepiness and decreased feeding, which is hard to distinguish from a fussy baby and why close monitoring in conjunction with the pediatrician is helpful.

ANTIDEPRESSANT USE IN PREGNANCY
A Challenging Literature

Antidepressants are the most commonly prescribed psychotropic medication during pregnancy.[35] Although other classes of medications, such as antipsychotics and lithium, are used as augmentation agents to treat depression, this review will focus on antidepressant use, nonpharmacological antidepressant treatments, and newer antidepressant agents. In general, the literature examining infant outcomes associated with antidepressant use in pregnancy is problematic due to the need to control for many confounding factors, including the underlying psychiatric illness and confounding risks and behaviors associated with the illness itself. Several older publications found associations between in utero antidepressant exposure and various negative infant outcomes. However, these studies failed to control for "confounding by indication" meaning controlling for risks and behaviors that are associated with the reason (indication) for the prescription medication exposure. Thus, in utero medication exposure was then associated with negative infant outcomes that were not due to the medication exposure itself but due to the risks and behaviors associated with underlying psychiatric illness. For example, smoking is more common in the psychiatric population-studies that did not control for having a psychiatric diagnosis or did not control for smoking might find an association between a negative infant outcome and in utero medication exposure that was actually due to the exposure to maternal smoking. Newer studies have taken pains to control for confounding by indication, and although some associations remain, most studies are reassuring and find only rare negative outcomes.

Major Organ Malformations

When looking at all the available literature, antidepressant use in pregnancy seems to not be clearly associated with major organ malformations. Despite at least one large epidemiologic study[36] citing an increased risk for selective serotonin reuptake inhibitors (SSRIs), 4 large meta-analyses reassuringly did not find a statistically significant increased risk.[37–40] There are limited data for other types of antidepressants, and the studies available have not found associations with major malformations with bupropion[41–43] or tricyclic antidepressant[44–48] exposure.

Cardiac Defects

The literature on cardiac defects and antidepressants is also peppered with problems. Early observational studies described an association between antidepressant exposure and cardiac defects (reviewed in ref[49]); however, most of these studies did not control for the underlying psychiatric illness or the risks that come with behaviors associated with MDD. Reassuringly, newer studies that attempt to control for the underlying illness and associated risks have not found an association between antidepressant use in the mother and cardiac malformations in the infant.[50,51]

Persistent pulmonary hypertension

Persistent pulmonary hypertension in the newborn (PPHN) carries a 10% to 20% mortality,[52] so the interest in identifying risk factors for the condition is large. The FDA published a public health advisory in 2006 based on a single study that reported PPHN was more common in babies if they were born to a mother taking an SSRI after 20 weeks of pregnancy.[53] This study did not control for the underlying depressive illness or its severity. In addition, several known risk factors for PPHN include obesity, gestational diabetes, smoking, and C-section, which are more common in the psychiatric population. One study found that a history of psychiatric hospitalization increased the risk of PPHN even when mothers did not take antidepressants in pregnancy, highlighting the many confounding factors.[54] In 2011, the FDA expanded their safety communication to note that there is conflicting data and that there is not sufficient evidence to conclude that SSRI use in pregnancy causes PPHN based on subsequent cohort and case-control studies.[55] The most recent cohort study by Huybrechts found a small increased odds ratio of 1.10 for PPHN in infants exposed to in utero SSRIs.[56] This study used propensity scores to decrease confounding factors, although this statistical adjustment used proxies for illness and severity of illness, again limiting generalization.[56] The authors concluded that there may be a small increased risk of PPHN but that the absolute risk was less than 1% of those exposed.[56]

Autism

A systematic review and meta-analysis found that psychiatric illness is a large confounding factor in the associations between SSRI exposure and autism and that there is not an increased risk for autism when studies controlled for maternal psychiatric illness.[57]

Spontaneous Abortion

This area of study is also plagued with problems because once again studies have not controlled for the underlying psychiatric illness or its risk factors. Four studies have published an increased risk of spontaneous abortion with odds ratios ranging from 1.4 to 1.6[58–61] but causation cannot be assumed. More controlled studies are needed.

Preterm Birth and Low Birth Weight

A 2016 systematic review and meta-analysis on this topic again underlines the importance of controlling for the underlying illness. This study examined preterm birth and low birth rate in women with MDD not receiving treatment versus in women without MDD and found untreated depression was associated with an increased risk of poor neonatal outcomes including preterm birth and low birth weight.[61]

Poor neonatal adaption syndrome

Poor neonatal adaption syndrome (PNAS) is a nonspecific syndrome that can include respiratory distress, cyanosis, apnea, seizures, temperature instability, feeding difficulty, vomiting, hypoglycemia, hypotonia, hypertonia, tremor, jitteriness, irritability, or constant crying.[62] Studying this syndrome and its association with antidepressants is challenging because the syndrome is not systematically defined or measured. Available data suggest that one-third of infants exposed to antidepressants will have at least mild symptoms (reviewed in ref[62]); however, more rigorous studies of the syndrome, particularly blinded studies, are needed.

New Treatments: Positive Allosteric Modulators of the Gamma-Aminobutyric Acid-A Receptor

Brexanolone was approved by the FDA in 2019 as the first antidepressant treatment specifically for PPD and has a unique mechanism of action compared to other types of antidepressants. Brexanolone is a synthetic intravenous form of the neuroactive steroid allopregnanolone and acts on the inhibitory gamma-aminobutyric acid (GABA) A receptor as a positive allosteric modulator to help restore the excitatory-inhibitory balance in the brain. The infusion is given during the course of 60 hours and generally requires an inpatient setting. Brexanolone's use in PPD is based on 4 published studies—an open label, proof of concept study, a small randomized controlled phase II trial, and 2 large randomized controlled phase III trials.[63–65] In the large randomized controlled trials (RCTs), the mean differences between Hamilton Depression Rating Scale (HAMD) scores of the placebo group versus both infusion rate groups were statistically different, and the separation from placebo occurred by 24 to 48 hours.[65] The rate of participants achieving remission was higher in brexanolone groups compared with placebo groups in both phase III trials. Brexanolone was well tolerated in the studies with headache, dizziness, and somnolence being the most reported adverse events.[65] Due to 5% of women experiencing sedation, including loss of consciousness, infusions now require a Risk Evaluation and Mitigation Strategy program and require continuous pulse-oximetry monitoring with a trained health-care provider to be available immediately to monitor the pulse-oximetry. In addition, a trained health-care provider, most likely nursing, has to assess the women for excessive sedation every 2 hours when awake and every 4 hours when asleep so that infusions can be stopped should an adverse event develop. Importantly, brexanolone is a novel therapeutic for PPD with a rapid 70% response rate and rapid 50% to 70% remission rate lasting up to 30 days after infusion, making it a breakthrough treatment of women with PPD.[63–65]

A recent study[66] used population pharmacokinetic modeling to describe a potential relative infant dose during breastfeeding in mothers receiving brexanolone. This was an open laboratory phase 1b study that collected allopregnanolone levels in breast milk and plasma after completion of a single continuous 60-hour infusion of brexanolone. Blood samples were collected at predetermined time points but breast milk was collected as mothers pumped and not at predetermined time points. The study found that allopregnanolone concentrations in breast milk were maximum between hour 24 and 48, and 95% of women had less than 10 ng/mL after 36 hours postcompletion of the infusion.[66] This result encourages more research to potentially support women restarting breastfeeding earlier than the current 7-day recommendation. In addition, the median relative infant dosing calculated was 0.69%, suggesting potential low infant exposure, if breastfeeding, but effects on infants are currently not described in the literature.

Zuranolone is an *oral* neuroactive steroid agent that is currently being considered for FDA approval for the treatment of PPD and MDD. There are 2 clinical trials evaluating its efficacy in PPD. The published "Robin" study is a phase III double-blind, randomized, placebo-controlled trial that enrolled women from third trimester to 4 weeks postpartum with a Hamilton Depression Rating (HAMD) score of 26 or higher.[67] The women received either placebo or zuranolone 30 mg. There was a statistically significant reduction in baseline HAMD scores in the zuranolone group versus the placebo group at the primary endpoint, day 15; however, greater reduction was seen even by day 3.[67] The response rate was approximately 70%, and the remission rate was approximately 50% in the active drug arm.[67] Zuranolone was generally well tolerated with common side effects of headache, dizziness, and somnolence, diarrhea, and sedation, similar to the placebo group and to side effects seen with brexanolone; however, no women experienced loss of consciousness.[67] Participants were not allowed to breastfeed during this trial, so the safety of breastfeeding while using zuranolone is currently unknown. As of this writing, the results of the second phase III trial of zuranolone 50 mg for treatment of PPD has not been published in a peer reviewed journal.

NONPHARMACOLOGIC TREATMENTS
Transcranial Magnetic Stimulation

A 2021 systematic review of noninvasive brain stimulation explored the role of transcranial magnetic stimulation (TMS) in peripartum depression.[68] There is only one RCT exploring TMS versus sham treatment in pregnancy[69] and one RCT of TMS versus sham in the postpartum period.[70] In these studies, TMS seems to decrease depression scores by the end of the treatment phase.[69,70] However, there were 3 preterm births reported in the pregnancy trial.[69] The preterm birth outcome needs to be further examined in larger trials because preterm birth is also noted to be higher in women with peripartum depression. Breastfeeding was not a defined outcome in these studies.

Electroconvulsive Therapy

Although electroconvulsive therapy (ECT) has been used longer than TMS in the treatment of depressive disorders, the use of ECT has only been described in the peripartum time-period in case reports and case series, which have a high risk of bias.[68] Patients would benefit from high-quality studies to evaluate safety and efficacy in this population in order to provide evidence-based treatment options. A review of the literature from 1960 to 2014 concluded that there are no absolute contraindications for the use of ECT in any trimester of pregnancy.[71] The review also found that non–life-threatening adverse events rates seem similar to the rates found in pregnant patients not receiving ECT and, as long as there is appropriate monitoring, ECT is a treatment modality that should be considered based on the history of the mother's psychiatric illness.[71]

Exercise

A systematic review and meta-analysis found that physical activity lowered depression symptoms in women with perinatal depression.[72] However, the analysis was limited by including studies in which attendance rates for exercise activities varied, only 2 studies included a clinical diagnosis of depression rather than depressive symptoms, and the exercise interventions were heterogenous ranging from education to observed aerobic exercise by a fitness specialist.[72] Future studies need to be completed to provide an evidence-based recommendation on type and duration of exercise. Overall, it is likely that exercise can be considered as having a positive effect on depressive symptoms in the perinatal period.

Light Box Therapy

Light box therapy (LBT) is an established treatment of MDD with seasonal onset and has also been studied with positive results in nonseasonal MDD as well as bipolar depression. Although LBT has shown mixed results in the perinatal population, this likely results from small sample sizes and not from a lack of effect. Epperson and colleagues, for example, conducted a randomized clinical trial of LBT at 7000 lux compared with placebo at 500 lux and found that those randomized to LBT had a 60% improvement in depression ratings compared with 41% in the placebo group.[73] However, the sample size was small (n = 10) and the results were not statistically different.[73] In a larger sample (n = 27), Wirz and colleagues found that LBT was superior to a control condition with 81% of the LBT sample responding compared with 45% in placebo condition.[74] In contrast, Bais and colleagues did not find a difference in treatment response between sham and active treatment during 6 weeks in 67 pregnant women due to a high response rate in the sham arm.[75] In contrast, Domnez and colleagues found a 75% response rate in the LBT arm compared with 18.2% in the placebo arm in 30 pregnant or postpartum women.[76] Similarly, Garbazza and colleagues found a 73% response rate in the LBT group compared with 27% in the placebo group in 22 pregnant or postpartum women.[77] Despite 2 statistically negative randomized trials, all studies found a robust response to LBT in pregnant and postpartum women (including in the statistically negative ones) and, in addition, demonstrated a quick response by week 1, highlighting a potential benefit over pharmacotherapy. Adverse events were also not different from the placebo group, underlining another potential benefit to this population of women. Overall the preponderance of the evidence supports using LBT in the perinatal population for the treatment of depressive symptoms.

Psychotherapy

Different modalities of psychotherapy have been used in the peripartum period for depression and is an important option to consider, especially for women with depression symptoms who are not interested in pursuing pharmacotherapy after a risk–

benefit discussion. The best-studied psychotherapeutic approaches have been inter-personal therapy (IPT) and cognitive behavioral therapy (CBT). A 2011 meta-analysis examining psychotherapy treatments of depression across the peripartum period found that psychotherapeutic approaches were efficacious at reducing depression symptoms in general, IPT had a greater effect size than CBT and that individual psychotherapy was more effective than group psychotherapy.[78] The review also noted that there were significant limitations in the literature including confounding factors such as the concurrent use of antidepressants, a lack of long-term outcomes, and differences in measurement of depressive symptoms.[78] Despite the lack of high-quality studies, the benefits of psychotherapy should be considered for this population, especially for those women against pharmacotherapy. Further research should be conducted to guide the types of psychological intervention recommended for this population.

SUMMARY

Perinatal depression continues to be an underrecognized and undertreated psychiatric condition. Screening for perinatal depression is key with initiation of or referral for treatment an important second step. Most antidepressant medications can be used during pregnancy and lactation, particularly when compared with the risks associated with maternal depression, which is associated with adverse pregnancy, infant and child outcomes. Nonpharmacological options such as TMS, LBT, ECT, and psychotherapy are available and should be used as well. New pharmacological agents are available or are soon to be available that treat PPD via modulation of the GABA-A receptor. In summary, a wide range of available treatments for perinatal depression are available and should be used to treat this potentially devastating illness.

CLINICS CARE POINTS

- Medication plans for pregnancy should be developed before pregnancy whenever possible and medication changes made before pregnancy.
- Ideally, the patient should be psychiatrically stable before attempting pregnancy.
- Use medications for which there are available data; older medications usually have more data than newer ones.
- Clinicians should no longer use the FDA Pregnancy categories to guide treatment decisions.
- Minimize the number of exposures for the baby including the number of medications and exposure to maternal psychiatric illness.
- Nonpharmacological interventions are available to treat perinatal depression and should be considered.
- Modulators of the GABA-A receptor are new therapeutic options for the treatment of PPD.

DISCLOSURE

Dr J.L. Payne reports research support from NIMH, United States and Janssen Pharmaceuticals, United States. Dr J.L. Payne has 2 patents: "Epigenetic Biomarkers of Postpartum Depression" and "Epigenetic Biomarkers of Premenstrual Dysphoric Disorder and SSRI Response." Dr J.L. Payne has received consulting fees from SAGE Therapeutics, Biogen, Flo Health, Dionysus Digital Health, Pure Tech, Brii Biosciences, and Merck. She receives royalties from UpToDate and Elsevier. She has produced content for and received honoraria from CMEToGo, Peerview Institute for Medical Education, Global Learning Collaborative, and Karuna Therapeutics. She owns Founder's Stock options from Dionysus Digital Health.

REFERENCES

1. Bajaj MA, Salimgaraev R, Zhaunova L, et al. Rates of self-reported postpartum depressive symptoms in the united states before and after the start of the COVID-19 pandemic. J Psychiatr Res 2022;151:108–12.
2. Mateus V, Cruz S, Costa R, et al. Rates of depressive and anxiety symptoms in the perinatal period during the COVID-19 pandemic: Comparisons between countries and with pre-pandemic data. J Affect Disord 2022;316:245–53.
3. Yonkers KA, Wisner KL, Stewart DE, et al. The management of depression during pregnancy: A report from the american psychiatric association and the american college of obstetricians and gynecologists. Gen Hosp Psychiatry 2009;31(5):403–13.
4. Li D, Liu L, Odouli R. Presence of depressive symptoms during early pregnancy and the risk of preterm delivery: A prospective cohort study. Hum Reprod 2009;24(1):146–53.
5. Steinig J, Nagl M, Linde K, et al. Antenatal and postnatal depression in women with obesity: A systematic review. Arch Womens Ment Health 2017;20(4):569–85.
6. Zuckerman B, Amaro H, Bauchner H, et al. Depressive symptoms during pregnancy: Relationship to poor health behaviors. Am J Obstet Gynecol 1989;160(5):1107.
7. Orr ST, Blazer DG, James SA, et al. Depressive symptoms and indicators of maternal health status during pregnancy. J Womens Health (Larchmt) 2007;16(4):535–42.
8. Osborne S, Biaggi A, Chua TE, et al. Antenatal depression programs cortisol stress reactivity in offspring through increased maternal inflammation and cortisol in pregnancy: The psychiatry research and motherhood - depression (PRAM-D) study. Psychoneuroendocrinology 2018;98:211–21.
9. Brennan PA, Pargas R, Walker EF, et al. Maternal depression and infant cortisol: Influences of timing, comorbidity and treatment. J Child Psychol Psychiatry 2008;49(10):1099–107.
10. Akman I, Kusçu K, Ozdemir N, et al. Mothers' postpartum psychological adjustment and infantile colic. Arch Dis Child 2006;91(5):417–9.
11. Grace SL, Evindar A, Stewart DE. The effect of postpartum depression on child cognitive development and behavior: A review and critical analysis of the literature. Arch Womens Ment Health 2003;6(4):263–74.
12. Lindahl V, Pearson JL, Colpe L. Prevalence of suicidality during pregnancy and the postpartum. Arch Wom Ment Health 2005;8(2):77–87.
13. Wilson RF, Klevens J, Williams D, et al. Infant homicides within the context of safe haven laws — united states, 2008–2017. MMWR (Morb Mortal Wkly Rep) 2020;69:1385–90.
14. Herman-Giddens ME, Smith JB, Mittal M, et al. Newborns killed or left to die by a parent: A population-based study. JAMA 2003;289(11):1425–9.
15. Siu AL, US Preventive Services Task Force (USPSTF), Bibbins-Domingo K, et al. Screening for depression in adults: US preventive services task force recommendation statement. JAMA 2016;315(4):380–7.
16. Jin J. Screening for depression and suicide risk in children and adolescents. JAMA 2022;328(15):1570.

17. Sangsawang B, Wacharasin C, Sangsawang N. Interventions for the prevention of postpartum depression in adolescent mothers: A systematic review. Arch Womens Ment Health 2019;22(2):215–28.

18. ACOG committee opinion no. 757 summary. Screening for perinatal depression. Obstet Gynecol 2018;132(5). Available at: https://journals.lww.com/greenjournal/Fulltext/2018/11000/ACOG_Committee_Opinion_No__757_Summary__Screening.37.aspx.

19. American Psychiatric Association. Position statement on screening and treatment of mood and anxiety disorders during pregnancy and postpartum. Available at: https://www.psychiatry.org/getattachment/c5db4e7b-6405-4655-aecb-bc79d5efb4ea/Position-Screening-and-Treatment-Mood-Anxiety-Disorders-During-Pregnancy-Postpartum.pdf. Accessed December 5.

20. Cox JL, Chapman G, Murray D, et al. Validation of the edinburgh postnatal depression scale (EPDS) in non-postnatal women. J Affect Disord 1996;39(3):185–9.

21. Spitzer RL, Kroenke K, Williams JB. Validation and utility of a self-report version of PRIME-MD: The PHQ primary care study. primary care evaluation of mental disorders. patient health questionnaire. JAMA 1999;282(18):1737–44.

22. Zigmond AS, Snaith RP. The hospital anxiety and depression scale. Acta Psychiatr Scand 1983;67(6):361–70.

23. Hirschfeld RM. The mood disorder questionnaire: A simple, patient-rated screening instrument for bipolar disorder. Prim Care Companion J Clin Psychiatry 2002;4(1):9–11.

24. Clark CT, Sit DKY, Driscoll K, et al. Does screening with the mdq and epds improve identification of bipolar disorder in an obstetrical sample? Depress Anxiety 2015;32(7):518–26.

25. Cohen LS, Altshuler LL, Harlow BL, et al. Relapse of major depression during pregnancy in women who maintain or discontinue antidepressant treatment. J Am Med Assoc 2006;295(5):499–507.

26. Viguera AC, Nonacs R, Cohen LS, et al. Risk of recurrence of bipolar disorder in pregnant and nonpregnant women after discontinuing lithium maintenance. Am J Psychiatry 2000;157(2):179–84.

27. Viguera AC, Whitfield T, Baldessarini RJ, et al. Risk of recurrence in women with bipolar disorder during pregnancy: Prospective study of mood stabilizer discontinuation. Am J Psychiatry 2007;164(12):1817–24.

28. Schoretsanitis G, Spigset O, Stingl JC, et al. The impact of pregnancy on the pharmacokinetics of antidepressants: A systematic critical review and meta-analysis. Expert Opin Drug Metab Toxicol 2020;16(5):431–40.

29. Food and Drug Administration. Content and format of labeling for human prescription drug and biological products; requirements for pregnancy and lactation labeling. Federalregister.gov Web site. Available at: https://www.federalregister.gov/documents/2014/12/04/2014-28241/content-and-format-of-labeling-for-human-prescription-drug-and-biological-products-requirements-for. 2014. Accessed 5 December, 2022.

30. Mosher WD, Bachrach CA. Understanding U.S. fertility: Continuity and change in the national survey of family growth, 1988-1995. Fam Plann Perspect 1996;28(1):4–12.

31. Finer LB, Zolna MR. Declines in unintended pregnancy in the united states, 2008-2011. N Engl J Med 2016;374(9):843–52.

32. World Health Organization. Health topics: Breastfeeding. Available at: www.who.int Web site. Available at: https://www.who.int/health-topics/breastfeeding#tab=tab_1. Accessed 3 November, 2022.

33. Dias CC, Figueiredo B. Breastfeeding and depression: A systematic review of the literature. J Affect Disord 2015;171:142–54.

34. Figueiredo B, Dias CC, Brandão S, et al. Breastfeeding and postpartum depression: State of the art review. J Pediatr 2013;89(4):332–8.

35. Hanley GE, Oberlander TF. The effect of perinatal exposures on the infant: Antidepressants and depression. Best Pract Res Clin Obstet Gynaecol 2014;28: 37–48.

36. Alwan S, Friedman JM, Chambers C. Safety of selective serotonin reuptake inhibitors in pregnancy: A review of current evidence. CNS Drugs 2016;30(6): 499–515.

37. Rahimi R, Nikfar S, Abdollahi M. Pregnancy outcomes following exposure to serotonin reuptake inhibitors: A meta-analysis of clinical trials. Reprod Toxicol 2006; 22(4):571–5.

38. Addis A, Koren G. Safety of fluoxetine during the first trimester of pregnancy: A meta-analytical review of epidemiological studies. Psychol Med 2000;30(1): 89–94.

39. Einarson TR, Einarson A. Newer antidepressants in pregnancy and rates of major malformations: A meta-analysis of prospective comparative studies. Pharmacoepidemiol Drug Saf 2005;14(12). https://doi.org/10.1002/pds.1084. Available at: https://pubmed-ncbi-nlm-nih-gov.proxy1.library.jhu.edu/15742359/. Accessed 15 April, 2021.

40. O'Brien L, Einarson TR, Sarkar M, et al. Does paroxetine cause cardiac malformations? J Obstet Gynaecol Can 2008;30(8):696–701.

41. Chun-Fai-Chan B, Koren G, Fayez I, et al. Pregnancy outcome of women exposed to bupropion during pregnancy: A prospective comparative study. Am J Obstet Gynecol 2005;192(3):932–6.

42. Cole JA, Modell JG, Haight BR, et al. Bupropion in pregnancy and the prevalence of congenital malformations. Pharmacoepidemiol Drug Saf 2007;16(5):474–84.

43. Alwan S, Reefhuis J, Botto LD, et al. Maternal use of bupropion and risk for congenital heart defects. Am J Obstet Gynecol 2010;203(1):52.e1–6.

44. Davis RL, Rubanowice D, McPhillips H, et al. Risks of congenital malformations and perinatal events among infants exposed to antidepressant medications during pregnancy. Pharmacoepidemiol Drug Saf 2007;16:1086–94.

45. Nulman I, Barrera M, Pulver A, et al. Neurodevelopment of children exposed in utero to venlafaxine: Preliminary results. Birth Defects Research Part A - Clinical and Molecular Teratology 2010;88(5):363.

46. Pastuszak A, Schick-Boschetto B, Zuber C, et al. Pregnancy outcome following first-trimester exposure to fluoxetine (prozac). JAMA 1993;269(17):2246–8.

47. Simon GE, Cunningham ML, Davis RL. Outcomes of prenatal antidepressant exposure. Am J Psychiatry 2002;159(12):2055–61.

48. Ramos E, St-Andre M, Rey E, et al. Duration of antidepressant use during pregnancy and risk of major congenital malformations. Br J Psychiatry 2008;192(5): 344–50.

49. Chisolm MS, Payne JL. Management of psychotropic drugs during pregnancy. BMJ 2016;532:h5918.

50. Huybrechts KF, Palmsten K, Avorn J, et al. Antidepressant use in pregnancy and the risk of cardiac defects. N Engl J Med 2014;370(25):2397.

51. Wang S, Yang L, Wang L, et al. Selective serotonin reuptake inhibitors (SSRIs) and the risk of congenital heart defects: A meta-analysis of prospective cohort studies. J Am Heart Assoc 2015;4(5). https://doi.org/10.1161/JAHA.114.001681.

52. Walsh-Sukys MC, Tyson JE, Wright LL, et al. Persistent pulmonary hypertension of the newborn in the era before nitric oxide: Practice variation and outcomes. Pediatrics 2000;105(1 Pt 1):14–20.

53. Chambers CD, Hernandez-Diaz S, Van Marter LJ, et al. Selective serotonin-reuptake inhibitors and risk of persistent pulmonary hypertension of the newborn. N Engl J Med 2006;354(6):579–87.

54. Kieler H, Artama M, Engeland A, et al. Selective serotonin reuptake inhibitors during pregnancy and risk of persistent pulmonary hypertension in the newborn: Population based cohort study from the five nordic countries. BMJ Br Med J (Clin Res Ed) 2012;344(7842):1.

55. Food and Drug Administration. FDA drug safety communication: Selective serotonin reuptake inhibitor (SSRI) antidepressant use during pregnancy and reports of a rare heart and lung condition in newborn babies. FDA.gov Web site. Available at: https://www.fda.gov/drugs/drug-safety-and-availability/fda-drug-safety-communication-selective-serotonin-reuptake-inhibitor-ssri-antidepressant-use-during. 2018. Accessed 5 December, 2022.

56. Huybrechts KF, Bateman BT, Palmsten K, et al. Antidepressant use late in pregnancy and risk of persistent pulmonary hypertension of the newborn. JAMA 2015; 313(21):2142–51.

57. Ross LE, Grigoriadis S, Mamisashvili L, et al. Selected pregnancy and delivery outcomes after exposure to antidepressant medication: A systematic review and meta-analysis. JAMA Psychiatr 2013;70(4):436–43.

58. Yonkers KA, Blackwell KA, Glover J, et al. Antidepressant use in pregnant and postpartum women. Annu Rev Clin Psychol 2014;10(1):369–92. Available at: https://search.datacite.org/works/10.1146/annurev-clinpsy-032813-153626.

59. Nakhai-Pour HR, Broy P, Berard A. Use of antidepressants during pregnancy and the risk of spontaneous abortion. CMAJ (Can Med Assoc J) 2010;182(10): 1031–7.

60. Pearlstein T. Use of psychotropic medication during pregnancy and the postpartum period. Womens Health (Lond Engl) 2013;9:605–15.

61. Jarde A, Morais M, Kingston D, et al. Neonatal outcomes in women with untreated antenatal depression compared with women without depression: A systematic review and meta-analysis. JAMA Psychiatr 2016;73(8):826–37.

62. Moses-Kolko E, Bogen D, Perel J, et al. Neonatal signs after late in utero exposure to serotonin reuptake inhibitors: Literature review and implications for clinical applications. JAMA, J Am Med Assoc 2005;293(19):2372.

63. Kanes SJ, Colquhoun H, Doherty J, et al. Open-label, proof-of-concept study of brexanolone in the treatment of severe postpartum depression. Hum Psychopharmacol 2017;32(2):e2576. Available at: https://search.datacite.org/works/10.1002/hup.2576.

64. Kanes S, Colquhoun H, Gunduz-Bruce H, et al. Brexanolone (SAGE-547 injection) in post-partum depression: A randomised controlled trial. Lancet 2017; 390(10093):480–9.

65. Meltzer-Brody S, Colquhoun H, Riesenberg R, et al. Brexanolone injection in postpartum depression: Two multicentre, double-blind, randomised, placebo-controlled, phase 3 trials. Lancet 2018;392(10152):1058–70.

66. Wald J, Henningsson A, Hanze E, et al. Allopregnanolone concentrations in breast milk and plasma from healthy volunteers receiving brexanolone injection,

with population pharmacokinetic modeling of potential relative infant dose. Clin Pharmacokinet 2022;61(9):1307–19.

67. Deligiannidis KM, Meltzer-Brody S, Gunduz-Bruce H, et al. Effect of zuranolone vs placebo in postpartum depression: A randomized clinical trial. JAMA Psychiatr 2021;78(9):951–9.

68. Pacheco F, Guiomar R, Brunoni AR, et al. Efficacy of non-invasive brain stimulation in decreasing depression symptoms during the peripartum period: A systematic review. J Psychiatr Res 2021;140:443–60.

69. Kim DR, Wang E, McGeehan B, et al. Randomized controlled trial of transcranial magnetic stimulation in pregnant women with major depressive disorder. Brain stimulation 2019;12(1). https://doi.org/10.1016/j.brs.2018.09.005. Available at: https://pubmed-ncbi-nlm-nih-gov.proxy1.library.jhu.edu/30249416/. Accessed 16 April, 2021.

70. Myczkowski ML, Dias AM, Luvisotto T, et al. Effects of repetitive transcranial magnetic stimulation on clinical, social, and cognitive performance in postpartum depression. Neuropsychiatr Dis Treat 2012;8:491–500.

71. Kim DR, Snell JL, Ewing GC, et al. Neuromodulation and antenatal depression: A review. Neuropsychiatr Dis Treat 2015;11:975–82.

72. Morres ID, Tzouma N, Hatzigeorgiadis A, et al. Exercise for perinatal depressive symptoms: A systematic review and meta-analysis of randomized controlled trials in perinatal health services. J Affect Disord 2022;298(Pt A):26–42.

73. Epperson CN, Terman M, Terman JS, et al. Randomized clinical trial of bright light therapy for antepartum depression: Preliminary findings. Journal of clinical psychiatry 2004;65(3). Available at: https://pubmed-ncbi-nlm-nih-gov.proxy1.library.jhu.edu/15096083/. Accessed 16 April, 2021.

74. Wirz-Justice A, Bader A, Frisch U, et al. A randomized, double-blind, placebo-controlled study of light therapy for antepartum depression. Journal of clinical psychiatry 2011;72(7). Available at: https://pubmed-ncbi-nlm-nih-gov.proxy1.library.jhu.edu/21535997/. Accessed 16 April, 2021.

75. Bais B, Kamperman AM, Bijma HH, et al. Effects of bright light therapy for depression during pregnancy: A randomised, double-blind controlled trial. BMJ Open 2020;10(10). Available at: https://pubmed-ncbi-nlm-nih-gov.proxy1.library.jhu.edu/33115894/. Accessed 16 April, 2021.

76. Donmez M, Yorguner N, Kora K, et al. Efficacy of bright light therapy in perinatal depression: A randomized, double-blind, placebo-controlled study. J Psychiatr Res 2022;149:315–22.

77. Garbazza C, Cirignotta F, D'Agostino A, et al. Sustained remission from perinatal depression after bright light therapy: A pilot randomised, placebo-controlled trial. Acta Psychiatr Scand 2022;146(4):350–6.

78. Sockol LE, Epperson CN, Barber JP. A meta-analysis of treatments for perinatal depression. Clin Psychol Rev 2011;31(5). https://doi.org/10.1016/j.cpr.2011.03.009. Available at: https://pubmed-ncbi-nlm-nih-gov.proxy1.library.jhu.edu/21545782/. Accessed 15 April, 2021.

Menopause and Mood

The Role of Estrogen in Midlife Depression and Beyond

Claudio N. Soares, MD, PhD, FRCPC, MBA*

KEYWORDS

- Depression • Perimenopause • Menopause • Estrogen • Treatments

KEY POINTS

- Depression is a prevalent, disabling condition.
- Midlife women are more vulnerable to develop depression (new onset or recurrent), often associated with vasomotor symptoms and sleep problems.
- Therapies should be tailored to alleviate all these symptoms and improve quality of life, while taking into consideration pharmacologic, behavioral, and/or hormonal options.

INTRODUCTION

The impact of mental illnesses (including substance use disorders) on the overall health of individuals and the society at large can no longer be disregarded or minimized. Recent estimates indicate that at least 1 billion individuals worldwide are affected by mental illnesses, a staggering number that represents approximately 15% of the world's adult population.[1] Depression is the most prevalent, disabling condition among all mental illnesses. The World Health Organization estimates that 300 million people suffer from depression worldwide, resulting in significant costs for individuals, their families, and their communities.[2]

Throughout the course of the COVID-19 pandemic, we have witnessed a dramatic increase in the prevalence of mental illnesses across all ages, with particularly high rates of depression, anxiety, and substance use disorders among both men and women. Data suggest that such increase was multifactorial, likely linked to the disruption of social support systems that are integral components of mental health services, the consequences of prolonged social isolation, financial concerns, food insecurity, grief, and bereavement, among others.[3]

Department of Psychiatry, Queen's University School of Medicine, Kingston, Ontario, Canada
* Department of Psychiatry, Providence Care Hospital, 752 King Street West, Kingston, Ontario K7L 4X3, Canada.
E-mail address: c.soares@queensu.ca

Psychiatr Clin N Am 46 (2023) 463–473
https://doi.org/10.1016/j.psc.2023.04.004
0193-953X/23/© 2023 Elsevier Inc. All rights reserved.

The enduring, adverse effects of COVID-19 on mental health of women across the lifespan will be examined for years to come; it is unquestionable though that women's mental health has been affected during the pandemic, with systematic reviews already signaling higher rates of depression and anxiety in women compared with men.[4] For example, increased rates of anxiety and depression were documented among women who experienced pregnancies or a postpartum period during the COVID-19 pandemic, particularly when subjected to social restrictions and prolonged lockdowns.[5] Elderly women also experienced the impact of the pandemic on various aspects of their health and well-being, including limited access to care (ie, getting routine care or timely access to appointments), difficulties in renewing prescriptions, or having access to in-person caregivers.[6]

Overall, it has been long known that women are more affected by depression and anxiety than men, with a 1.5- to 2.0-fold increased risk (point prevalence) for either of these disorders. The burden and disability associated with these conditions have also grown disproportionally among women over the past few decades.[1] Clinicians and researchers have documented an increased risk for developing depression (new onset and/or recurrent) among some women at certain points in time across their reproductive life cycle. This observation has led to the conceptual framework of *reproductive-related windows of vulnerability* for depression. Essentially, hormonal changes could be contributing to the emergence of mood symptoms and/or influencing their clinical presentation and severity. This would be the case, for example, of women experiencing mood symptoms and dysphoria during the luteal phase of their menstrual cycles, the emergence of depressive symptoms during puerperium or depression associated with the menopausal transition.[7]

The worsening of other mental health conditions has been associated with periods of intense, sometimes chaotic hormonal changes across the female lifecycle. Premenstrual worsening of symptoms has been documented among women with diagnosis of anxiety disorders, psychotic disorders, depression, and borderline personality disorder[8,9]; suicidality can also increase premenstrually.[10]

During the midlife transition, women may experience the compounding effects of psychological stressors and physical changes, the latter including metabolic issues, cardiovascular diseases, diabetes, osteoporosis, osteoarthritis, chronic pain, and so forth. In addition, the emergence of menopause-related problems such as vasomotor symptoms (VMS) and sleep disruptions may ultimately affect a woman's quality of life and overall functioning.[11–13]

Menopause and Depression

Depressive symptoms are characterized by low mood, reduced motivation, poor engagement in usual activities, limited enjoyment, and disrupted sleep; depressive symptoms seem to increase during the menopause transition and are often associated with psychosocial impairment and poorer quality of life.[14–16] A high prevalence of depressive symptoms among midlife women has now been confirmed by cross-sectional and longitudinal studies, even among those who had never been diagnosed with depression before. Major depressive episodes (MDDs), although less common than depressive symptoms, are also more commonly observed during midlife years. Previous studies indicated a 2- to 4-fold increased risk for MDD during the menopause transition compared with the premenopausal or postmenopausal years. The occurrence of depression (rather than depressive symptoms) was documented in cohort studies that followed women throughout the menopause transition and early postmenopausal years, and the increased risk was particular high for recurrent depressive episodes, that is, among those with prior history of depression.[17,18]

One could examine the occurrence of depression (MDD or depressive symptoms) during midlife years through the lens of 2 clusters of factors: continuum-related factors and window-related factors. *Continuum-related* factors are those that are pervasive in nature and may "follow" a woman throughout her life journey—they include socioeconomic conditions, psychosocial stressors, and their overall health, just to name a few. The strongest predictor for the occurrence MDD during midlife years is, however, a previous diagnosis of MDD, which means depression is more likely to reoccur during midlife years, rather than emerging as a new condition, for the first time.

Window-related factors are, on the other hand, more time related or context related; they are usually understood as mediating or precipitating factors for the occurrence of MDD among midlife women. Among window-related factors we consider the occurrence of significant hormone variations and the emergence of menopause-related symptoms (sleep problems, vasomotor symptoms); the experience of stressful life events, particularly when those occur closely in time to the menopause transition; and the presence of chronic medical conditions that might worsen during midlife years.[19–24] Health care professionals should be able to recognize moderating (continuum-related) and mediating (window-related) factors in order to better prevent, detect, and/or effectively treat depression during midlife years and beyond.

The Effects of Estrogen on Mood

Estrogen (E) has neuromodulatory effects, primarily through its interactions with monoaminergic systems that involved in mood regulation, such as serotonin (5-hydroxytryptamine [5-HT]) and noradrenaline (NE). Such effects are, overall, deemed to be beneficial to mood.[25–27] The administration of estradiol (E2), for example, may result in a net increase in 5-HT synthesis; this increase occurs through various mechanisms, including the reduction of enzymes involved in 5-HT degradation and an increase in tryptophan hydroxylase, the enzyme that is necessary for serotonin synthesis. Estradiol also increases 5-HT availability by downregulating $5HT_{1a}$ autoreceptors and upregulating $5HT_{2a}$ receptors in the synaptic cleft, thus increasing 5-HT availability for postsynaptic transmission.[28,29]

Estrogen also increases NE synthesis through similar mechanisms to those described for serotonin and likely has neuroprotective effects by stimulating the release of brain-derived neurotrophic factor.[30,31]

Consistent with the aforementioned neuromodulatory effects of E2, there are now several studies that correlate intense fluctuations in E2 levels with the development of perimenopausal depression. There are at least 3 studies that documented a relationship between greater, wider fluctuations in E2 levels and an increased risk for developing depressive symptoms.[21,22] Schmidt and colleagues also demonstrated such association in an experiment in which they produced an E2 withdrawal after administering E2 (transdermal) to women with a history of perimenopausal depression that had been responsive to E2.[32]

The GABAergic deficit hypothesis for depression has gained increasing attention. The serotonergic and GABAergic systems are known to be interconnected; with that, it has been postulated that deficiencies in GABAergic neural inhibition could contribute to the occurrence depressive symptoms across a woman's reproductive life cycle; conversely, the restoration of the GABAergic neurotransmission could produce antidepressant effects—this seems to be one of the plausible mechanisms for the antidepressant effects exerted by estrogen and allopregnanolone (ALLO).[33]

There is now strong evidence suggesting a mediating effect of ALLO (ie, heightened sensitive to ALLO fluctuations) for the association between changes in reproductive steroid hormones and mood in the context of PMDD[34] and postpartum depression.[35]

However, it has yet to be determined the extent to which a similar sensitivity may play a role in the development of perimenopausal depression. In one study involving late perimenopausal and early postmenopausal women (n = 140), a negative correlation was found between serum ALLO levels and feelings of guilt among the early postmenopausal women, likely coinciding with a hypogonadal state.[36]

Estrogen-Based Therapy for Depression

Despite accumulated, preclinical evidence demonstrating the antidepressant properties of estrogen therapy (ET), its use in clinical practice has been limited. Two randomized controlled trials[37,38] demonstrated the efficacy and safety of transdermal estradiol for the treatment of MDD and led to the inclusion of E2 therapy into the 2016 Clinical Guidelines of the Canadian Network for Mood and Anxiety Treatments (CANMAT), as a second-line treatment (level 2) for the management of MDD during perimenopause.[39] Both studies used standardized procedures to confirm the diagnosis of depression and to properly characterize menopausal staging; antidepressant effects were significant—similar to those observed with conventional antidepressants—and mood improvements were documented among women with new or recurrent depression, with and without concomitant vasomotor symptoms. It is important to note that the use of similar intervention (transdermal E2) for depression in late *postmenopausal* women failed to show positive results,[40] reinforcing the notion that the menopause transition might be not only a critical window for the occurrence of depression but a *window of opportunity* for the antidepressant use of ET.[41] It is undeniable, however, that the knowledge dissemination regarding the promising antidepressant benefits of E2 therapy for midlife depression and the development of further clinical investigations in this field were for years curtailed by the negative views, lack of nuanced analyses, and misconceptions on estrogen therapies that were generated by the Women's Health Initiative study; some of these misconceptions have lasted for a decade, despite numerous efforts by clinicians and researchers to provide some context to the study analyses and their limitations.[42]

Estrogen has been studied as a prophylactic approach to prevent the development of depressive symptoms in midlife women.[43] The use of transdermal estradiol (100 μg) plus intermittent oral micronized progesterone for 12 months led to a reduction in the risk of developing depressive symptoms compared with the use of placebo (32.3% vs 17.3%, respectively), when administered to women in early perimenopause. Interestingly, prophylactic E2 effects were more pronounced among women who had experienced stressful life events in the preceding 6 months of the study.

Based on existing data and accumulated clinical experience, it is reasonable to consider E2 as part of the treatment armamentarium for midlife depression; clinicians should consider a brief trial with E2 (4–6 weeks), particularly for women in the menopause transition who present with depressive symptoms and concomitant VMS. The evidence is also supportive of the use of transdermal E2, rather than other formulations or routes of administration. The use of E2 should be considered as an option for symptomatic midlife women suffering from depression who are unable or unwilling to initiate treatment with antidepressants or other therapies.[24]

Menopause, Anxiety, and Estrogens

Despite being identified as a significant contributing factor to poorer quality of life and impaired functioning among midlife women, anxiety does not often receive the same attention of studies and clinical trials compared with that dedicated to depression. Longitudinal studies revealed an increase of anxiety and its various components (eg, irritability, nervousness or tension, fearfulness, and heart racing) across different menopausal staging. In the SWAN study, women with high anxiety at baseline (ie, pre-menopausal) experienced a peak in anxiety during late perimenopausal years, with a subsequent decline in the postmenopausal period; anxiety was experienced by women even in the absence of other menopause-related symptoms, which reiterates the importance of proper screening and disease awareness among clinicians.[44]

For a significant number of midlife women, anxiety is strongly associated with the presence and severity of hot flashes. In the Penn Ovarian Aging Cohort, somatic anxiety (eg, chest pain, fatigue, dizziness) was found to be significantly associated with hot flashes in the menopause transition, even after adjusting for factors such as age, menopausal staging, reproductive hormone levels, history of depression, and others. Importantly, somatic anxiety *preceded* the occurrence of hot flashes.[45] A recent Japanese study also revealed independent associations between VMS and anxiety and distressing burden caused by rapid or irregular heartbeats (palpitations).[46]

The association between E2 fluctuations and symptoms of anxiety and anhedonia were examined in a recent study in which 73 women (aged 49 ± 3 years) were submitted to a social anxiety test (Trier social stress tests [TSST]) at study entry, at week 8 and week 16. Study participants were randomly assigned to receive 8 weeks of trans-dermal estradiol (0.1 mg per24 hours) or placebo. Hormone measurements were collected for 8 weeks before the treatment allocation (E2 or placebo) and throughout the experiment. Greater E2 fluctuations over the initial 8-week period (ie, before treatment allocation) predicted the presence of greater symptoms of anxiety and a higher cortisol reactivity to TSST. Moreover, transdermal E2 was effective in improving symptoms of anxiety and anhedonia. Therapy with E2 was particularly helpful for those who exhibited high baseline E2-anxiety sensitivity. If further confirmed, this intervention could be particularly beneficial for midlife women with somatic symptoms and for those who seem to be more vulnerable to develop anxiety in the context of E2 fluctuations.[47]

Managing Midlife Depression—a Treatment Framework

Antidepressants and behavioral interventions remain the first-line treatment of depression across the life span. The use of antidepressants should be prioritized for women who experienced multiple depressive episodes in the past (ie, not exclusively hormone related) and/or those reporting severe depressive symptoms, functional impairment, or suicidal ideation.

A frequently asked question by patients and health care providers is whether there could be a preferred option or choice of a particular agent for the management of depression in midlife women; to address this question, an important distinction needs to be made between new-onset and recurrent episodes. For recurrent episodes, a previous response to a specific antidepressant (agent, class) should influence the decision on what to try first—if a particular medication was helpful in the past, this should be considered. For those who are experiencing depression for the first time during midlife years, those who are treatment-naive, or those presenting with partial or no response to antidepressants in the past, there is evidence of the efficacy and safety of various agents—at usual doses compared with other stages in life. That includes the use of fluoxetine, sertraline, venlafaxine, citalopram, escitalopram, duloxetine, desvenlafaxine, and vortioxetine for depressed, menopausal women.[48–56] Overall, there no evidence to support a superior efficacy of a particular antidepressant agent or class over the others for the management of midlife depression. In a randomized, double-blind study of *postmenopausal* women (aged 40–70 years) with diagnosis of MDD, both desvenlafaxine (100–200 mg/d) and escitalopram (10–20 mg/d) led to significant and comparable results, either after an 8-week acute treatment or during a 6-

month continuation phase. These results did not support the hypothesis that serotonin and norepinephrine reuptake inhibitors (SNRIs) could have an efficacy advantage for the treatment of MDD in postmenopausal women.[55] The study, unfortunately, did not include more accurate information on time since menopause to better explore the hypothesis that the lack of superior efficacy of an SNRI over an selective serotonin reuptake inhibitor observed in this study could have been due to the timing of the antidepressant intervention—that is, depressive women in the menopausal transition and early postmenopausal years could have benefited more from SNRIs due to the occurrence of wide estrogen fluctuations during this period and the putative impact of these hormone changes on mood and behavior.

In one recent study, venlafaxine was found to be superior to fluoxetine for the treatment of MDD in postmenopausal women (average 57 years of age); the study, however, include a wide dose range for venlafaxine (75–225 mg/d) and fluoxetine (20–60 mg/d), which could have affected both norepinephrine effects of venlafaxine (when administered at lower doses) and the tolerability of fluoxetine (when used at higher doses).[57]

Information on tolerability should be part of the discussion for the selection of antidepressants for midlife women, particularly when sexual dysfunction and changes in weight are of concern. Existing data on the efficacy of some agents for menopause-related symptoms (VMS, pain, disrupted sleep) and quality-of-life improvement could also help guide clinicians. Drug-drug interactions need to be considered, given that perimenopausal and postmenopausal women tend to be on multiple medications for comorbid conditions.[24]

Behavior-based interventions such as cognitive behavioral therapy (CBT) have shown to be effective not only for depression but also for the management of other menopause-related problems, including anxiety, sleep problems, and VMS.[58,59] Evidence shows that patients are more likely to adhere to treatments and have more favorable outcomes when provided with choices to pursue medication, behavioral therapies, or both.[60]

γ-Aminobutyric Acid Type A Modulators

With the increasing evidence of the role of GABAergic systems for the development of depression and anxiety, a greater attention has been paid to the potential value of neurosteroids such as allopregnanolone for the management of these conditions, given it can positively modulate γ-aminobutyric acid type A (GABAA) receptors. Enhancing the inhibitory effects on GABAA receptors may lead to rapid decreases in anxiety levels and reduction in depression symptoms.

Among those, zuranolone and brexanolone are promising treatments due to their effects as positive allosteric modulators of GABAA receptors—brexanolone is already Food and Drug Administration–approved for the management of postpartum depression,[61] whereas zuranolone is in late stage of clinical development.[62] It remains to be seen whether the antidepressant properties of GABAA modulators will be further applied to midlife-related mood and anxiety symptoms.

SUMMARY

The transition to menopause and early postmenopausal years may be quite challenging for some women, with the increased risk for developing depressive symptoms (new, recurrent) and anxiety, along with vasomotor complaints, sleep problems, and other menopause-related health conditions. It is fundamental that health professionals providing care for women during midlife years are prepared to recognize this window of vulnerability and to manage it accordingly. Importantly, neither depression nor anxiety during midlife years should be managed in isolation. Sleep problems, cognitive complaints, sexual dysfunction as well as the occurrence of context-related life stressors should be taken into consideration for the development of comprehensive, effective treatment plans.

It is now well established that estrogen plays an important neuromodulatory role—on the one hand, E2 fluctuations may contribute to the emergence of depression and anxiety symptoms; on the other hand, E2-based therapies may in fact alleviate these conditions, particularly when administered to symptomatic women in the menopausal transition and early postmenopausal years and/or experiencing increasing anxiety and stress during times of intense E2 fluctuations.

Antidepressants and behavioral therapies remain, however, the treatments of choice for depression and anxiety across the life span, including midlife years.

CLINICS CARE POINTS

- Some women may experience a 'window of vulnerability' for the development of mood and anxiety symptoms during the menopause transition.
- The presence and severity of vasomotor symptoms, sleep disturbances and cognitive changes should be taken into consideration when reviewing treatment options for symptomatic midlife women suffering from depression.
- Evidence-based treatments include pharmacologic, hormonal and behavioural options; treament should be tailored to patients' needs, taking into account efficacy, safety and tolerability.

DISCLOSURE

Dr C.N. Soares has received honoraria as an advisory board member/consultant and/or received research funds from Eisai, Japan, Bayer, Germany, Otsuka, United States, Lundbeck, Denmark, Ontario Brain Institute, Canada, and CAN-BIND Solutions.

REFERENCES

1. Rehm J, Shield KD. Global Burden of Disease and the Impact of Mental and Addictive Disorders. Curr Psychiatry Rep 2019;21(2):10.
2. Available at: https://www.who.int/news-room/fact-sheets/detail/depression. Consulted on September 24, 2022.
3. Available at: https://www.who.int/news/item/02-03-2022-covid-19-pandemic-triggers-25-increase-in-prevalence-of-anxiety-and-depression-worldwide. Consulted on October 1, 2022.
4. Ettman CK, Fan AY, Subramanian M, et al. Prevalence of depressive symptoms in U.S. adults during the COVID-19 pandemic: A systematic review. SSM Popul Health 2023;21:101348.
5. Hessami K, Romanelli C, Chiurazzi M, et al. COVID-19 pandemic and maternal mental health: a systematic review and meta-analysis. J Matern Fetal Neonatal Med 2022;35(20):4014–21.
6. Wong E, Franceschini N, Tinker LF, et al. Continuity of Care Among Postmenopausal Women With Cardiometabolic Diseases in the United States Early During the COVID-19 Pandemic: Findings From the Women's Health Initiative. J Gerontol A Biol Sci Med Sci 2022;77(Suppl 1):S13–21.

7. Soares CN, Zitek B. Reproductive hormone sensitivity and risk for depression across the female life cycle: a continuum of vulnerability? J Psychiatry Neurosci 2008;33(4):331–43.

8. Nolan LN, Hughes L. Premenstrual exacerbation of mental health disorders: a systematic review of prospective studies. Arch Womens Ment Health 2022; 25(5):831–52.

9. Eisenlohr-Moul TA, Schmalenberger KM, Owens SA, et al. Perimenstrual exacerbation of symptoms in borderline personality disorder: evidence from multilevel models and the Carolina Premenstrual Assessment Scoring System. Psychol Med 2018;48(12):2085–95 [published correction appears in Psychol Med. 2018 Sep;48(12):2100].

10. Yan H, Ding Y, Guo W. Suicidality in patients with premenstrual dysphoric disorder-A systematic review and meta-analysis. J Affect Disord 2021;295: 339–46.

11. Soares CN. Mood disorders in midlife women: understanding the critical window and its clinical implications. Menopause 2014;21(2):198–206.

12. Kase NG, Gretz Friedman E, Brodman M, et al. The midlife transition and the risk of cardiovascular disease and cancer I: magnitude and mechanisms. Am J Obstet Gynecol 2020;223(6):820–33.

13. El Khoudary SR, Greendale G, Crawford SL, et al. The menopause transition and women's health at midlife: a progress report from the Study of Women's Health Across the Nation (SWAN). Menopause 2019;26(10):1213–27.

14. Pietrzak RH, Kinley J, Afifi TO, et al. Subsyndromal depression in the United States: prevalence, course, and risk for incident psychiatric outcomes. Psychol Med 2013;43(7):1401–14.

15. Bromberger JT, Matthews KA, Schott LL, et al. Depressive symptoms during the menopausal transition: the Study of Women's Health Across the Nation (SWAN). J Affect Disord 2007;103(1–3):267–72.

16. de Kruif M, Spijker AT, Molendijk ML. Depression during the perimenopause: A meta-analysis. J Affect Disord 2016;206:174–80.

17. Cohen LS, Soares CN, Vitonis AF, et al. Risk for new onset of depression during the menopausal transition: the Harvard study of moods and cycles. Arch Gen Psychiatry 2006;63(4):385–90.

18. Bromberger JT, Kravitz HM. Mood and menopause: findings from the Study of Women's Health Across the Nation (SWAN) over 10 years. Obstet Gynecol Clin North Am 2011;38(3):609–25.

19. Shea AK, Sohel N, Gilsing A, et al. Depression, hormone therapy, and the menopausal transition among women aged 45 to 64 years using Canadian Longitudinal Study on aging baseline data. Menopause 2020;27(7):763–70.

20. Bromberger JT, Schott L, Kravitz HM, et al. Risk factors for major depression during midlife among a community sample of women with and without prior major depression: are they the same or different? Psychol Med 2015;45:1653–64.

21. Freeman EW, Sammel MD, Lin H, et al. Associations of hormones and menopausal status with depressed mood in women with no history of depression. Arch Gen Psychiatry 2006;63:375–82.

22. Gordon JL, Rubinow DR, Eisenlohr-Moul TA, et al. Estradiol variability, stressful life events, and the emergence of depressive symptomatology during the menopausal transition. Menopause 2016;23(3):257–66.

23. Bromberger JT, Kravitz HM, Youk A, et al. Patterns of depressive disorders across 13 years and their determinants among midlife women: SWAN mental health study. J Affect Disord 2016;206:31–40.

24. Soares CN, Shea AK. The Midlife Transition, Depression, and Its Clinical Management. Obstet Gynecol Clin North Am 2021;48(1):215–29.
25. McEwen BS, Alves SE. Estrogen actions in the central nervous system. Endocr Rev 1999;20(3):279–307.
26. Lokuge S, Frey BN, Foster JA, et al. Depression in women: windows of vulnerability and new insights into the link between estrogen and serotonin. J Clin Psychiatry 2011;72(11):e1563–9.
27. Rubinow DR, Johnson SL, Schmidt PJ, et al. Efficacy of estradiol in perimenopausal depression: so much promise and so few answers. Depress Anxiety 2015;32(8):539–54.
28. Cyr M, Bosse R, Di Paolo T. Gonadal hormones modulate 5-hydroxytryptamine2A receptors: emphasis on the rat frontal cortex. Neuroscience 1998;83(3):829–36.
29. Hiroi R, McDevitt RA, Neumaier JF. Estrogen selectively increases tryptophan hydroxylase-2 mRNA expression in distinct subregions of rat midbrain raphe nucleus: association between gene expression and anxiety behavior in the open field. Biol Psychiatry 2006;60(3):288–95.
30. Pau KY, Hess DL, Kohama S, et al. Oestrogen upregulates noradrenaline release in the mediobasal hypothalamus and tyrosine hydroxylase gene expression in the brainstem of ovariectomized rhesus macaques. J Neuroendocrinol 2000;12(9):899–909.
31. Srivastava DP, Woolfrey KM, Evans PD. Mechanisms underlying the interactions between rapid estrogenic and BDNF control of synaptic connectivity. Neuroscience 2013;239:17–33.
32. Schmidt PJ, Ben Dor R, Martinez PE, et al. Effects of estradiol withdrawal on mood in women with past perimenopausal depression: a randomized clinical trial. JAMA Psychiatr 2015;72:714–26.
33. Schweizer-Schubert S, Gordon JL, Eisenlohr-Moul TA, et al. Steroid Hormone Sensitivity in Reproductive Mood Disorders: On the Role of the GABA$_A$ Receptor Complex and Stress During Hormonal Transitions. Front Med 2021;7:479646.
34. Schiller CE, Johnson SL, Abate AC, et al. Reproductive steroid regulation of mood and behavior. Compr Physiol 2016;6:1135.
35. Kanes S, Colquhoun H, Gunduz-Bruce H, et al. Brexanolone (SAGE-547 injection) in post-partum depression: a randomised controlled trial. Lancet 2017;390:480–9.
36. Slopien R, Pluchino N, Warenik-Szymankiewicz A, et al. Correlation between allopregnanolone levels and depressive symptoms during late menopausal transition and early postmenopause. Gynecol Endocrinol 2018;34:144–7.
37. Schmidt PJ, Nieman L, Danaceau MA, et al. Estrogen replacement in perimenopause-related depression: a preliminary report. Am J Obstet Gynecol 2000;183(2):414–20.
38. Soares CN, Almeida OP, Joffe H, et al. Efficacy of estradiol for the treatment of depressive disorders in perimenopausal women: a double-blind, randomized, placebo-controlled trial. Arch Gen Psychiatry 2001;58(6):529–34.
39. MacQueen GM, Frey BN, Ismail Z, et al. Canadian Network for Mood and Anxiety Treatments (CANMAT) 2016 Clinical Guidelines for the Management of Adults with Major Depressive Disorder: Section 6. Special Populations: Youth, Women, and the Elderly. Can J Psychiatry 2016;61(9):588–603.
40. Morrison MF, Kallan MJ, Ten Have T, et al. Lack of efficacy of estradiol for depression in postmenopausal women: a randomized, controlled trial. Biol Psychiatry 2004;55(4):406–12.

41. Maki PM, Kornstein SG, Joffe H, et al. Guidelines for the evaluation and treatment of perimenopausal depression: summary and recommendations. Menopause 2018;25(10):1069–85.
42. Manson JE, Bassuk SS, Kaunitz AM, et al. The Women's Health Initiative trials of menopausal hormone therapy: lessons learned. Menopause 2020;27(8):918–28.
43. Gordon JL, Rubinow DR, Eisenlohr-Moul TA, et al. Efficacy of Transdermal Estradiol and Micronized Progesterone in the Prevention of Depressive Symptoms in the Menopause Transition: A Randomized Clinical Trial. JAMA Psychiatr 2018; 75(2):149–57.
44. Bromberger JT, Kravitz HM, Chang Y, et al. Does risk for anxiety increase during the menopausal transition? Study of women's health across the nation. Menopause 2013;20(5):488–95.
45. Freeman EW, Sammel MD. Anxiety as a risk factor for menopausal hot flashes: evidence from the Penn Ovarian Aging Cohort. Menopause 2016;23(90):942–9.
46. Enomoto H, Terauchi M, Odai T, et al. Independent association of palpitation with vasomotor symptoms and anxiety in middle-aged women. Menopause 2021; 28(7):741–7.
47. Lozza-Fiacco S, Gordon JL, Andersen EH, et al. Baseline anxiety-sensitivity to estradiol fluctuations predicts anxiety symptom response to transdermal estradiol treatment in perimenopausal women.A randomized clinical trial. Psychoneuroendocrinology 2022;143:105851.
48. Freeman MP, Cheng LJ, Moustafa D, et al. Vortioxetine for major depressive disorder, vasomotor, and cognitive symptoms associated with the menopausal transition. Ann Clin Psychiatry 2017;29(4):249–57.
49. Frey BN, Haber E, Mendes GC, et al. Effects of quetiapine extended release on sleep and quality of life in midlife women with major depressive disorder. Arch Womens Ment Health 2013;16(1):83–5.
50. Gambacciani M, Ciaponi M, Cappagli B, et al. Effects of low-dose, continuous combined estradiol and noretisterone acetate on menopausal quality of life in early postmenopausal women. Maturitas 2003;44(2):157–63.
51. Joffe H, Groninger H, Soares CN, et al. An open trial of mirtazapine in menopausal women with depression unresponsive to estrogen replacement therapy. J Womens Health Gend Based Med 2001;10(10):999–1004.
52. Joffe H, Soares CN, Petrillo LF, et al. Treatment of depression and menopauserelated symptoms with the serotonin-norepinephrine reuptake inhibitor duloxetine. J Clin Psychiatry 2007;68(6):943–50.
53. Kornstein SG, Jiang Q, Reddy S, et al. Short-term efficacy and safety of desvenlafaxine in a randomized, placebo-controlled study of perimenopausal and postmenopausal women with major depressive disorder. J Clin Psychiatry 2010;71(8): 1088–96.
54. Soares CN, Kornstein SG, Thase ME, et al. Assessing the efficacy of desvenlafaxine for improving functioning and well-being outcome measures in patients with major depressive disorder: a pooled analysis of 9 double-blind, placebocontrolled, 8-week clinical trials. J Clin Psychiatry 2009;70(10): 1365–71.
55. Soares CN, Thase ME, Clayton A, et al. Desvenlafaxine and escitalopram for the treatment of postmenopausal women with major depressive disorder. Menopause 2010;17(4):700–11.
56. Soares CN, Frey BN, Haber E, et al. A pilot, 8-week, placebo lead-in trial of quetiapine extended release for depression in midlife women: impact on

mood and menopause-related symptoms. J Clin Psychopharmacol 2010;30(5): 612–5.

57. Zhou J, Wang X, Feng L, et al. Venlafaxine vs. fluoxetine in postmenopausal women with major depressive disorder: an 8-week, randomized, single-blind, active-controlled study. BMC Psychiatr 2021;21(1):260.

58. Green SM, Donegan E, McCabe RE, et al. Objective and subjective vasomotor symptom outcomes in the CBT-Meno randomized controlled trial. Climacteric 2020;23(5):482–8.

59. Diem SJ, LaCroix AZ, Reed SD, et al. Effects of pharmacologic and nonpharmacologic interventions on menopause-related quality of life: a pooled analysis of individual participant data from four MsFLASH trials. Menopause 2020;27(10): 1126–36.

60. McCurry SM, Guthrie KA, Morin CM, et al. Telephone-Based Cognitive Behavioral Therapy for Insomnia in Perimenopausal and Postmenopausal Women With Vasomotor Symptoms: A MsFLASH Randomized Clinical Trial. JAMA Intern Med 2016; 176(7):913–20.

61. Edinoff AN, Odisho AS, Lewis K, et al. Brexanolone, a GABA$_A$ Modulator, in the Treatment of Postpartum Depression in Adults: A Comprehensive Review. Front Psychiatry 2021;12:699740.

62. Gunduz-Bruce H, Silber C, Kaul I, et al. Trial of SAGE-217 in Patients with Major Depressive Disorder. N Engl J Med 2019;381(10):903–11.

Schizophrenia in Women
Clinical Considerations

Mary V. Seeman, OC, MDCM, DSc

KEYWORDS

- Schizophrenia • Sex/gender • Risks • Reproductive needs • Violence
- Antipsychotics adverse effects

KEY POINTS

- Men and women, for biologic and sociocultural reasons, differ in the nature of their risks for schizophrenia and also in their care needs.
- Clinicians need to be alert to these differences.
- Differences, however, are based on averages and, thus, are not seen in all individuals.

INTRODUCTION

Depending on many confounding factors, such as age and hormone level, women with schizophrenia show sex-specific health care risks and needs that are different from those of men. This article addresses the current evidence for difference.

RISKS

Genes on sex chromosome X (of which women have two) influence neurodevelopment by altering neuronal differentiation, protein encoding, and synaptic transmission (**Box 1**).[1] This means that X chromosome aneuploidy (Turner syndrome [TS]), where one X chromosome is either completely or partially lost, a condition that occurs in 1 out of 2500 female births, becomes a risk factor for schizophrenia. TS is at least three times more prevalent in women with schizophrenia than it is in the general population.[2] Most women with TS show 45,X0 monosomy, but, interestingly, the mosaic (45,X0/46/XX) is more frequent among those who develop schizophrenia.[3] Treatment of girls with TS consists of growth hormone for height and sex hormones to induce puberty because there is some evidence that early puberty is preventive against schizophrenia.[4,5]

Polycystic ovary syndrome, which is characterized by hyperandrogenism, chronic anovulation, and polycystic ovaries seen on ultrasound, affects from 5% to 20% of women[6] and increases schizophrenia risk via metabolic dysfunction and hormonal imbalance.[7,8]

Department of Psychiatry, University of Toronto, Toronto, Ontario M5P3L6, Canada
E-mail address: mary.seeman@utoronto.ca

Psychiatr Clin N Am 46 (2023) 475–486
https://doi.org/10.1016/j.psc.2023.04.005
0193-953X/23/© 2023 Elsevier Inc. All rights reserved.

> **Box 1**
> **Schizophrenia: women-specific risks**
>
> - Turner syndrome
> - Polycystic ovary syndrome
> - Eating disorders
> - Autoimmune disorders
> - Specific hormone-induced disorders

Eating disorders, much more prevalent in women than in men, have been associated with schizophrenia,[9,10] especially when they present during adolescence, a critical period for brain structural, neurochemical, and molecular change.[11]

Autoimmune disease is also considerably more prevalent in women than in men and is seen in approximately 3.6% of individuals with schizophrenia.[12] The degree of this association seems to differ in people of different ethnic origins[13] and is stronger for some autoimmune diseases than for others.[14] On genome-wide association studies, immunity genes have consistently been shown to associate with schizophrenia.[15] There is another connection. The treatment of autoimmune disease (corticosteroids) can also precipitate psychosis.[16]

Hyperthyroid and hypothyroid conditions (not only ones of autoimmune origin) are more common in women than in men and are known to be associated with psychosis. Thyroid disease poses a particular risk for schizophrenia in women during the postpartum period.[17,18] Thyroid screening is important at this time.

Hormones prescribed for infertility or to increase breast milk during lactation can lower estrogen levels sufficiently to induce transient psychotic symptoms in women, which need to be differentiated from those of schizophrenia.[19,20]

DIAGNOSIS AND EARLY TREATMENT

The diagnosis of schizophrenia is based on identical criteria for men and women and, as such, may delay effective treatment of women because women present somewhat differently. For instance, many women retain social skills and a broad range of affect. The delusions and hallucinations, in women, may be attributed to posttraumatic stress disorder or borderline personality (both more commonly seen, outside of veterans' services, in women). Later in life, when many women with schizophrenia first present, the initial diagnostic impression may be psychotic depression,[21–24] leading to a treatment delay that makes recovery less likely.

REPRODUCTION-RELATED NEEDS
Menstruation

Many women treated with antipsychotic (AP) drugs have irregular periods and stretches of amenorrhea.[25] As estrogen levels fluctuate over the course of the menstrual month, many experience changes in symptom severity (more intense psychotic symptoms when estrogen levels are low).[26] It is often helpful to increase AP doses temporarily for several days a month should this occur.[27]

Contraception

It is important to address contraception with all women with schizophrenia; many become pregnant against their wishes, with no means and no support for child care. Before prescribing hormonal contraception, there are potential interactions between psychotropic medications and contraceptives that must be considered.[28] Progesterone-only contraception in the form of intrauterine devices or long-acting injections may be the easiest for women to take, and perhaps the safest.[29,30] The rates of abortion in women with schizophrenia are not precisely known, but are higher than in the general population.[31] Addressing the need for contraception and educating patients about safe sex and contraceptive options is an important and often neglected part of comprehensive treatment of women with schizophrenia.

Fertility

Some women with schizophrenia want to have children and do have sufficient family support to do this well. The issue then becomes ensuring fertility in the face of treatment with prolactin-raising APs.[32] This can mean changing APs or lowering the dose, perhaps trying brief drug holidays. Ensuring good prenatal care and monitoring changing dosage needs throughout pregnancy is vital. Lack of or sporadic prenatal care results in psychotic relapse and hospitalizations during pregnancy. In one study of 98 pregnancies in women with schizophrenia, approximately 40% required hospital admission, most often during the first trimester,[33] a critical time for fetal development.

Sexual Exploitation

Because women with schizophrenia are usually poor, sometimes homeless, and often hungry, they are easy targets for sexual exploitation and sex trafficking.[34–36] This has now been reported in many parts of the globe.[37] A recent review of 16 studies that explored the sexual experiences of women with diagnoses of serious mental illness[38] concluded that sexual exploitation of women with psychotic illness leads to unwanted pregnancy, abortion, addiction, and the spread of sexually transmitted disease. Sexual abuse of seriously mentally ill women has even been reported in settings whose intent is to provide safety and healing (eg, psychiatric hospitals).[39]

Assortative Mating

Women with schizophrenia are reported to preserve their social skills much more frequently than men with the same disorder, and to form intimate partnerships far more readily.[40] The danger for women with schizophrenia when they marry is that they often meet potential spouses in mental health settings, which could lead to unstable marriages, with genetic and environmental risks for offspring. Two people with severe mental illness living together constitutes a potential risk for domestic abuse and violence at home.[41,42] Premarriage counseling, always useful, may be vital for this population. Despite a large literature on family therapy in the context of schizophrenia, I could not find any literature on marriage counseling despite the fact that the prevalence of poor marital adjustment was judged to be 60% in studies from India.[43,44] The literature on marriage and schizophrenia mostly comes from India where, in many families, marriage is considered a potential cure for mental illness. Not only it is not a cure, but it can lead to serious domestic abuse, especially notable during pregnancy.[45] Partner abuse needs to be specifically inquired about because it is rarely spontaneously revealed.

Pregnancy

Pregnancy in women with schizophrenia deserves greater priority than it currently receives in terms of stigma prevention, quality prenatal care, and preparation for motherhood. A further necessity is effective psychiatric monitoring to prevent symptom exacerbation.[46,47]

Women with schizophrenia who become pregnant, especially but not only single women, suffer criticism from family and from health care providers. They feel stigmatized for bringing babies into the world who may inherit schizophrenia genes and who may, consequently, become a burden on society. Current opinion is that women with schizophrenia will not be good mothers because of their illness, their poverty, their frequent hospitalizations, and the lack of support they receive from their families and from the health and welfare systems.[48,49]

There are pregnancy-associated delusions in the context of schizophrenia, which are not uncommon. One is the false conviction that one is pregnant and occurs in women who very much want to be mothers or to women who very much fear they are pregnant when that is not what they want.[50] The delusion is reinforced by the hyperprolactinemia that accompanies APs, giving rise to amenorrhea, galactorrhea, and swollen, tender breasts, mimicking pregnancy. Women who believe they are pregnant are reluctant to take drugs and may need involuntary hospitalization. Another delusion is the denial of pregnancy,[51] which may also require hospitalization to protect the fetus from ill effects, such as substance use.

Ensuring good prenatal care and monitoring changing dose needs of APs throughout pregnancy is considered vital. Depending on the drug used, doses may need to be raised or lowered in pregnancy to maintain wellness.[47,49] Getting the dose right is essential, to protect the mother from psychotic relapse and to minimize the potential negative effects of APs on the growing fetus.[52–56] This is also necessary during breastfeeding.[57]

Children of women with schizophrenia are at demonstrated risk for many physical and mental conditions. This is not necessarily caused by APs taken by their mothers during pregnancy but this potential contributory cause needs further investigation.[58]

Postpartum

Children's Aid workers may take infants away from mothers with schizophrenia at birth if they have an indication that the mother could be harmful to or neglectful of her child. Clinicians need to prepare mothers to help prevent this eventuality. If the mother's illness is severe, clinicians can help mothers organize family support so that the child is placed with a close relative.[59,60] Grandmothers, either maternal or paternal, are usually the ones who can be counted on to shelter and nurture the children.[61]

Exacerbation of psychosis postpartum is a widespread phenomenon precipitated by the stress of labor and delivery and the sudden drop in neuroprotective estrogens.[62] Mothers with schizophrenia sometimes stop their AP for fear of sleeping through their infants' cries and also, mistakenly, wanting to show Children's Aid that they do not need drugs and are, therefore, well enough to look after their child.[63] The probability of symptom exacerbation postpartum needs to be explained beforehand. Daily home visits after birth and summoning family support are essential because postpartum psychosis can have disastrous results for mother and child.

Parenting

Mothers with schizophrenia often feel that they are not good enough parents to their children.[64–66] They are often single parents and are eight times more likely to be involved with the child welfare system and 25 times more likely to have their children removed from the home compared with peers in the general population.[67]

Although this is so, some, especially those with close family support and a multidisciplinary care team that provides effective treatment, help at home, appropriate housing, respite provision, and parent training groups, are very good mothers.[68–71]

At this time, there is insufficient evidence as to specific interventions that have improved child and mother outcomes. Children's services and adult services do not always agree on the best course of support and treatment; working in collaboration to keep families safe and to provide an optimal environment for children is an essential service for women with schizophrenia.[72,73]

MENOPAUSE

The years leading up to menopause are difficult for women with schizophrenia. Parents are aging; children are leaving home; or, when there are no children, there is the realization that there never will be. Physical health may start to deteriorate at this time. Once menopause comes, there are hot flushes and other difficult-to-tolerate menopausal symptoms. Importantly, APs seem to lose their effect and, when doses are raised, adverse effects set in.[74–77] At this stage in life, it is important to attend to comorbidities, psychosocial issues that all women face at menopause, and to ensure optimal antipsychotic treatment: choice of drug, appropriate dose, and appropriate route of administration.

NEUROINFLAMMATION

Numerous studies show that, in later life, women are more likely than men to be diagnosed with schizophrenia for the first time.[78] There are potential hormonal explanations for this[79,80] but recent research suggests another player, neuroinflammation, which needs to be taken seriously. Women, postmenopause, are known to show more inflammatory markers than men.[81] Therapeutics aimed at modulating microglia activation are now being developed.[82]

VIOLENCE/ABUSE/SUICIDE

Women with schizophrenia can at times be perpetrators of violence, but, more often, they are at the receiving end of physical and psychological violence and financial exploitation. This is reported from many different parts of the world.[83–87] With respect to the perpetration of violence, findings from a systematic review of 24 studies spanning 35 years show this behavior occurring in approximately one in four men with schizophrenia and 1 in 20 in women. The female/male risk ratio of acting aggressively, relative to that of the general population, however, was higher.[88] This parallels the gender difference in suicide rate in schizophrenia. More men than women with schizophrenia commit suicide but the risk relative to the population at large is higher in women.[89] This means that, in the schizophrenia population, potential violence to oneself or others has to be suspected and prevented in women and men.

HOUSING

Women with schizophrenia can become homeless as a result of many factors, especially illness severity, lack of family support, and substance abuse.[90] Safe and appropriate housing is especially important for women who are mothers[91] for whom available supported housing is often not suitable.

ADVERSE EFFECTS OF ANTIPSYCHOTICS

Treatment of schizophrenia centers on AP, the kinetics and dynamics of which, although individual and dependent to a large degree on personal genetics, differ, on average, between women and men. There are male/female differences in absorption, distribution, metabolism, and elimination of drugs, and access to and effects at molecular target sites. On average, this means that, until menopause, women are overdosed when given doses appropriate for men and, as a consequence, suffer more side effects. Women are particularly vulnerable to osteoporosis, weight gain, metabolic disturbances, and certain cardiovascular complications. Breast cancer may be a risk.[92] These adverse effects need to be prevented (by appropriate drug choice, avoidance of polypharmacy, and low doses whenever possible), screened for, and rapidly treated should they emerge.[29]

Women with schizophrenia are also more prone than men to medical illnesses that result, at least in part, from long-term AP. Obesity is a major side effect, which can lead to reproductive problems and potential later problems for offspring. Seven of 16 categories of birth defects have been attributed to overweight mothers during pregnancy, most tied to undiagnosed gestational diabetes.[93] Obesity contributes to diabetes and cardiovascular disease. The blockade of cardiac potassium channels by APs and the subsequent prolongation of ventricular repolarization as shown by the length of the QTc (rate corrected QT interval on the electrocardiogram) is a prime example of sex difference in response to AP.[94] More than 80% of psychiatric patients receive at least one QT-prolonging drug during their hospital stay, and in almost 50% of cases, two or more such drugs are co-prescribed.[95] Two-thirds of cases of drug-induced torsades de pointes, a rare, drug-induced ventricular arrhythmia caused by QTc prolongation, occur in women.[96] APs can induce a hypercoagulability state that raises the risk for venous thromboembolism, pulmonary embolism, and cerebrovascular accident, for which women are at risk in the immediate postpartum period. Contraceptives, hormone-replacement, pregnancy, and obstetrical complications are additional thromboembolism risk factors for women.

APs can raise prolactin levels up to10-fold. Prolactin elevation, defined as a level above 18.77 ng/mL for males and above 24.20 ng/mL for females, is seen in almost half of postmenopausal women on AP, but in more than 65% of reproductive-age women. Women are, as a consequence, at risk for hirsutism, acne, amenorrhea, loss of fertility, osteoporosis, potential prolactinoma, and breast cancer.[97]

Box 2
Schizophrenia: clinical tips when treating women

- Women's presentations may be atypical
- Drug doses may need to change over the menstrual period
- Drug doses may need to change over the course of pregnancy
- Contraception is important and must not interact with therapeutic drugs
- Prenatal care and frequent visits are vital during pregnancy and lactation
- Sexual exploitation and domestic abuse are risks
- Premarriage counseling is important
- Be aware of pregnancy-related delusions
- Postpartum is a vulnerable time for symptom relapse
- Mothers need support, training, respite
- Menopause usually needs drug review and psychosocial intervention
- Appropriate housing is critical, especially for mothers and children
- Antipsychotics have many women-specific side effects and sequelae

Compared with sex-matched control subjects, the odds ratio for sexual dysfunction as a result of AP is 15.2 for women and 3.7 for men,[97] which is perhaps a surprising statistic to many clinicians. Switching to prolactin-sparing AP drugs alleviates hyperprolactinemia but, consequently, reproductive-age women not on contraceptives must be warned that they can now more readily become pregnant.[98] Hyperprolactinemia is also associated with autoimmune diseases, such as systemic lupus erythematosus, rheumatoid arthritis, Sjögren syndrome, Hashimoto thyroiditis, celiac disease, type 1 diabetes mellitus, Addison disease, and multiple sclerosis. Schizophrenia has been associated with a nearly 50% higher lifetime prevalence of one or more autoimmune disorders, most more prevalent in women than in men.[92] Autoimmune conditions may, however, precede treatment and, thus, cannot be attributed to AP.

DISCUSSION

The differences described in the literature between men and women are based on averages and do not pertain to everyone. Guidelines, however, are usually still slanted toward average male presentations so that it is important for clinicians to recognize that the average woman differs from the average man. There are also profound cultural differences that always need attention when formulating a differential diagnosis and deciding on optimal interventions.

SUMMARY

Women with schizophrenia have several reproduction-associated risks and care needs that require special clinical consideration (**Box 2**). They also have several specific risks related to AP and gender-associated needs not necessarily related to biology. These require clinicians' diagnostic acumen, treatment skills, cultural sensitivity, and advocacy know-how.

CLINICS CARE POINTS

- Men and women, for biologic and sociocultural reasons, differ in the nature of their risks for schizophrenia and also in their care needs.
- Clinicians need to be alert to these differences when they take histories, entertain provisional diagnoses, prescribe treatment, make referrals, talk to families, and advocate for services.
- All differences, however, are based on averages and, thus, may or may not pertain to a specific patient.

REFERENCES

1. Zhang X, Yang J, Li Y, et al. Sex chromosome abnormalities and psychiatric diseases. Oncotarget 2017;8:3969–79.
2. Gravholt CH, Viuff M, Just J, et al. The changing face of Turner syndrome. Endocrine Rev 2022. https://doi.org/10.1210/endrev/bnac016. bnac016.
3. Jung SY, Park JW, Kim DH, et al. Mosaic Turner syndrome associated with schizophrenia. Ann Pediatr Endocrinol Metab 2014;19:42–4.
4. Cohen RZ, Seeman MV, Gotowiec A, et al. Earlier puberty as a predictor of later onset of schizophrenia in women. Am J Psychiatry 1999;156:1059–64.

5. Damme KSF, Ristanovic I, Vargas T, et al. Timing of menarche and abnormal hippocampal connectivity. in youth at clinical-high risk for psychosis. Psychoneuroendocrinology 2020;117:104672. https://doi.org/10.1016/j.psyneuen.2020.104672.

6. Escobar-Morreale HF. Polycystic ovary syndrome: definition, aetiology, diagnosis and treatment. Nat Rev Endocrinol 2018;14:270–84.

7. Chen SF, Yang YC, Hsu CY, et al. Risk of schizophrenia in patients with polycystic ovary syndrome: a nationwide population-based cohort study from Taiwan. J Psychosom Obstet Gynecol 2021;42:272–8.

8. Doretto L, Chaves Mari F, Chaves AC. Polycystic ovary syndrome and psychotic disorder. Front Psychiatry 2020;11:543.

9. Lu C, Jin D, Palmer N, et al. Large-scale real-world data analysis identifies comorbidity patterns in schizophrenia. Transl Psychiatry 2022;12:154.

10. Seeman MV. Eating disorders and psychosis: seven hypotheses. World J Psychiatry 2014;4:112–9.

11. Jia JM, Zhao J, Hu Z, et al. Age-dependent regulation of synaptic connections by dopamine D2 receptors. Nat Neurosci 2013;16:1627–36.

12. Eaton WW, Byrne M, Ewald H, et al. Association of schizophrenia and autoimmune diseases: linkage of Danish national registers. Am J Psychiatry 2006;163:521–8.

13. Srinivas L, Vellichirammal NN, Nair IV, et al. Contribution from MHC-mediated risk in schizophrenia can reflect a more ethnic-specific genetic and comorbid background. Cells 2022;11:2695.

14. Wang LY, Chen SF, Chiang JH, et al. Autoimmune diseases are associated with an increased risk of schizophrenia: a nationwide population-based cohort study. Schizophr Res 2018;202:297–302.

15. Merikangas AK, Shelly M, Knighton A, et al. What genes are differentially expressed in individuals with schizophrenia? A systematic review. Mol Psychiatry 2022;27:1373–83.

16. Niebrzydowska A. Grabowski J. Medication-induced psychotic disorder. A review of selected drugs side effects. Psychiatr Danub 2022;34:11–8.

17. Keshavan MS, Kaneko Y. Secondary psychoses: an update. World Psychiatr 2013;12:4–15.

18. Sharif K, Tiosano S, Watad A, et al. The link between schizophrenia and hypothyroidism: a population-based study. Immunol Res 2018;66:663–7.

19. González-Rodríguez A, Cobo J, Soria V, et al. Women undergoing hormonal treatments for infertility: a systematic review on psychopathology and newly diagnosed mood and psychotic disorders. Front Psychiatry 2020;11:479.

20. Seeman MV. Transient psychosis in women on clomiphene, bromocriptine, domperidone and related endocrine drugs. Gynecol Endocrinol 2015;31:751–4.

21. Brand BA, de Boer JN, Dazzan P, et al. Towards better care for women with schizophrenia-spectrum disorders. Lancet Psychiatr 2022;9:330–6.

22. Díaz-Pons A, González-Rodríguez A, Ortiz-García de la Foz V, et al. Disentangling early and late onset of psychosis in women: identifying new targets for treatment. Arch Womens Ment Health 2022;25:335–44.

23. Sommer IE, Tihonen J, van Mourik A, et al. The clinical course of schizophrenia in women and men: a nation-wide cohort study. npj Schizophrenia 2020;6:12.

24. Vanasse A, Courteau J, Courteau M, et al. Multidimensional analysis of adult patients' care trajectories before a first diagnosis of schizophrenia. Schizophr 2022;8:52.

25. Gleeson PC, Worsley R, Gavrilidis E, et al. Menstrual cycle characteristics in women with persistent schizophrenia. Austral NZ J Psychiatry 2016;50:481–7.

26. Seeman MV. Menstrual exacerbation of schizophrenia symptoms. Acta Psychiatrica Scand 2012;125:363–71.

27. Nolan NL, Hughes L. Premenstrual exacerbation of mental health disorders: a systematic review of prospective studies. Arch Womens Ment Health 2022;25:831–52.

28. Berry-Bibee EN, Kim MJ, Simmons KB, et al. Drug interactions between hormonal contraceptives and psychotropic drugs: a systematic review. Contraception 2016;94:650–67.

29. Brand BA, Haveman YRA, de Beer F, et al. Antipsychotic medication for women with schizophrenia spectrum disorders. Psychol Med 2022;52:649–63.

30. Seeman MV, Ross R. Prescribing contraceptives for women with schizophrenia. J Psychiat Pract 2011;17:258–69.

31. Brown HK, Dennis C-L, Kurdyak P, et al. A population-based study of the frequency and predictors of induced abortion among women with schizophrenia. Br J Psychiatr 2019;215:736–43.

32. Edinoff AN, Silverblatt NS, Vervaeke HE, et al. Hyperprolactinemia, clinical considerations, and infertility in women on antipsychotic medications. Psychopharmacol Bull 2021;51:131–48.

33. Harris EL, Frayne J, Allen S, et al. Psychiatric admission during pregnancy in women with schizophrenia who attended a specialist antenatal clinic. J Psychosom Obstet Gynecol 2019;40:211–6.

34. Boysen GA, Isaacs RA. Perceptions of people with mental illness as sexually exploitable. Evolutionary Behav Sci 2022;16:38–52.

35. Goodman LA, Salyers MP, Mueser KT, et al. Recent victimization in women and men with severe mental illness: prevalence and correlates. J Trauma Stress 2001;14:615–32.

36. Seeman MV. Sexual exploitation of a woman with schizophrenia. J Clin Cases 2018;1:1–6.

37. Tumwakire E, Arnd H, Gavamukulya Y. A qualitative exploration of Ugandan metal health care workers' perspectives and experiences on sexual and reproductive health of people living with mental illness in Uganda. BMC Pub Health 2022;22:1722.

38. Grachev K, Santoro Lamelas V, Gresle AS, et al. Feminist contributions on sexual experiences of women with serious mental illness: a literature review. Arch Womens Ment Health 2022;25:853–70.

39. Wu KK, Cheng JP, Leung J, et al. Patients' reports of traumatic experience and postraumatic stress in psychiatric settings. East Asian Arch Psychiatry 2020;30:3–11.

40. Caqueo-Urízar A, Fond G, Urzúa A, et al. Gender differences in schizophrenia: a multicentric study from three Latin-America countries. Psychiatry Res 2018;266:65–71.

41. Seeman MV. Assortative mating. Psychiatr Serv 2012;63:174–5.

42. Seeman MV. Bad, burdened or ill? Characterizing the spouses of women with schizophrenia. Int J Soc Psychiatry 2013;59:805–10.

43. Kumar P, Sharma N, Ghai S, et al. Perception about marriage among caregivers of patients with schizophrenia and bipolar disorder. Indian J Psychol Med 2019;41:440–7.

44. Muke SS, Ghanawat GM, Chaudhury S, et al. Marital adjustment of patients with substance dependence, schizophrenia and bipolar affective disorder. Med J Dr Vidyapeeth 2014;7:133–8.
45. Suparare L, Watson SJ, Binns R, et al. Is intimate partner violence more common in pregnant women with severe mental illness? A retrospective study. Int J Soc Psychiatry 2020;66:225–31.
46. Etchecopar-Etchart D, Mignon R, Boyer L, et al. Schizophrenia pregnancies should be given greater health priority in the global health agenda: results from a large-scale meta-analysis of 43,611 deliveries of women with schizophrenia and 40,948,272 controls. Mol Psychiatry 2022. https://doi.org/10.1038/s41380-022-01593-9.
47. Seeman MV. Clinical interventions for women with schizophrenia: pregnancy. Acta Psychiatrica Scand 2012;127:12–22.
48. Dolman C, Jones I, Howard LM. Pre-conception to parenting: a systematic review and meta-synthesis of the qualitative literature on motherhood for women with severe mental illness. Arch Womens Ment Health 2013;16:173–96.
49. Howard LM, Khalifeh H. Perinatal mental health: a review of progress and challenges. World Psychiatr 2020;19:313–27.
50. Seeman MV. Pseudocyesis, delusional pregnancy, and psychosis: the birth of a delusion. World J Clin Cases 2014;2:338–44.
51. Dua D, Grover S. Delusion of denial of pregnancy: a case report. Asian J Psychiatry 2019;45:72–3.
52. Heinonen E, Forsberg L, Nörby U, et al. Neonatal morbidity after fetal exposure to antipsychotics: a national register-based study. BMJ Open 2022;12:e061328.
53. Nguyen T, Frayne J, Watson S, et al. Long-acting injectable antipsychotic treatment during pregnancy: outcomes for women at a tertiary maternity hospital. Psychiatry Res 2022;313:114614.
54. Viguera AC. Accumulation of reproductive safety data for second-generation atypical antipsychotics: a call to accelerate the process. J Clin Psychiatry 2022;83:22com14489.
55. Wang Z, Chan AYL, Coghill D, et al. Association between prenatal exposure to antipsychotics and attention-deficit/hyperactivity disorder, autism spectrum disorder, preterm birth, and small for gestational age. JAMA Intern Med 2021;181:1332–40.
56. Yakuwa N, Takahashi K, Anzai T, et al. Pregnancy outcomes with exposure to second-generation antipsychotics during the first trimester. J Clin Psychiatry 2022;83:21m14081.
57. Kronenfeld N, Berlin M, Shaniv D, et al. Use of psychotropic medications in breastfeeding women. Birth Defects Res 2017;109:957–97.
58. Toufeili A, Cohen E, Ray JG, et al. Complex chronic conditions among children born to women with schizophrenia. Schizophr Res 2022;241:24–35.
59. Seeman MV. Preventing unnecessary loss of child custody. In: Reupert A, Maybery D, Nicholson J, et al, editors. Parental psychiatric disorder: distressed parents and their families. Cambridge, UK: Cambridge University Press; 2015. p. 333–42.
60. Taylor CL, Munk-Olsen T, Howard LM, et al. Schizophrenia around the time of pregnancy: leveraging population-based health data and electronic health record data to fill knowledge gaps. BJPsych Open 2020;6:e97. https://doi.org/10.1192/bjo.2020.78.
61. Cowling V, Seeman MV, Göpfert MJ. Grandparents as primary caregivers. Parental psychiatric disorder: distressed parents and their families. In: Reupert A, Maybery D,

Nicholson J, et al, editors. Ch. 23. Cambridge, UK: Cambridge University Press; 2015. p. 248–58.

62. Sharma V, Mazmanian D, Palagini L, et al. Postpartum psychosis: revisiting the phenomenology, nosology, and treatment. J Affect Disord Rep 2022;10:100378.

63. Seeman MV. Antipsychotic-induced somnolence in mothers with schizophrenia. Psychiatr Q 2012;83:83–9.

64. Chan SYY, Ho GWK, Bressington D. Experiences of self-stigmatization and parenting in Chinese mothers with severe mental illness. Int J Ment Health Nurs 2019;28:527–37.

65. Shettima FB, Rabbebe IB, Wakawa IA, et al. Internalized stigma and stigmatizing cultural beliefs on parenting with mental illness among female patients with schizophrenia: a comparison of female parent versus non parent. Global J Health Sci 2022;7:1–17.

66. Strand J, Boström P, Grip K. Parents' descriptions of how their psychosis affects parenting. J Child Family Stud 2020;29:620–31.

67. Kaplan K, Brusilovskiy E, O'Shea AM, et al. Child protective service disparities and serious mental illnesses: results from a national survey. Psychiatr Serv 2019;70:202–8.

68. Niemelä M, Kalunki H, Jokinen J, et al. Collective impact on prevention: let's talk about children service model and decrease in referrals to child protection services. Front Psychiatry 2019;10:64.

69. Radley J, Grant C, Barlow J, et al. Parenting interventions for people with schizophrenia or related serious mental illness. Cochrane Database Syst Rev 2021;10: CD013536.

70. Radley J, Sivarajah N, Moltrecht B, et al. A scoping review of interventions designed to support parents with mental illness that would be appropriate for parents with psychosis. Front Psychiatry 2022;12:787166.

71. Seeman MV. Parenting issues in mothers with schizophrenia. Curr Womens Health Rev 2010;6:51–7.

72. Lauritzen C, Reedtz C, Rognmo K, et al. Identification of and support for children of mentally ill parents: a 5 year follow-up study of adult mental health services. Front Psychiatry 2018;9:507.

73. Nicholson J, de Girolamo G, Schrank B. Parents with mental and/or substance use disorders and their children. Front Psychiatry 2019;10:915.

74. Culbert KM, Thakkar KN, Klump KL. Risk for midlife psychosis in women: critical gaps and opportunities in exploring perimenopause and ovarian hormones as mechanisms of risk. Psychol Med 2022;52:1612–20.

75. Fisher VL, Ortiz LS, Powers AR. A computational lens on menopause-associated psychosis. Front Psychiatry 2022;13:906796.

76. González-Rodríguez A, Monreal JA, Seeman MV. The effect of menopause on antipsychotic response. Brain Sci 2022;12:1342.

77. Sommer IE, Brand BA, Gangadin S, et al. Women with schizophrenia-spectrum disorders after menopause: a vulnerable group for relapse. Schizophr Bull 2022;sbac139. https://doi.org/10.1093/schbul/sbac139.

78. Johnstone S, Dela Cruz GA, Girard TA, et al. Potential explanatory models of the female preponderance in very late onset schizophrenia. Women 2022;2:353–70.

79. Hwang WJ, Lee TY, Kim NS, et al. The role of estrogen receptors and their signaling across psychiatric disorders. Int J Mol Sci 2021;22:373.

80. Vegeto E, Villa A, Della Torre S, et al. The role of sex and sex hormones in neurodegenerative diseases. Endocrine Rev 2020;41:273–319.

81. Villa A, Della Torre S, Maggi A. Sexual differentiation of microglia. Front Neuroen-docrinology 2019;52:156–64.
82. Miller S, Blanco M-J. Small molecule therapeutics for neuroinflammation-mediated neurodegenerative disorders. RSC Medicinal Chem 2021;12:871–86.
83. Bhattacharya A. The day I die is the day I will find my peace:" narratives of family, marriage, and violence among women living with serious mental illness in India. Violence Against Women 2022;8:966–90.
84. Doyle KW, Knetig JA, Iverson KM. Practical implications of research on intimate partner violence experiences for the mental health clinician. Curr Treat Options Psych 2022;9:280–300.
85. El Missiry A, Meguid M, Abourayah A, et al. Rates and profile of victimization in a sample of Egyptian patients with major mental illness. Int J Soc Psychiatry 2019; 65:183–93.
86. Ünlü İİ, Baykara Acar Y. Violence against patients with schizophrenia from their surrounding environment: a qualitative study in Turkey. J Psychosoc Rehabil Ment Health 2022;9:159–67.
87. Yosep I, Mediani HS, Lindayani L, et al. How patients with schizophrenia "as a victim" cope with violence in Indonesia: a qualitative study. Egypt J Neurol Psychiatry Neurosurg 2021;57:71.
88. Whiting D. disorders and violence perpetration in adults and adolescents from 15 countries: a systematic review and meta-analysis. JAMA Psychiatr 2022;79: 120–32.
89. Pan CH, Chen PH, Chang HM, et al. Incidence and method of suicide mortality in patients with schizophrenia: a nationwide cohort study. Soc Psychiatry Psychiatr Epidemiol 2021;56:1437–46.
90. Caton CL, Shrout PE, Dominguez B, et al. Risk factors for homelessness among women with schizophrenia. Am J Pub Health 1995;85:1153–6.
91. Perlman S, Cowan B, Gewirtz A, et al. Promoting positive parenting in the context of homelessness. Am J Orthopsychiatry 2012;82:402–12.
92. Solmi M, Murru A, Pacchiarotti I, et al. Safety, tolerability, and risks associated with first- and second-generation antipsychotics: a state-of-the-art clinical review. Ther Clin Risk Manag 2017;13:757–77.
93. Gaillard R. Maternal obesity during pregnancy and cardiovascular development and disease in the offspring. Eur J Epidemiol 2015;30:1141–52.
94. Elliott A, Mørk T, Højlund M, et al. QTc interval in patients with schizophrenia receiving antipsychotic treatment as monotherapy or polypharmacy. CNS Spectr 2018;23:278–83.
95. Hefner G, Hahn M, Hiemke C. Pharmacodynamic drug–drug interactions of QT-prolonging drugs in hospitalized psychiatric patients. J Neural Transm 2021; 128:243–52.
96. Peirlinck M, Sahli Costabal F, Kuhl E. Sex differences in drug-induced arrhythmo-genesis. Front Physiology 2021;12:7084.
97. Lu Z, Sun Y, Zhang Y, et al. Pharmacological treatment strategies for antipsychotic-induced hyperprolactinemia: a systematic review and network meta-analysis. Transl Psychiatry 2022;12:267.
98. Seeman MV. Loss of libido in a woman with schizophrenia. Am J Psychiatry 2013; 170:471–5.

Substance Use Disorders in Women

Kathryn Polak, PhD[a],*, Nancy A. Haug, PhD[b],
Pamela Dillon, PharmD[c], Dace S. Svikis, PhD[d]

KEYWORDS

- Gender differences • Women • Female • Addiction • Substance use disorder
- Treatment outcomes • Pregnancy • Risk factors

KEY POINTS

- SUDs in women and men differ with regard to cause, course, comorbidities, and treatment uptake and retention.
- Women experience more adverse medical, psychiatric, and social consequences associated with substance use, and they are of greater severity compared with men.
- Universal screening is important for identifying women with SUD, and attention must be given to language in screening instruments to minimize stigmatizing women with SUD. This is especially important for pregnant women with SUDs.
- A gender gap exists in SUD treatment with women being less likely to engage and remain in treatment compared with men, and gender-specific treatments may help address this gap.

Substance use disorders (SUDs) are a chronic, relapsing condition in which the "recurrent use of alcohol and/or drugs causes clinically significant impairment, including health problems, disability, and failure to meet major responsibilities at work, school, or home."[1] Alcohol, tobacco, and other drug use disorders (DUDs) impose significant health, economic, and social burdens and are among the leading causes of premature morbidity and mortality. According to the diagnostic and statistical manual of mental disorders (DSM-5-TR), SUDs are diagnosed based on 11 criteria that assess physical dependence, risky use, social problems, and impaired control.[2] The 2020 National Survey on Drug Use and Health (NSDUH) reports more than 40 million people

[a] Department of Psychiatry, Virginia Commonwealth University, 806 West Franklin Street, PO Box 842018, Richmond, VA 23284, USA; [b] Department of Psychology, Palo Alto University, 1791 Arastradero Road, Palo Alto, CA 94304, USA; [c] Wright Center for Clinical and Translational Research, Virginia Commonwealth University, 1200 East Clay Street, Richmond, VA 23298, USA; [d] Department of Psychology, Institute for Women's Health, Virginia Commonwealth University, 806 West Franklin Street, PO Box 842018, Richmond, VA 23284, USA
* Corresponding author.
E-mail address: polakkm@vcu.edu

Psychiatr Clin N Am 46 (2023) 487–503
https://doi.org/10.1016/j.psc.2023.04.006
0193-953X/23/© 2022 Elsevier Inc. All rights reserved.

psych.theclinics.com

(14.5%), in the United States, aged 12 years and older had a DSM-5-defined SUD in the past year, with 44.8% (>18 million) of them were women.[3]

EPIDEMIOLOGY OF SUBSTANCE USE DISORDERS IN WOMEN

Prevalence rates for SUDs vary widely based on substance, with alcohol use disorders being reported most often for men and women. Polysubstance use is common in both genders, although it is reported more frequently in men. In general, men also have higher rates of substance use and SUDs but the gap seems to be narrowing.[3] In younger cohorts (aged 12–20 years), rates of alcohol misuse and binge drinking are slightly higher in women compared with men,[4] and men and women have similar rates of amphetamine use and stimulant medication misuse.[5]

Globally, in 2020, more than 1.3 billion people (22.8%) aged 15 years and older reported past-year alcohol consumption in amounts that increased their health risks beyond that of nondrinkers. This included 1.03 billion men (35.1%) and 312 million women (10.5%).[6] For other drugs, per the 2020 World Drug Report, more than 284 million people (5.6%) worldwide aged between 15 and 64 years reported past year use of a psychoactive substance.[5] Finally, 1.3 billon people worldwide (22.3%) use tobacco with its use being 4 times more prevalent in men compared with women (36.7% and 7.8%, respectively).[5]

In the United States, according to the 2020 NSDUH, more than 28 million people (10.2%) $\geq$ 12 years of age reported past year AUD, with more than 12.6 million (8.8%) women reporting AUD. In addition, more than 18 million people (6.6%) reported illicit DUD, with more than 8 million (5.7%) of them women. This included 14.2 million people (5.1%) who used cannabis, 3.5 million (1.3%) who misused a prescription drug, and 2.7 million (1.0%) who used opioids. In addition, approximately 70.7 million people aged 12 years and older reported past year tobacco use.[3]

SEX AND GENDER DIFFERENCES IN SUBSTANCE USE DISORDERS

A significant body of research shows that, in addition to gender distinctions in SUD prevalence, there are significant gender differences in SUD etiology, course, comorbidities, and treatments. Reasons for these differences are multifold and certainly include biologic, genetic, environmental, and behavioral factors. Research consistently shows pharmacokinetic differences, including disparate metabolic enzyme activity and total body water, between women and men that affects the distribution, degradation, and effects of many substances of abuse. Women have lower levels of alcohol dehydrogenase and total body water compared with men resulting in higher blood alcohol concentrations and greater impairment with consumption of equivalent amounts of alcohol.[7] Nicotine is metabolized more quickly and addiction risk is higher in women compared with men, likely due to nicotine's breakdown by the CYP2A6 enzyme, which is induced by estrogen.[8] In addition, research has shown the effects of substances of abuse vary as ovarian hormone levels fluctuate across the menstrual cycle. The data are most consistent with stimulants and show that women have greater plasma concentrations of cocaine and subjective reinforcing responses to cocaine and methamphetamine during the follicular phase when estrogen levels are relatively higher than during the luteal phase when progesterone levels are relatively higher.[9]

Although changes in brain structure and function are seen in both women and men with SUDs, the alterations observed in women are distinct. Both women and men have decreased gray matter volume in response to drug use (eg, cocaine, alcohol, nicotine) but women may be more sensitive to the resultant functional effects.[7] Moreover, women are more susceptible to the dysregulation of neural pathways following cocaine use, whereas men seem to respond to alcohol, nicotine, and stimulant use with increased activation of brain reward pathways compared with women. In cocaine dependence, women show greater neural activation in response to stress cues compared with drug cues for men, and with alcohol and nicotine use, women show greater sensitivity to stress-induced craving compared with men.[9]

The heritability of AUD and other SUDs is well documented, and genetic factors are responsible for about 50% of SUD risk.[10,11] Genetic influences predispose to SUDs in general as well as to risk for using specific substances.[12] However, much less is known about the heritability of substance use by gender. This is mostly due to the large samples required for such evaluations but also due to challenges in disentangling the impact of environmental factors, especially stress, on the development of SUDs. The few studies that have evaluated by-gender heritability show mixed results. A twin study showed similar genetic risk for SUDs between men and women,[12] whereas other research suggests some differences including less heritability for women compared with men in cocaine use disorder and the identification of a significant sex-specific locus that may affect gender differences in the risk of opioid dependence.[13]

Socio-environmental factors also affect substance use and vary between women and men. Women are more likely than men to use substances of abuse in order to have increased energy for work and family responsibilities and to self-treat physical and psychiatric conditions (eg, opioids for pain; opioids and nicotine for anxiety and stress; nicotine and stimulants for weight loss).[14] In addition, women with SUDs are more likely to have family members with SUDs, substance-using partners, experienced physical or sexual violence, and experienced trauma compared with women in the general population.[15] Moreover, women more often experience social stigma associated with their substance use than do men.[9]

Not surprising then, the presentation of SUDs is unique between men and women. With drugs including alcohol, cannabis, cocaine, and opioids, women generally experience a telescoping effect, progressing more quickly from substance use initiation to dependence.[16] Compared with men, women report greater craving and, with substances including nicotine, cannabis, cocaine, and methamphetamines, withdrawal symptoms with abstinence, which may lead to higher rates of relapse in women compared with men. Moreover, women with SUDs experience more functional impairment, decreased quality of life, and increased medical and psychiatric comorbidities, and these comorbidities may be more severe than in men.[17]

COMORBIDITIES ASSOCIATED WITH SUBSTANCE USE DISORDERS IN WOMEN

Medical and psychiatric comorbidities with SUDs are common and increase the burden of both diseases. NSDUH data show that more than 6.7% (17 million) of US adults reported both a SUD and past-year psychiatric disorder.[3] Although men are more likely to have SUDs, women are 2 to 3 times more likely to have a comorbid psychiatric disorder including depression, anxiety, eating disorders, posttraumatic stress disorder (PTSD), and general psychological distress, and the presentation is often more severe.[9,16]

Some researchers postulate that substance use may make the brain more susceptible to psychiatric disorders, whereas others suggest patients use alcohol and other drugs to relieve symptoms associated with psychiatric disorders.[18] Compared with men, women are more likely to use alcohol and drugs to self-medicate for stress and mood and eating disorders, and conversely, to report anxiety and mood disorders associated with substance use, especially opiates, cocaine, and cannabis.[14] In women, SUD and trauma are inextricably linked. Women with SUDs are more likely to have substance-using partners, have experienced intimate partner violence (IPV; 40%–70% of women with SUDs), and been diagnosed with PTSD (up to 80% of women with SUDs) compared with the women without SUDs.[14] This may be especially true for sexual minorities who experience higher rates of SUDs and trauma than the general population.[9]

Often comorbid psychiatric disorders and SUDs go undetected, which can hamper access to appropriate treatment of both illnesses. When diagnosed, the co-occurrence of these disorders can complicate treatment, and this may be more significant in women than in men.

Medical comorbidities are also common in patients with SUDs. Due to physiologic differences in absorption, distribution, and metabolism between women and men, women with SUDs develop adverse physical health conditions such as cirrhosis, cardiovascular disease, diabetes, and gastrointestinal disorders at higher rates and with lower levels of substance intake and shorter periods of use than men.[15] Compared with men, women are more likely to develop neurologic deficits and the impairment occurs more quickly after initiation of substance use.[14] In addition, women with SUDs are at greater risk for gender-specific conditions such as breast and cervical cancer, vaginal infections, infertility, and pregnancy-related complications than women without SUDs.[15] Women with SUDs also report poorer overall quality of life compared with men.[7] Women with SUDs are more likely than men to experience other adverse health outcomes including violence, particularly IPV and infection with HIV and HCV.[14] Further, binge drinking and illicit drug use in women have been associated with sexual assault, unintended pregnancy, engagement in risky sexual behavior, physical injury, and overdose.[7]

SCREENING FOR SUBSTANCE USE DISORDERS IN WOMEN

Universal screening to identify risk for hazardous/problem substance use is essential.[19,20] Screening additionally provides an opportunity to educate patients about the risks of substance use and prevent the progression to SUDs. As shown in **Table 1**, there are multiple standardized screening tools available.

These screeners vary in length, mode of administration (interview or survey), target population (eg, pregnant women), and target substance(s) (alcohol, drugs, alcohol, and drugs). For alcohol, the 10-item Alcohol Use Disorders Identification Test (AUDIT) is well known and examines quantity and frequency of use as well as alcohol-related problems.[21] Shorter screeners include the 4-item Cut down, Annoyed, Guilty, and Eyeopener (CAGE)[22] and the 3-item Alcohol Use Disorders Identification Test Consumption screening tool (AUDIT-C).[23]

For other drugs, the time required for screening can increase substantively if each class of drug is examined separately. For example, the Alcohol, Smoking and Substance Involvement Screening Test (ASSIST) is a structured interview, taking approximately 5 to 15 minutes to complete, and consists of 8 to 57 questions screening for problem or hazardous use of 10 psychoactive substances. Responses produce a score and subsequent substance-specific risk stratification for each substance (eg, low-moderate- or high-risk category).[24] An alternative approach is to screen across all drug categories, using a tool such as the 10-item Drug Abuse Screening Test (DAST).[25]

Instrument-based screening practices can be subject to major barriers to implementation such as lack of space, time, training, and resources to support such procedures.[26,27] To address the research to practice gap, the Tobacco, Alcohol,

Table 1
Screening instruments for alcohol and other drugs

Substance	Screener	Target Population	Description	Scoring
Alcohol	CAGE	Adults	4-item screen for at-risk drinking	≥2 is positive
	AUDIT	Adults	10-item screen for at-risk alcohol use; constructed by the World Health Organization	≥8 is positive
	AUDIT-C	Adults	3-item screen assessing alcohol consumption to screen for risk for hazardous/problem drinking; shortened version of the 10-item AUDIT	≥4 is positive in men; ≥3 is positive in women
	T-ACE	Adults, pregnant women	4-item screen for hazardous/problem drinking	≥2 is positive
	TWEAK	Adults, pregnant women	5-item screen for hazardous/problem drinking	≥2 is positive
Alcohol and other medications	DAST	Adolescents, adults	10-item screen of drug use, including prescribed or over-the-counter drugs in excess of directions and any nonmedical use of drugs	≥3 warrants further assessment
	ASSIST	Adults	8-item screen with questions covering tobacco, alcohol, cannabis, cocaine, amphetamine-type stimulants, inhalants, sedatives, hallucinogens, opioids and 'other drugs'	Scores calculated into 3 subgroups: low risk, moderate risk, high risk
	TAPS tool	Adults	Consists of 2 parts: TAPS-1 is a 4-item screen for alcohol and other drug use; TAPS-2 is a brief assessment with substance-specific questions to determine risk level (initiated when TAPS-1 is positive)	0 = No use in past 3 mo; 1 = Problem use; 2+ = Higher risk

(continued on next page)

Table 1
(continued)

Substance	Screener	Target Population	Description	Scoring
	NIDA Quick Screen	Adults	3-item screen with questions about use of alcohol, tobacco, and other drugs. If the patient says "Yes" to use of illegal drugs or prescription drugs for nonmedical reasons, the NIDA-Modified ASSIST is completed	An answer of "Yes" to one or more days of heavy drinking or any current use of tobacco = at risk. For each other drug, a Substance Involvement score is calculated and used to identify risk level. 0–3 = Lower risk; 4–26 = Moderate risk; 27+ = High risk
	WIDUS	Pregnant women	6-indirect item screen that identifies risk in the perinatal period by asking about correlates of drug use	A cut score of 3 is considered to result in the best overall classification but different cut scores can be used to maximize either sensitivity or specificity

Prescription medication, and other Substance use (TAPS) tool was developed with the goal of more easily becoming part of routine clinical practice. This 2-stage screener includes all commonly used substances and both interviewer and computer-administered versions are available.[28] A recent study of the TAPS-1 initial screener found it identified unhealthy substance use in primary care patients with a high level of accuracy, thereby providing an opportunity for rapid triage in busy primary care settings.[29]

Similarly, the NIDA Quick Screen has been recommended as an alternative approach to traditional screening that only requires asking 3 open-ended questions about patient use of alcohol, tobacco, and other drugs: "In the past year how many times have you drunk greater than 4 alcoholic drinks per day? Used tobacco products? Taken illegal drugs or prescription drugs for nonmedical reasons?"[30] This approach is thought to demonstrate good sensitivity and specificity and requires less time and administrative support than instrument-based screening.

Screening for substance use disorders in pregnancy

The American College of Obstetricians and Gynecologists recommends universal screening for alcohol and drug use during pregnancy to promote early identification and referral to treatment when appropriate.[31,32] Screening should be conducted at the first prenatal visit. For those who screen positive, screening should be repeated throughout pregnancy to monitor use.[32]

Identification of substance use among pregnant women is hindered by the potential consequences of disclosing use.[33] SUD is associated with greater stigma compared with other mental health concerns,[34] with pregnant women representing a particularly affected subgroup.[35] This stigma extends to the care system. For example, providers often have negative attitudes toward pregnant women with SUD, which contributes to suboptimal treatment.[36] Correspondingly, punitive measures (eg, incarceration, civil commitment, loss of parental rights/custody) are common, and consequently, pregnant women who use drugs often avoid accessing care or underreport substance use for fear of repercussions.[35,37] Additionally, pregnant women may misreport the timing of substance use as occurring earlier in the pregnancy.[38] Therefore, clinician-administered instruments may result in patients feeling uncomfortable disclosing their use to a provider.

In an effort to address these barriers to care, the wording of screening items and mode of instrument administration with pregnant women has been explored. The Tolerance, Annoyed, Cut down, and Eye-Opener (T-ACE)[39] and Tolerance, Worried, Eye-opener, Amnesia, and K/Cut Down (TWEAK)[40] are brief screeners developed specifically to identify hazardous/problem drinking among pregnant women. Indirect screening approaches (eg, Wayne Indirect Drug Use Screener [WIDUS][41]) that focus on correlates of substance use (eg, mental health, demographics) have been found to more accurately predict toxicology results compared with direct screening measures. Screeners with increased time windows (eg, NIDA Quick Screen) beyond pregnancy could minimize fears of the negative repercussions of disclosure of substance use during pregnancy.[32] Moreover, using self-administered screening tools instead of face-to-face interviews may help to mitigate concern regarding the stigma of substance use[42] and have been linked with more accurate reporting and higher rates of disclosure than face-to-face interviews.[43] Technology can help address barriers to care and provide opportunities for tailoring treatment to better meet an individual's needs. For example, computerized screeners/assessments have shown higher rates of self-report of stigmatized behaviors (eg, Newman and colleagues, 2002),[44] sensitivity, and specificity when compared with pencil-and-paper administered screeners.[45]

Across all screening approaches, providers are responsible for ensuring the appropriate steps are taken following a positive screen for risky substance use, including patient education, motivational interviewing around behavior change, brief intervention, and referral to treatment as needed.[31] Discussions focused on substance use with patients should be conducted in a nonjudgmental manner, with providers serving as a source of support for positive change. In addition to screening for problem/hazardous substance use, women should be screened for commonly occurring comorbid conditions, including mood disorders, trauma, psychosocial issues (eg, IPV), and other medical issues.[42]

DIAGNOSIS OF SUBSTANCE USE DISORDERS IN WOMEN

Screening tools are not diagnostic instruments. A positive screen does not confirm the presence or absence of an SUD but signifies that further assessment is warranted. To diagnose SUDs, it is necessary to use DSM-5 criteria assessed by a knowledgeable provider. In the classification of SUDs, the DSM-5 eliminated the distinct abuse and dependence disorders in favor of a single, dimensional SUD diagnosis, characterized as mild, moderate, or severe based on the number of symptoms endorsed.[46]

The implementation and dissemination of screening and testing procedures should be linked to evidence-based interventions. To determine the appropriate level of care for individuals with SUD, the American Society of Addiction Medicine (ASAM) Criteria uses a multidimensional assessment to provide outcome-oriented and results-based care. ASAM Criteria treatment plans include 5 levels of treatment and account for the patient's needs, strengths, barriers, resources, and risk factors.[47]

TREATMENT AND MANAGEMENT OF SUBSTANCE USE DISORDERS IN WOMEN

Despite nearly equal prevalence, a gender gap remains at the level of addiction treatment. The overall proportion of men to women who present for the treatment of SUDs has remained constant from 2010 to 2020 at an overall ratio of 2:1 according to the Treatment Episode Data Set of publicly funded substance use treatment facilities.[48] In 2020, women (aged 12 years or older) represented 30.6% of treatment admissions for primary use of alcohol, 33.2% of heroin, 42.5% of opioids other than heroin, 31.6% of cannabis, 32.1% of cocaine, and 43.2% of methamphetamine admissions. Of note, the rate of women admitted for methamphetamine treatment has significantly increased in recent years compared with men, particularly among adults aged 18 to 44 years.[49]

Several factors have been identified to explain why women are less likely to utilize treatment services in comparison to men. Gender-related barriers include work and family responsibilities such as childcare,[16,50] lack of family support,[51] and co-occurring psychiatric disorders and history of trauma.[52] Shame and stigma may also contribute to women's willingness to attend treatment.[53,54] Women with children may have concerns about jeopardizing child custody by seeking SUD treatment.[55] Not only are women less likely to seek treatment of SUD but they are also more likely to leave treatment, particularly when women-only services are not available.[56] Treatment seeking and utilization is even lower among pregnant women with an estimated 8.7% obtaining specialized treatment.[57]

In contrast to the TEDS, a recent study examined data from the National Epidemiologic Survey on Alcohol and Related Conditions-III to determine whether women are more or less likely than men to receive any care for SUDs.[58] The cross-sectional sample included noninstitutionalized civilians aged 18 years or older in the United States. Those in correctional facilities or hospitals were excluded, and specific substances were not examined (ie, alcohol and substances are combined). Overall results showed no significant difference, such that 10.7% of women with SUDs received treatment of SUD compared with 9.9% of men with SUDs. Correlates of service use for women included being separated or divorced, annual income less than US$20,000, homelessness, previous incarceration or legal difficulties, trauma exposure, and co-occurring psychiatric diagnoses. The low rates of treatment service utilization suggest that more outreach and intervention are needed to engage women with SUDs.

A study of private, residential treatment of individuals with co-occurring psychiatric disorders and SUDs indicated that women had greater severity of problems on the Addiction Severity Index medical, employment/support, family/social relationships and psychiatric domains compared with men. In addition, women stayed in treatment longer and had higher rates of treatment retention at 30 days compared with men.[50] The funding source may have affected retention among this sample of women, in contrast to the TEDS population drawn from publicly funded programs. In addition to trauma, depression, and anxiety disorders, high rates of eating disorders have been reported in patients in privately funded addiction treatment programs.[59]

Treatment Outcomes

In terms of treatment outcomes, results are mixed but most large-scale clinical trials have not found evidence of gender differences in pharmacologic treatment with a few exceptions.[7] Women perform equally well compared with men on behavioral treatments such as motivational interviewing, cognitive-behavioral therapies, contingency management, and behavioral couples therapy.[60–63] Mutual-help groups (eg, Alcoholics Anonymous) are also effective for women and may be associated with treatment seeking.[58]

Clearly, women with SUDs who present for treatment are a heterogenous population who may require comprehensive services tailored to their specific needs. Several treatment protocols have been developed for specific subpopulations of women with SUDs, including pregnant and postpartum women, women with co-occurring trauma, and women in correctional facilities.[64] Gender-specific and gender-responsive treatments are associated with better treatment outcomes (eg, substance use, criminal justice) than mixed-gender programs.[7]

Gender-Specific Treatment

A recent systematic review of gender-responsive and integrated SUD treatment programs for women with co-occurring psychiatric disorders identified 24 studies from 10 distinct programs.[15] A description of each of these treatment programs from the systematic review can be found in **Table 2**. The findings indicated benefits in both substance use and psychiatric disorders when women's specific needs, trauma, and mental health were integrated into the intervention. Women in the gender-informed treatment groups reported high client satisfaction and were more likely to stay in treatment. Significant improvements on clinical outcomes related to trauma and other psychiatric symptoms were seen in protocols that addressed these issues (ie, Seeking Safety, Trauma Recovery and Empowerment Model [TREM], Breaking the Cycle and VOICES, Women's Recovery Group). The authors noted a lack of interventions to address the needs of women with serious psychiatric disorders including psychosis.

Treatment of Pregnant Women

Smoking cessation has been a target for treatment in pregnant women given the adverse effects of smoking on maternal and fetal health. Contingency management

Table 2
Gender-responsive and integrated substance use disorder treatment programs for women with co-occurring disorders

Intervention	Description	Manual or Reference
A Woman's Path to Recovery (WPR)	• Based on self-help A Woman's Addiction Workbook • 12 sessions focused on gender-based psychoeducation for addiction and co-occurring disorders • Topics include body and sexuality, stress, relationships, trauma and violence, and thrill-seeking	Najavits, L. M. (2002). A Woman's Addiction Workbook: Your Guide to In-Depth Healing. Oakland, CA: New Harbinger. Najavits LM, Enggasser J, Brief D, Federman E. A randomized controlled trial of a gender-focused addiction model vs 12-step facilitation for women veterans. The American Journal on Addictions. 2018;27:210–16.
Breaking the Cycle (BC)	• Relationship-focused intervention for mother and child dyads • Weekly sessions cover basic needs support, addiction counseling and mental health	Espinet SD, Espinet SD, Motz M, Jeong JJ, Jenkins JM. (2016). 'Breaking the Cycle' of maternal substance use through relationships: a comparison of integrated approaches. Addiction Research & Theory, 24, 375–88.
Female-Specific Cognitive Behavioral Therapy (FS-CBT)	• Manualized treatment based on CBT, relapse prevention and Motivational Enhancement Therapy • 12 sessions; female-specific modules include social support, interpersonal functioning, coping with negative affect, and psychoeducation about women and alcohol	Epstein EE, McCrady BS, Hallgren KA, Cook S, Jensen NK, Hildebrandt T. A randomized trial of female-specific cognitive behavior therapy for alcohol dependent women. Psychol Addict Behav. 2018 Feb;32(1):1-15.
Helping Women Recover (HWR) and Beyond Trauma (BT)	• Combined intervention for adult women with addiction and trauma history • 32 sessions organized into 7 modules focused on relapse prevention and healing from trauma.	Covington, S. (1999, rev. 2008 and 2019). Helping Women Recover: A program for treating addiction. John Wiley & Sons, Inc. Covington, S. (2003, rev. 2016). Beyond Trauma: A healing journey for women. Hazelden.
Moment by Moment in Women's Recovery (MMWR)	• Mindfulness-based intervention focused on the needs of women in residential treatment (ie, parenting, trauma, interpersonal conflict) • Delivered twice weekly for a total of 12 group sessions • Combines stress reduction with relapse prevention; aimed at reducing treatment drop-out	Vallejo Z, Amaro H. Adaptation of mindfulness-based stress reduction program for addiction relapse prevention. The Humanistic Psychologist. 2009;37(2):192–206. Black DS, Amaro H. Moment-by-Moment in Women's Recovery (MMWR): mindfulness-based intervention effects on residential substance use disorder treatment retention in a randomized controlled trial. Behav Res Ther. 2019;120:103437.

Program	Description	Reference
Seeking Safety	• Integrated treatment program targeting co-occurring PTSD and SUD in women • 25 topics addressing cognitive, behavioral and interpersonal domains with a focus on safe coping skills	Najavits, L. M. (2002). Seeking Safety: A Treatment Manual for PTSD and Substance Abuse. New York: Guilford.
TREM and Boston Consortium Model (modified TREM)	• Manualized group intervention for women with substance use, trauma and mental health conditions • 24–29 sessions using cognitive–behavioral, skills training, and psychoeducational techniques	Harris, M., & The Community Connections Working Group. (1998). Trauma Recovery and Empowerment: A clinician's guide to working with women in groups. The Free Press.
Understanding and Overcoming Substance Misuse (UOSM)	• Integrated treatment of women with serious mental illness in a forensic setting • 14–20 group sessions based on cognitive–behavioral therapy and relapse prevention	Long, C. G., Fulton, B., & Hollin, C. R. (2008). The development of a 'best practice' service for women in a medium-secure psychiatric setting: Treatment components and evaluation. Clinical Psychology and Psychotherapy, 15, 304-319.
VOICES	• Program of self-discovery and empowerment for girls ages 12–24 y based on HWR • Group intervention with 4 modules, 18 sessions	Covington, S. (2012). Curricula to support trauma-informed practice with women. In N. Poole, & L. Greaves (Eds). Becoming trauma informed. Toronto, Ontario, Canada: Centre for Addiction and Mental Health (CAMH).
Women's Recovery Group (WRG)	• Relapse-prevention group therapy based on CBT skills • 12 sessions and 14 flexible modules with women-specific content on substance use, violence and abuse, mood, anxiety eating disorders, stigma and shame, partners, caregiving, and achieving balance	Greenfield, S.F., Crisafulli, M.A., Kaufman, J.S., Freid, C.M., Bailey, G.L., Connery, H.S.,Rapoza, M., Rodolico, J., 2014. Implementing substance abuse group therapy clinical trials in real-world settings: challenges and strategies for participant recruitment and therapist training in the Women's Recovery Group Study. Am.J. Addict. 23, 197–204.

and psychosocial interventions are effective behavioral treatments to address smoking among pregnant women.[65] Computer-delivered brief interventions may also improve smoking abstinence during pregnancy.[41] Pharmacotherapy, such as nicotine replacement, has shown less efficacy in treating pregnant women who smoke and is associated with some risks to infants.[66,67]

For pregnant women with opioid use disorder, both methadone and buprenorphine are well-established pharmacologic treatments, with some evidence for better infant outcomes with buprenorphine.[68] Contingency management in the form of behavioral incentives (eg, vouchers for maternal or infant-related items) also demonstrated improved attendance and retention in the treatment of pregnant women who use substances such as opioids and cocaine.[69–71] In contrast, Motivational Enhancement Therapy for pregnant substance users did not show improved retention or substance use outcomes in comparison to treatment as usual in a Clinical Trials Network study with 4 treatment sites,[72] although it may be beneficial for minority women.[73]

There is a lack of research on treatment of alcohol problems in pregnant women, particularly in the use of pharmacotherapies for AUD and detoxification.[7] Brief interventions for reducing alcohol during pregnancy have demonstrated efficacy for women with higher baseline levels of alcohol consumption and when a partner participated.[74] A brief intervention consisting of 10 to 15-minute sessions of counseling by a nutritionist in a community setting resulted in higher abstinence from alcohol and better birth outcomes compared with an assessment-only condition.[75] Another study showed that brief advice on the risks of substance use during pregnancy was comparable to a combined MET-CBT intervention for perinatal women.[76]

SOCIOCULTURAL CONSIDERATIONS FOR WOMEN WITH SUBSTANCE USE DISORDERS

Sociocultural considerations should be included in every facet of care for women with SUD. Assessments should be conducted in the patient's preferred language and should be sensitive to ethnic and cultural differences. Treatment should align with the patient's cultural lens and be administered by providers who are trained in culturally responsive care. SAMHSA published guidelines for the treatment of women in specific racial and ethnic populations.[42] However, little research has been done to examine the effectiveness of treatments in diverse ethnocultural populations.[77]

SUMMARY

Overall, the gap between men and women in prevalence of SUDs seems to be narrowing, with women accounting for 45% of SUDs in 2020. Biological, genetic, and environmental factors contribute to the unique presentation of SUDs in women, including the telescoping effect. Compared with men, women experience more functional impairment, decreased quality of life, and higher medical and psychiatric disorders including depression, anxiety, PTSD, and eating disorders. Universal screening for alcohol, substance use, and associated comorbid symptoms is an important component of quality care for women, especially in pregnancy and postpartum. Women with SUDs are a heterogenous population who may benefit most from gender-specific and gender-responsive treatments tailored to their specific needs and settings. Interventions include pharmacologic, psychosocial, behavioral, trauma-informed, and culturally sensitive treatment approaches. Future research is needed to increase service utilization rates and treatment retention among women with SUDs.

DISCLOSURE

The authors have nothing to disclose.

REFERENCES

1. Substance Abuse and Mental Health Services Administration. (2022, November 22). Mental health and substance use disorders. Mental Health and Substance Use Disorders. Available at: https://www.samhsa.gov/find-help/disorders. Accessed November 28, 2022.
2. American Psychiatric Association. (2022). Diagnostic and statistical manual of mental disorders (5th ed., text rev.). Available at: https://doi.org/10.1176/appi.books.9780890425787. Accessed November 28, 2022.
3. Substance Abuse and Mental Health Services Administration. (n.d.). 2020 National Survey of Drug Use and Health (NSDUH) releases. SAMHSA.gov. Available at: https://www.samhsa.gov/data/release/2020-national-survey-drug-use-and-health-nsduh-releases. Accessed November 29, 2022.
4. Substance Abuse and Mental Health Services Administration. (2020). Key substance use and mental health indicators in the United States: Results from the 2019 National Survey on Drug Use and Health (HHS Publication No. PEP20-07-01-001, NSDUH Series H-55). Rockville, MD: Center for Behavioral Health Statistics and Quality, Substance Abuse and Mental Health Services Administration. Available at: https://www.samhsa.gov/data. Accessed December 15, 2022.
5. United Nations Office on Drugs and Crime. World Drug Report 2022. Available at: https://www.unodc.org/res/wdr2022/MS/WDR22_Booklet_1.pdf. Published 2022. Accessed December 28, 2022.
6. GBD 2020 Alcohol Collaborators. Population-level risks of alcohol consumption by amount, geography, age, sex, and year: a systematic analysis for the Global Burden of Disease Study 2020. Lancet 2022;400(10347):185–235 [published correction appears in Lancet. 2022 Jul 30;400(10349):358].
7. McHugh RK, Votaw VR, Sugarman DE, et al. Sex and gender differences in substance use disorders. Clin Psychol Rev 2018;66:12–23.
8. Benowitz NL, Lessov-Schlaggar CN, Swan GE, et al. Female sex and oral contraceptive use accelerate nicotine metabolism. Clin Pharmacol Ther 2006;79(5):480–8.
9. Polak K, Haug NA, Drachenberg HE, et al. Gender Considerations in Addiction: Implications for Treatment. Curr Treat Options Psychiatry 2015;2(3):326–38.
10. Prom-Wormley EC, Ebejer J, Dick DM, et al. The genetic epidemiology of substance use disorder: A review. Drug Alcohol Depend 2017;180:241–59.
11. Edwards AC, Svikis DS, Pickens RW, et al. Genetic influences on addiction. Prim Psychiatry 2009;16(8):40–6.
12. Kendler KS, Myers J, Prescott CA. Specificity of genetic and environmental risk factors for symptoms of cannabis, cocaine, alcohol, caffeine, and nicotine dependence. Arch Gen Psychiatry 2007;64(11):1313–20.
13. Datta U, Schoenrock SE, Bubier JA, et al. Prospects for finding the mechanisms of sex differences in addiction with human and model organism genetic analysis. Genes Brain Behav 2020;19(3):e12645.
14. Fonseca F, Robles-Martínez M, Tirado-Muñoz J, et al. A Gender Perspective of Addictive Disorders. Curr Addict Rep 2021;8(1):89–99.
15. Johnstone S, Dela Cruz GA, Kalb N, et al. A systematic review of gender-responsive and integrated substance use disorder treatment programs for women with co-occurring disorders. Am J Drug Alcohol Abuse 2023;49(1):21–42.

16. Kliewer W, Svikis DS, Yousaf N, et al. Psychosocial Interventions for Alcohol and/or Drug Misuse and Use Disorders in Women: A Systematic Review. J Womens Health (Larchmt) 2022;31(9):1271–304.

17. Moran-Santa Maria MM, Flanagan J, Brady K. Ovarian hormones and drug abuse. Curr Psychiatry Rep 2014;16(11):511.

18. Ross S, Peselow E. Co-occurring psychotic and addictive disorders: neurobiology and diagnosis. Clin Neuropharmacol 2012;35(5):235–43.

19. Svikis DS, Reid-Quiñones K. Screening and prevention of alcohol and drug use disorders in women. Obstet Gynecol Clin North Am 2003;30(3):447–68.

20. Moyer VA. Screening and behavioral counseling interventions in primary care to reduce alcohol misuse: U.S. Preventive Services Task Force recommendation statement. Ann Intern Med 2013;159:210–8.

21. Saunders JB, Aasland OG, Babor TF, et al. Development of the Alcohol Use Disorders Identification Test (AUDIT): WHO Collaborative Project on Early Detection of Persons with Harmful Alcohol Consumption–II. Addiction 1993;88(6):791–804.

22. Ewing JA. Detecting alcoholism: the CAGE questionnaire. JAMA 1984;252:1905–7.

23. Bush K, Kivlahan DR, McDonell MB, et al. The AUDIT alcohol consumption questions (AUDIT-C): an effective brief screening test for problem drinking. Ambulatory Care Quality Improvement Project (ACQUIP). Alcohol Use Disorders Identification Test. Arch Intern Med 1998;158(16):1789–95.

24. WHO ASSIST Working Group. The Alcohol, Smoking and Substance Involvement Screening Test (ASSIST): Development, reliability and feasibility. Addiction 2002;97(9):1183–94.

25. Skinner HA. The drug abuse screening test. Addict Behav 1982;7:363–71.

26. Bentley SM, Melville JL, Berry BD, et al. Implementing a clinical and research registry in obstetrics: overcoming the barriers. Gen Hosp Psychiatry 2007;29:192–8.

27. Johnson M, Jackson R, Guillaume L, et al. Barriers and facilitators to implementing screening and brief intervention for alcohol misuse: A systematic review of qualitative evidence. Journal of Public Health 2011;33(3):412–21.

28. McNeely J, Wu LT, Subramaniam G, et al. Performance of the tobacco, alcohol, prescription medication, and other substance use (TAPS) tool for substance use screening in primary care patients. Ann Intern Med 2016;165(10):690–9.

29. Gryczynski J, McNeely J, Wu LT, et al. Validation of the TAPS-1: A Four-Item Screening Tool to Identify Unhealthy Substance Use in Primary Care. J Gen Intern Med 2017;32(9):990–6.

30. National Institute on Drug Abuse. Screening for drug use in general medical settings: Resource guide. n.d. Available at: https://nida.nih.gov/sites/default/files/resource_guide.pdf. Accessed September 16, 2022.

31. American College of Obstetricians and Gynecologists (ACOG). Opioid use and opioid use disorder in pregnancy. 2017. Available at: https://www.acog.org/-/media/Committee-Opinions/Committee-on-Obstetric-Practice/co711.pdf?dmc=1&ts=20180720T1132299400, Accessed September 16, 2022.

32. Wright TE, Terplan M, Ondersma SJ, et al. The role of screening, brief intervention, and referral to treatment in the perinatal period. Am J Obstet Gynecol 2016;215:539–47.

33. Polak K, Kelpin S, Terplan M. Screening for substance use in pregnancy and the newborn. Semin Fetal Neonatal Med 2019;24(2):90–4.

34. Corrigan PW, Lurie BD, Goldman HH, et al. How adolescents perceive the stigma of mental illness and alcohol abuse. Psychiatr Serv 2005;56(5):544–50.

35. Terplan M, Kennedy-Hendricks A, Chisolm MS. Prenatal Substance Use: Exploring Assumptions of Maternal Unfitness. Subst Abuse 2015;9(Suppl 2):1–4.
36. van Boekel LC, Brouwers EP, van Weeghel J, et al. Stigma among health professionals towards patients with substance use disorders and its consequences for healthcare delivery: systematic review. Drug Alcohol Depend 2013;131(1–2): 23–35.
37. Haug NA, Osomo RA, Yanovitch MA, et al. Biopsychosocial approach to the management of drug and alcohol use in pregnancy. In: Edozien LC, Shaughn O'Brien PM, editors. Biopsychosocial factors in Obstetrics and Gynecology. New York: Cambridge University Press; 2017. p. 280–91.
38. Yonkers KA, Howell HB, Gotman N, et al. Self-report of illicit substance use versus urine toxicology results from at-risk pregnant women. J Subst Use 2011;16: 372–89.
39. Sokol RJ, Martier SS, Ager JW. The T-ACE questions: practical prenatal detection of risk-drinking. Am J Obstet Gynecol 1989;160:863–70.
40. Russell M. New assessment tools for risk drinking during pregnancy: T-ACE, TWEAK, and others. Alcohol Res 1994;18:55.
41. Ondersma SJ, Svikis DS, LeBreton JM, et al. Development and preliminary validation of an indirect screener for drug use in the perinatal period. Addiction 2012;107:2099–106.
42. SAMHSA. Addressing the specific needs of women for treatment of substance use disorders. 2021. Available at: https://store.samhsa.gov/sites/default/files/SAMHSA_Digital_Download/PEP20-06-04-002.pdf. Accessed September 16, 2022.
43. Butler SF, Villapiano A, Malinow A. The effect of computer-mediated administration on self-disclosure of problems on the Addiction Severity Index. J Addiction Med 2009;3:194–203.
44. Newman JC, Des Jarlais DC, Turner CF, et al. The differential effects of face-to-face and computer interview modes. Am J Public Health 2002;92(2):294–7.
45. Chan-Pensley E. Alcohol-Use Disorders Identification Test: a comparison between paper and pencil and computerized versions. Alcohol Alcohol 1999; 34(6):882–5.
46. American Psychiatric Association. Diagnostic and statistical manual of mental disorders. 5th edition. Arlington: American Psychiatric Publishing; 2013.
47. American Society of Addiction Medicine. (2022). About the ASAM Criteria. ASAM Criteria. Available at: https://www.asam.org/asam-criteria/about-the-asam-criteria. Accessed December 22, 2022.
48. Substance Abuse and Mental Health Services Administration. Center for behavioral health Statistics and quality. Treatment Episode data Set (TEDS): 2020. Admissions to and Discharges from publicly funded substance Use treatment facilities. Rockville (MD): Substance Abuse and Mental Health Services Administration; 2022.
49. Jones CM, Olsen EO, O'Donnell J, et al. Resurgent Methamphetamine Use at Treatment Admission in the United States, 2008-2017. Am J Public Health 2020;110(4):509–16.
50. Choi S, Adams SM, Morse SA, et al. Gender differences in treatment retention among individuals with co-occurring substance abuse and mental health disorders. Subst Use Misuse 2015;50(5):653–63.
51. Greenfield SF, Brooks AJ, Gordon SM, et al. Substance abuse treatment entry, retention, and outcome in women: a review of the literature. Drug Alcohol Depend 2007;86(1):1–21.

52. Grella CE. Effects of gender and diagnosis on addiction history, treatment utilization, and psychosocial functioning among a dually-diagnosed sample in drug treatment. J Psychoactive Drugs 2003;35(Suppl 1):169–79.
53. Stone R. Pregnant women and substance use: fear, stigma, and barriers to care. Health Justice 2015;3:2.
54. Verissimo AD, Grella CE. Influence of gender and race/ethnicity on perceived barriers to help-seeking for alcohol or drug problems. J Subst Abuse Treat 2017;75:54–61.
55. Powis B, Gossop M, Bury C, et al. Drug-using mothers: social, psychological and substance use problems of women opiate users with children. Drug Alcohol Rev 2000;19:171–80.
56. McCrady BS, Epstein EE, Fokas KF. Treatment Interventions for Women with Alcohol Use Disorder. Alcohol Res 2020;40(2):08.
57. Terplan M, McNamara EJ, Chisolm MS. Pregnant and non-pregnant women with substance use disorders: the gap between treatment need and receipt. J Addict Dis 2012;31(4):342–9.
58. Falker CG, Stefanovics EA, Rhee TG, et al. Women's Use of Substance Use Disorder Treatment Services: Rates, Correlates, and Comparisons to Men. Psychiatr Q 2022;93(3):737–52.
59. Killeen TK, Greenfield SF, Bride BE, et al. Assessment and treatment of co-occurring eating disorders in privately funded addiction treatment programs. Am J Addict 2011;20(3):205–11.
60. Burch AE, Rash CJ, Petry NM. Sex effects in cocaine-using methadone patients randomized to contingency management interventions. Exp Clin Psychopharmacol 2015;23(4):284–90.
61. Campbell AN, Nunes EV, Pavlicova M, et al. Gender-based Outcomes and Acceptability of a Computer-assisted Psychosocial Intervention for Substance Use Disorders. J Subst Abuse Treat 2015;53:9–15.
62. DeVito EE, Babuscio TA, Nich C, et al. Gender differences in clinical outcomes for cocaine dependence: randomized clinical trials of behavioral therapy and disulfiram. Drug Alcohol Depend 2014;145:156–67.
63. Rash CJ, Petry NM. Contingency management treatments are equally efficacious for both sexes in intensive outpatient settings. Exp Clin Psychopharmacol 2015; 23(5):369–76.
64. Greenfield SF, Sugarman DE, Freid CM, et al. Group therapy for women with substance use disorders: results from the Women's Recovery Group Study. Drug Alcohol Depend 2014;142:245–53.
65. Chamberlain C, O'Mara-Eves A, Porter J, et al. Psychosocial interventions for supporting women to stop smoking in pregnancy. Cochrane Database Syst Rev 2017;2(2):CD001055.
66. Blanc J, Tosello B, Ekblad MO, et al. Nicotine Replacement Therapy during Pregnancy and Child Health Outcomes: A Systematic Review. Int J Environ Res Public Health 2021;18(8):4004.
67. Cooper S, Lewis S, Thornton JG, et al. The SNAP trial: a randomised placebo-controlled trial of nicotine replacement therapy in pregnancy–clinical effectiveness and safety until 2 years after delivery, with economic evaluation. Health Technol Assess 2014;18(54):1–128.
68. Jones HE, O'Grady KE, Johnson RE, et al. Infant neurobehavior following prenatal exposure to methadone or buprenorphine: results from the neonatal intensive care unit network neurobehavioral scale. Subst Use Misuse 2010;45(13): 2244–57.

69. Svikis DS, Lee JH, Haug NA, et al. Attendance incentives for outpatient treatment: effects in methadone- and nonmethadone-maintained pregnant drug dependent women. Drug Alcohol Depend 1997;48(1):33–41.
70. Jones HE, Haug NA, Stitzer ML, et al. Improving treatment outcomes for pregnant drug-dependent women using low-magnitude voucher incentives. Addict Behav 2000;25(2):263–7.
71. Svikis DS, Silverman K, Haug NA, et al. Behavioral strategies to improve treatment participation and retention by pregnant drug-dependent women. Subst Use Misuse 2007;42(10):1527–35.
72. Winhusen T, Kropp F, Babcock D, et al. Motivational enhancement therapy to improve treatment utilization and outcome in pregnant substance users. J Subst Abuse Treat 2008;35(2):161–73.
73. Greenfield SF, Rosa C, Putnins SI, et al. Gender research in the National Institute on Drug Abuse National Treatment Clinical Trials Network: a summary of findings. Am J Drug Alcohol Abuse 2011;37(5):301–12.
74. Chang G, McNamara TK, Orav EJ, et al. Brief intervention for prenatal alcohol use: a randomized trial. Obstet Gynecol 2005;105(5 Pt 1):991–8.
75. O'Connor MJ, Whaley SE. Brief intervention for alcohol use by pregnant women. Am J Public Health 2007;97(2):252–8.
76. Yonkers KA, Forray A, Howell HB, et al. Motivational enhancement therapy coupled with cognitive behavioral therapy versus brief advice: a randomized trial for treatment of hazardous substance use in pregnancy and after delivery. Gen Hosp Psychiatry 2012;34(5):439–49.
77. Venner KL, Hernandez-Vallant A, Hirchak KA, et al. A scoping review of cultural adaptations of substance use disorder treatments across Latinx communities: Guidance for future research and practice. J Subst Abuse Treat 2022;137:108716.

Body Dysmorphic Disorder in Women

Katharine A. Phillips, MD[a],*, Leah C. Susser, MD[b]

KEYWORDS

- Body dysmorphic disorder • Women • Gender • Clinical features • Diagnosis
- Treatment • Reproduction • Perinatal

KEY POINTS

- Body dysmorphic disorder (BDD) is a common but underrecognized disorder that occurs more often in women than in men.
- BDD is associated with marked impairment in functioning, poor quality of life, and high rates of suicidality.
- Most women obtain cosmetic treatment for BDD concerns, but such treatment virtually never improves BDD symptoms and can make them worse.
- Serotonin-reuptake inhibitors, often at high doses, and cognitive-behavioral therapy that is tailored to BDD's unique symptoms are the first-line treatments for BDD and are often effective.
- Susceptible women may be at high risk of BDD during reproductive transitions, such as the perinatal period and menarche.

INTRODUCTION

Body dysmorphic disorder (BDD) is a common yet underrecognized disorder that is more common in women than in men. BDD usually causes marked impairment in functioning and poor quality of life, and it is associated with high rates of suicidality. BDD was first described in the 1800s but has been systematically studied for only the past few decades. During this time, knowledge about BDD has dramatically increased, and effective treatments have been developed and studied.

In this article, the authors provide a clinically focused overview of BDD, noting aspects of BDD that are particularly relevant to women, although research data on women specifically are limited. Studies on reproductive aspects of BDD, in particular,

[a] New York-Presbyterian/Weill Cornell Medical Center and Weill Cornell Medical College, Weill Cornell Psychiatry Specialty Center, 315 East 62nd Street, New York, NY 10065, USA; [b] New York-Presbyterian/Weill Cornell Medical Center and Weill Cornell Medical College, Outpatient Department, 21 Bloomingdale Road, White Plains, NY 10605, USA
* Corresponding author. Weill Cornell Psychiatry Specialty Center, 315 East 62nd Street, New York, NY 10065.
E-mail address: kap9161@med.cornell.edu

Psychiatr Clin N Am 46 (2023) 505–525
https://doi.org/10.1016/j.psc.2023.04.007
0193-953X/23/© 2023 Elsevier Inc. All rights reserved.

psych.theclinics.com

are scarce, but the authors include a discussion of reproductive issues that may be relevant to women with BDD.

In recent years, a plethora of poorly defined constructs that overlap with BDD has emerged in both the lay press and the scientific literature—for example, "body dysmorphia," "skin dysmorphia," "acne dysmorphia," "snapchat dysmorphia," and "zoom dysmorphia." It is often unclear whether these terms are synonymous with the disorder BDD, as defined in *Diagnostic and Statistical Manual of Mental Disorders* (Fifth Edition) (*DSM-5*), or instead reflect more common, nonpathologic body image dissatisfaction. In this article, the authors focus on the disorder BDD.

CLINICAL FEATURES OF BODY DYSMORPHIC DISORDER
Definition of Body Dysmorphic Disorder

BDD is defined in *DSM-5* as a preoccupation with perceived defects in one's physical appearance that to other people appear nonexistent or only slight. The appearance preoccupations trigger excessive repetitive behaviors (such as mirror checking, excessive grooming, skin picking) or repetitive mental acts (such as comparing one's appearance with that of other people). To qualify for a diagnosis of BDD, the preoccupation must cause clinically significant distress or clinically significant impairment in functioning. This criterion differentiates the disorder BDD from more normative, nonpathologic body image dissatisfaction and concerns. In an individual with an eating disorder diagnosis, preoccupation with perceived excessive body fat or weight counts toward the eating disorder diagnosis rather than a diagnosis of BDD.[1]

DSM-5 classifies BDD in the chapter of obsessive-compulsive and related disorders, reflecting BDD's similarities to obsessive-compulsive disorder (OCD).[1] However, BDD and OCD have important differences. For example, BDD is associated with higher rates of suicidality, poorer insight, more frequent comorbidity with major depressive disorder and substance use disorder, and differences in cognitive-behavioral treatment approaches.[2]

Appearance Preoccupations

Appearance preoccupations can focus on any body area but most often involve perceived defects of the face or head. Concern with multiple body areas is common. Skin, hair, and nose concerns are most common—for example, perceived facial acne or scarring, "uneven" hair length, or a "misshapen" nose.[3,4] Girls and women are more likely than boys and men to be preoccupied with "excessive" body/facial hair; with their breasts/chest, hips, or legs; and with being overweight.[5] Girls and women are also preoccupied with more body areas than boys and men.[5]

Patients often describe disliked areas as looking "ugly"; other common terms are "deformed," "defective," abnormal," "unattractive," or "hideous." Appearance preoccupations occur for an average of 3 to 8 hours a day. They are intrusive, unwanted, distressing, and usually difficult to resist and control.[4]

Body Dysmorphic Disorder-Related Insight

BDD-related insight is usually absent or poor. In other words, most patients (before treatment) are completely or mostly certain that their view of their perceived defects is accurate—that they really do, or probably do, look abnormal or ugly.[6] This distorted view likely reflects visual processing abnormalities (see later discussion). Thus, it is not effective to try to talk people with BDD out of their belief about how they look. It may be more difficult to engage people with poor or absent insight in psychiatric treatment.

Individuals with absent insight should be diagnosed with "BDD with absent insight/delusional beliefs specifier" rather than a psychotic disorder.[1]

Repetitive Behaviors

Appearance preoccupations trigger excessive repetitive behaviors (ie, rituals, compulsions). These behaviors typically aim to check, fix, or obtain reassurance about the perceived appearance flaws. Although these behaviors intend to alleviate emotional distress, they often increase distress. If they relieve distress, the relief is usually short-lived. Patients feel strong urges to perform these behaviors; they are usually difficult to resist or control. They occur for an average of 3 to 8 hours a day.[3,4]

Table 1 lists common repetitive behaviors.[3,4] Girls and women are more likely than boys and men to check mirrors, frequently change their clothes to find a more flattering or concealing outfit, and pick their skin.[5] Patients may also engage in repetitive behaviors not listed in **Table 1**, such as compulsively taking selfies, shopping for skin products, or searching online for information about cosmetic surgery. Repetitive behaviors may be a clue that a person has BDD. Some behaviors, however, such as comparing with others, are mental rituals that others cannot observe.

Table 1 Common repetitive behaviors (rituals, compulsions) and camouflaging behaviors in body dysmorphic disorder[a]	
Behavior	**Percentage of Individuals with Behavior[b]**
Repetitive behaviors	
Comparing one's appearance with that of other people	88
Checking perceived flaws in mirrors and other reflecting surfaces	87
Excessive grooming (applying makeup, hair combing, hair removal, face washing, and so forth)	59
Reassurance seeking about appearance	54
Touching perceived flaws to check them	52
Excessive clothes changing (to find a more flattering or more concealing outfit)	46
Dieting	39
Skin picking (to try to improve skin's appearance)	38
Tanning (to try to improve appearance, for example, "pale" skin)	22
Excessive exercise	21
Excessive weightlifting	18
Camouflaging	91
With body position or posture	65
With clothing	63
With makeup	55
With hand	49
With hair	49
With hat	29

[a] This is a partial listing of common repetitive behaviors; others include such behaviors as taking excessive selfies, videotaping perceived flaws, altering one's appearance with apps, comparing photographs of oneself to one another, and seeking information about cosmetic procedures.
[b] Lifetime (past or current) behaviors; sample size = 507.

Camouflaging

More than 90% of patients attempt to camouflage their perceived defects.[3,4] Women are more likely than men to camouflage, and to camouflage with makeup or by covering disliked areas with their hand.[5] Camouflaging aims to hide perceived defects from others, or at least minimize them, to avoid ridicule and rejection. **Table 1** lists common camouflaging behaviors.[3,4] Camouflaging is sometimes done repeatedly (for example, repeatedly reapplying makeup to cover "skin marks") and thus may constitute a repetitive behavior.[4]

Distressing Emotions

Appearance preoccupations trigger an array of distressing emotions, such as embarrassment, self-consciousness, shame, social anxiety, depressed mood, anxiety, or hostility. BDD is associated with high levels of these emotions as well as high rejection sensitivity, neuroticism, and perceived stress. It is associated with low extraversion, assertiveness, and self-esteem.[4]

Referential Thinking

Many people with BDD have BDD-related referential thinking-inaccurately believing that other people take special notice of them in a negative way because of how they look (for example, mock them or stare at them).[3] Referential thinking can worsen social avoidance and trigger hostility and anger toward others.

IMPAIRMENT IN PSYCHOSOCIAL FUNCTIONING AND QUALITY OF LIFE

BDD is associated with markedly impaired psychosocial functioning (**Table 2**).[7] Although degree of functional impairment varies—with more severe BDD associated with greater impairment—inability to work, school dropout, and social avoidance are common. Patients may be housebound to avoid being seen by others.[7] Girls and women may be somewhat less functionally impaired than boys and men.[5]

In an inpatient study, patients with BDD had significantly lower scores on the Global Assessment of Functioning (GAF) scale than patients without BDD.[8] In a prospective observational study, psychosocial functioning remained consistently poor over 1 to 3 years of follow-up; the cumulative probability of attaining functional remission on the Social and Occupational Functioning Scale (score >70 for at least 2 consecutive months) was only 10.6%.[9]

Table 2	
Functional impairment in individuals with body dysmorphic disorder	
Functioning Domain	**Percentage**
Work impairment due to BDD (current)	90
Did not work for ≥1 wk in past month due to psychopathology (BDD was primary diagnosis for most)	39
Receiving disability payments (current)	23
Dropped out of school temporarily or permanently due to BDD	25
Housebound due to BDD (≥1 wk)	29
Psychiatrically hospitalized	60
Psychiatrically hospitalized primarily for BDD	24

All variables reflect lifetime (past or current) functioning except where noted.
Sample sizes: n = 141, 200, and 507.

BDD is also associated with markedly poor quality of life.[8] **Fig. 1** shows quality of life and psychosocial functioning scores on standardized measures in a broadly ascertained BDD sample. Scores on all measures reflect poor functioning/quality of life compared with community norms, with very large effect sizes (higher scores on the Social Adjustment Scale-SR reflect poorer social functioning).

SUICIDALITY

BDD is associated with high rates of suicidality (**Table 3**).[10] Furthermore, suicidality appears more common in BDD than in a range of other often-severe psychiatric disorders. For example, in one study, inpatients with BDD had twice as many suicide attempts as inpatients without BDD.[8] Among US veterans, the lifetime suicide attempt rate in those with BDD (58%) was significantly higher than in veterans without BDD (19%).[11]

In a 2016 systematic review and meta-analysis of 17 studies that compared BDD with other groups (for example, healthy controls, OCD, eating disorders, any anxiety disorder), individuals with BDD were nearly four times more likely to have had suicidal ideation (pooled odds ratio [OR] = 3.87) and 2.6 times more likely to have attempted suicide (pooled OR = 2.57).[12] A subsequent study in a partial hospital setting (n = 498) found that in multivariate analyses (after adjusting for age, gender, and other psychiatric disorders), BDD had a significant association with suicidal ideation (OR = 6.62) and suicidal behaviors (OR = 2.45).[13] These odds ratios were higher than for any other psychiatric disorders examined, including major depressive disorder, bipolar depression, OCD, and posttraumatic stress disorder (PTSD; **Table 4**).[13]

Greater BDD severity predicts suicidal ideation and suicide attempts, independent of comorbidity, but certain comorbidities may further strengthen the relationship with suicidality, such as comorbid major depressive disorder, PTSD, and a substance use disorder.[13] Conversely, in other psychiatric disorders, the presence of comorbid BDD may increase risk of suicidality.[14]

Completed suicide in BDD has been only minimally studied, but the rate appears markedly elevated.[10]

PREVALENCE

BDD occurs around the world. In nationwide epidemiologic studies conducted in the United States and Europe, BDD has a current (point) prevalence of 1.7% to 2.9%, with a higher prevalence in girls and women (~60%) than in boys and men (~40%). In these studies, individuals with BDD had less education, lower income, and more unemployment and sick days than those without BDD.[15]

BDD is more common than this in clinical settings among both youth and adults. For example, 13% to 16% of US psychiatric inpatients have BDD.[8,15] In a systematic review, BDD's estimated weighted prevalence was 11.3% in dermatology outpatient settings, 13.2% in general cosmetic surgery settings, 11.2% in orthognathic surgery settings, 5.2% in orthodontics/cosmetic dentistry settings, and 20.1% in rhinoplasty settings.[16]

Might BDD's prevalence be increasing? The answer is unknown, but BDD's prevalence was higher in the most recent nationwide epidemiologic study of BDD than in previous studies.[15] Also, it is plausible that increases in use of image-focused social media might contribute to an increased risk of developing BDD in individuals with other risk factors for the disorder.

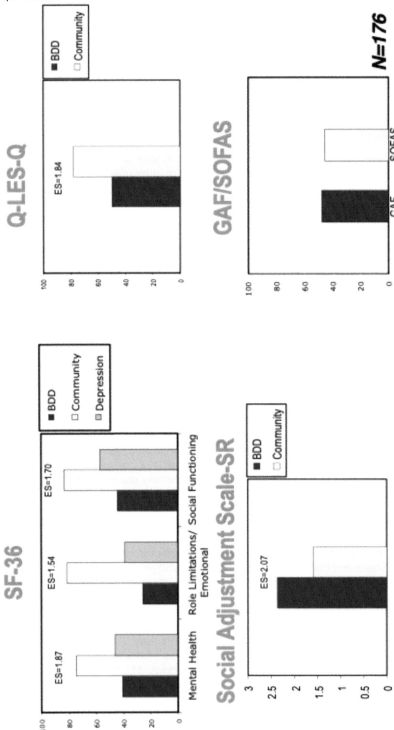

Fig. 1. Functioning and quality of life in individuals with BDD. On the SF-36 and Q-LESQ-Q, lower scores reflect poorer functioning/quality of life; on the Social Adjustment Scale-SR, higher scores reflect poorer social functioning; on the GAF and SOFAS, mean BDD scores

AGE AT ONSET AND COURSE OF ILLNESS

BDD can onset as early as age 4 years and as late as the 40s. The most common age at onset is 12 to 13 years, and two-thirds experience onset before age 18. Those with BDD onset before age 18 have more comorbidity, and they are more likely to have been psychiatrically hospitalized and to have attempted suicide.[17] BDD is usually a chronic illness unless evidence-based treatment is received. Gender does not predict course of illness.[18]

COMORBIDITY

Major depressive disorder is the most common comorbid disorder, occurring in about three-quarters of individuals with BDD (lifetime rate). Lifetime rates of substance use disorders (30%–50%), social anxiety disorder (nearly 40%), and OCD (about one-third) are also high.[3,19] Nearly 70% of individuals with BDD with a substance use disorder attribute their substance use at least in part to the distress caused by BDD.[20] Women are less likely than men to have a substance use disorder but more likely to have an eating disorder.[5]

CAUSE AND PATHOPHYSIOLOGY
Genetics

Heritability of BDD is estimated to be 37% to 49% and may be higher in women.[21] BDD and OCD have shared genetic vulnerability, but there are genetic determinants that are specific to BDD.[22] BDD is more common in first-degree relatives of OCD probands than control probands.[23]

Visual Processing Abnormalities and Other Neurobiological Findings

Visual processing abnormalities in BDD consist of a bias for analyzing and encoding details of faces and nonface objects (such as houses) as well as for disrupted holistic ("big picture") visual processing.[24,25] Thus, details of the face and body override the "big picture," gestalt view of the whole. Studies have found widespread compromised white matter in the brain (reduced organization); hyperactivity in left orbitofrontal cortex and bilateral head of the caudate when viewing one's own face (vs a familiar face), which may reflect obsessional preoccupation; and abnormalities in brain connectivity.[26,27]

Cognitive and Emotional Processing

BDD is characterized by abnormalities in executive functioning, emotion recognition (for example, facial expressions), attention, and neurocognition. For example, individuals with BDD have a bias toward interpreting neutral faces as contemptuous and angry, and misinterpreting ambiguous scenarios as threatening; these findings are consistent with referential thinking in BDD.[28]

---

reflect serious symptoms and serious impairment in functioning. The sample (n = 176) is a broadly ascertained sample of convenience of individuals with current *DSM-IV* BDD. ES, effect size compared with community norms; GAS/SOFAS, global assessment of functioning scale and social and occupational functioning scale; Q-LES-Q, quality of life enjoyment and satisfaction questionnaire; SF-36, medical outcomes study 36-item short-form health survey; Social Adjustment Scale-SR, social adjustment scale–self report.

Table 3
Suicidal ideation and suicide attempts in body dysmorphic disorder[a]

Suicidality Variable	Epidemiologic Studies			Clinical Samples[b] and Samples of Convenience[b]								Youth Studies	
	Rief et al n = 2552 BDD = 42	Buhlmann et al n = 2510 BDD = 45	Shieber et al n = 2129 BDD = 62	Phillips et al[b] n = 307	Phillips et al[c] n = 200	Veale et al[c] n = 50	Perugi et al[b] n = 58	Altamura et al[b] n = 487 BDD=30	Conroy et al[b] n = 100 BDD = 16	Pope et al[c,d] n = 200M MD = 14	Kelly et al[b] n = 100BD BDD = 12	Albertini & et al[b,e] n = 33[d]	Phillips et al[c,d] n = 200 Youth=36
Suicidal ideation	—	—	31%	81%	78%	—	—	50%	100%	—	—	67%	81%
Suicidal ideation attributable primarily to BDD[f]	19%	31%	—	68%	55%	—	45% (current)	—	13%[g]	—	—	—	—
Attempted suicide	—	—	—	24%	28%	24%	—	—	94%	50%	58%	21%	44%
Attempted suicide primarily due to BDD[f]	7%	22%	—	15%	13%	—	—	—	7%[g]	—	—	—	—
Number of suicide attempts[h]	—	—	—	2.1 ± 1.4	3.2 ± 4.1	—	—	—	—	—	—	—	—
Number of suicide attempts due to BDD[f,h]	—	—	—	1.2 ± 1.4	1.2 ± 3.0	—	—	—	—	—	—	—	—

—, the variable was not assessed.

[a] All percentages reflect lifetime (ie, past or current) rates, except for the Perugi et al study, which reported a current rate; Rief et al and Buhlmann et al did not specify a period of time during which suicidality occurred.

[b] Clinical samples: All clinical samples consisted of outpatients except for the Conroy et al study, which consisted of inpatients. Participants in the Altamura study were seeking cosmetic treatment, whereas the other studies ascertained individuals for BDD. The Phillips et al sample is an expansion of previously reported samples (eg, Refs.[17,51]).

[c] Broad samples of convenience that ascertained individuals with BDD.

[d] The muscle dysmorphia study (Pope et al) and the Phillips et al youth study used the same sample of convenience as Phillips et al (n = 200).

[e] The Albertini and Phillips youth study was a subset of the Phillips et al clinical sample (n = 307).

[f] BDD was the primary reason, in the subject's and interviewer's view.

[g] BDD was the major reason or "somewhat of a reason" (as opposed to a "minor reason" or "not a reason") for 50% of suicide attempts and 33% of suicide attempts.

[h] Among suicide attempters.

From Phillips KA. Suicidality and aggressive behavior in body dysmorphic disorder. In: Body Dysmorphic Disorder: Advances in Research and Clinical Practice.

Table 4
Psychiatric disorders predicting suicidality in partial hospital program

	n (%)	Bivariate[a] OR (95% CI)	P	Multivariate OR (95% CI)	P
Suicidal ideation[b]					
Major depressive episode	224 (73.4)	3.02 (2.05–4.44)	<.000	3.00 (1.95–4.63)	<.000
Unipolar depression	160 (71.1)	1.84 (1.25–2.70)	.002	1.82 (1.20–2.74)	.005
Bipolar depression	57 (80.3)	2.64 (1.42–4.90)	.002	2.71 (1.36–5.40)	.005
Panic disorder	65 (69.9)	1.32 (0.81–2.17)	.275	1.99 (0.92–4.31)	.081
Agoraphobia	41 (62.1)	0.84 (0.49–1.46)	.537	0.43 (0.18–1.00)	.050
Social anxiety disorder	116 (71.2)	1.60 (1.06–2.41)	.027	1.18 (0.74–1.88)	.484
Obsessive-compulsive disorder	60 (65.9)	1.14 (0.70–1.86)	.603	0.78 (0.43–1.39)	.391
Posttraumatic stress disorder	39 (66.1)	1.08 (0.60–1.94)	.791	0.74 (0.38–1.42)	.367
Generalized anxiety disorder	135 (64.3)	1.07 (0.73–1.58)	.717	0.92 (0.60–1.42)	.709
Body dysmorphic disorder	33 (91.7)	6.51 (1.95–21.67)	.002	6.62 (1.92–22.79)	.003
Suicidal behavior[c]					
Major depressive episode	59 (20.1)	2.60 (1.45–4.65)	.001	2.11 (1.12–3.98)	.021
Unipolar depression	35 (16.1)	1.08 (0.65–1.79)	.766	1.28 (0.73–2.22)	.392
Bipolar depression	21 (30.0)	2.94 (1.62–5.31)	<.000	2.02 (0.09–4.13)	.054
Panic disorder	20 (21.7)	1.66 (0.92–2.98)	.091	1.56 (0.67–3.61)	.302
Agoraphobia	11 (15.3)	1.09 (0.53–2.23)	.814	0.58 (0.21–1.65)	.308
Social anxiety disorder	28 (17.6)	1.23 (0.73–2.09)	.438	0.85 (0.46–1.58)	.608
Obsessive-compulsive disorder	17 (19.3)	1.38 (0.75–2.55)	.298	0.92 (0.44–1.94)	.824
Posttraumatic stress disorder	11 (19.0)	1.36 (0.66–2.82)	.405	0.90 (0.39–2.09)	.804
Generalized anxiety disorder	29 (14.1)	0.98 (0.57–1.68)	.938	0.92 (0.52–1.64)	.781
Body dysmorphic disorder	10 (27.8)	2.34 (1.05–5.18)	.037	2.45 (1.05–5.71)	.038

Abbreviation: CI, confidence interval.
[a] Adjusted for age and gender.
[b] Suicidal ideation = a score of at least 1 on the suicide ideation scale.
[c] Actual, aborted, or interrupted suicide attempt or preparatory behavior imminently preceding an attempt.
From Snorrason I, Beard C, Christensena K, et al. Body dysmorphic disorder and major depressive episode have comorbidity independent associations with suicidality in an acute psychiatric setting. J Affect Disord 2019;259:266-70.

Environmental Factors

A history of bullying or teasing is a possible risk factor for developing BDD. Studies also suggest high rates of childhood neglect and/or abuse (higher than in OCD) and other types of trauma. Sociocultural influences that emphasize the importance of appearance likely play a role in BDD's development.[29] Greater use of image-focused social media appears associated with body image dissatisfaction more generally[30]; one study also found this to be the case for BDD,[31] although causality has not been determined.

HOW TO ASSESS AND DIAGNOSE BODY DYSMORPHIC DISORDER

BDD is common but underdiagnosed in mental health settings.[15] Patients typically do not spontaneously reveal their appearance concerns because of embarrassment, shame, fear that the clinician will negatively judge them (eg, consider them vain) or not understand their concerns, or their belief that cosmetic treatment rather than mental health treatment will help.[15] To detect BDD, clinicians usually need ask about BDD symptoms using questions such as those in **Box 1**.

BDD can also be missed because it is confused with another disorder. BDD must be differentiated from OCD, major depressive disorder, social anxiety disorder, avoidant personality disorder, generalized anxiety disorder, agoraphobia, a psychotic disorder, gender dysphoria, and olfactory reference disorder. It is also important that BDD not be misdiagnosed as excoriation (skin-picking) disorder or trichotillomania (hair-pulling disorder) in patients who pick their skin or remove their hair to try to improve their appearance.

Box 1
Diagnostic questions for body dysmorphic disorder[a]

Preoccupation with perceived appearance defects or flaws:
- "Are you very worried about your appearance in any way?" *OR:* "Are you unhappy with how you look?"
- "Can you tell me about your concern?" *OR* "What don't you like about how you look?"
- "How much time would you estimate that you spend each day thinking about your appearance, if you add up all the time you spend?" (*About 1 hour a day or more is compatible with a BDD diagnosis.*)

Repetitive behaviors:
- "Is there anything you do over and over again in response to your appearance concerns?" (*Give examples of repetitive behaviors.*)

Clinically significant distress or impairment in functioning:
- "How much distress do your appearance concerns cause you?" (*Ask about emotions such as depressed mood, anxiety, social anxiety, embarrassment, suicidal thinking.*)
- "Do your appearance concerns interfere with your life or cause problems for you in any way?" (*Ask about interference in areas such as school, work, role functioning [for example, managing a household], social activities, relationships, intimacy.*)

Appearance concerns are not better explained by an eating disorder:
- *If body image concerns focus on being overweight or having excessive fat in nonfacial body areas, ask diagnostic questions for anorexia nervosa, bulimia nervosa, and binge eating disorder. In patients with an eating disorder diagnosis, preoccupation with these areas does not count toward a diagnosis of BDD.*

[a]Questions to assess BDD diagnostic specifiers (the muscle dysmorphia form of BDD and level of insight) are not included here.

TREATMENT
Pharmacotherapy

Box 2 lists key points about treating BDD with medication.

First-line medication
Serotonin-reuptake inhibitors (SRIs; selective serotonin reuptake inhibitors [SSRIs]) at adequately high doses are the first-line medication for BDD.[32,33] They appear more efficacious than non-SRI antidepressants or other medications.[32,33] Gender does not predict SRI response.[34]

SRIs significantly improve BDD symptoms in a majority of patients, and they are as efficacious for patients with delusional BDD beliefs as for those with nondelusional beliefs.[32,33] Symptoms such as depression, anxiety, and anger-hostility, as well as functioning and quality of life, usually also improve.[32] SRIs decrease suicidal ideation, and they protect against suicidality worsening compared with placebo in adults with BDD.[32,33]

Serotonin-reuptake inhibitors dosing
High SRI doses are usually needed;[32,33] Many patients require doses over the Food and Drug Administration (FDA) maximum doses.[32,33] However, the FDA maximum dose should not be exceeded for citalopram (because of the potential for QTc interval prolongation) or clomipramine (a tricyclic antidepressant with a low therapeutic index).[32,33]

Table 5 shows FDA maximum doses of SRIs and maximum doses sometimes used for BDD. The maximum doses for BDD are supported by an international consensus paper on pharmacotherapy of BDD,[33] the American Psychiatric Association's practice

---

Box 2
Key points about treating body dysmorphic disorder with medication

- Serotonin reuptake inhibitors (SRIs, SSRIs) are the first-line medication for BDD and are often effective.

- All SRIs are probably equally effective for BDD, but an SSRI is usually used before the SRI clomipramine for tolerability reasons. In the first author's experience, fluoxetine, sertraline, or escitalopram may be better tolerated than other SSRIs.

- High SRI doses are usually needed.

- Many patients require SSRI doses that exceed the FDA maximum dose, but maximum FDA doses should not be exceeded for citalopram or clomipramine.

- An adequate SRI trial should be at least 12 to 16 weeks to determine treatment response, with about 4 of these weeks on the maximum FDA dose (but 30 mg/d for escitalopram), unless a lower dose is improving symptoms.

- Certain medications may be helpful when added to an SRI, such as an atypical neuroleptic (perhaps aripiprazole in particular), buspirone, or possibly N-acetylcysteine.

- The SRI clomipramine can be added to an SSRI (or vice versa), but clomipramine plus desmethylclomipramine levels must be checked during dose titration, as SSRIs can increase levels of clomipramine, which has a low therapeutic index.

- If an adequate SRI trial is not helpful enough, another SRI should be tried.

- If several SSRI trials have not improved symptoms sufficiently, the SRI clomipramine is a good option (assuming the patient is willing to have blood levels drawn and electrocardiograms checked).

- Cognitive behavioral therapy for BDD can be added to medication at any time.

Table 5
Serotonin-reuptake inhibitor doses

Medication	Maximum FDA Daily Dose (mg)	Maximum Daily Dose Sometimes Used for BDD (mg)[a]
Fluoxetine[a]	80	120
Escitalopram	20	60
Sertraline	200	400
Fluvoxamine	300	450
Clomipramine	250	250
Paroxetine	60	100
Citalopram (no longer recommended)[b]	40	40 (20 mg/d if over age 60)

[a] Lower maximum doses should be considered for the elderly and younger youth, especially pre-teens. It is generally recommended that the FDA maximum dose not be exceeded when treating younger youth.
[b] Because the revised FDA maximum dose is usually too low to effectively treat BDD.

guideline on OCD,[35] and a paper by OCD experts on pharmacotherapy of OCD.[36] OCD dosing guidelines are mentioned here because medication treatment for BDD appears very similar to that for OCD.[2]

Lower initial and maximum doses should be considered for youth and the elderly, and doses exceeding FDA maximums are not recommended for preteens. Clomipramine dosing is determined by serum levels of clomipramine plus desmethylclomipramine. An electrocardiogram should be obtained when prescribing clomipramine and at escitalopram doses of 40 mg/d[33] (or 30 mg/d)[33] and higher and can be considered when prescribing high doses of other SSRIs.

Serotonin-reuptake inhibitor trial duration
An SRI trial of 12 to 16 weeks is needed to determine whether an SRI is effective.[32] The FDA maximum dose (but 30 mg/d for escitalopram) should be reached and used for at least 4 of the 12 to 16 weeks unless symptoms have improved on a lower dose. The mean time for SRI response is 4 to 9 weeks.[32,33]

Next steps
If the above approach yields less than full remission and remaining symptoms are mild, an SRI could be continued at the same dose for a period of time, as more than one-third of patients experience further improvement with 6 more months of treatment.[37] For more problematic remaining symptoms, the first author's preferred approach is to gradually increase the SRI dose above the FDA limit, if tolerated (excluding clomipramine and citalopram).[32]

Alternatively, the SRI can be augmented with an atypical neuroleptic, such as aripiprazole, buspirone (mean dose of 50–60 mg/d), or N-acetylcysteine (up to 1800 mg twice a day), although data are very limited.[32,33] Augmenting an SSRI with clomipramine (or vice versa) is discussed in **Box 2**. If one SRI is not effective, another should be tried.[32,33]

Cognitive-Behavioral Therapy

First-line therapy
Cognitive-behavioral therapy (CBT) that is tailored to BDD's unique clinical features is the best-studied psychotherapy for BDD. It is more efficacious than a waiting list control or several other types of therapy.[38,39] CBT is effective for most patients.[38] Gender does not predict CBT response.[40]

It can be helpful for therapists to use a BDD-specific CBT treatment manual, which provides detailed guidance. Two CBT treatment manuals with published evidence of their efficacy are available.[41,42]

Components of cognitive-behavioral therapy for body dysmorphic disorder

The treatment developed by the first author and her colleagues has the following components.[39,42] **Box 3** describes of each treatment component. Completion of daily structured homework assignments is essential.

- Foundation for treatment
- Cognitive restructuring
- Exposure
- Ritual (response) prevention
- Perceptual (mirror) retraining
- Advanced cognitive strategies
- Relapse prevention
- Optional treatment modules are used with patients who have symptoms addressed by the module:
  ○ Habit reversal training (for skin picking and hair plucking/pulling)

Box 3
Components of cognitive-behavioral therapy for body dysmorphic disorder

- *Treatment Foundation*: The first three or four sessions focus on developing an understanding of the patient's symptoms, providing psychoeducation, building an individualized cognitive-behavioral model of the patient's symptoms, and setting meaningful treatment goals. *Motivational interviewing* is often needed early and later in treatment to enhance motivation for treatment.

- *Cognitive restructuring* teaches patients to identify and evaluate negative appearance-related thoughts and beliefs, identify cognitive errors, and develop more accurate and helpful appearance-related beliefs.

- *Exposure* teaches patients how to gradually face avoided situations (which are usually social situations). Behavioral experiments are done during exposures.

- *Ritual (response) prevention* teaches patients to stop excessive repetitive behaviors, such as mirror checking.

- *Perceptual (mirror) retraining* teaches patients to develop a more holistic, rather than a detail-oriented, view of their appearance as well as a less-judgmental view. It includes mindfulness techniques.

- *Advanced cognitive strategies* help patients identify and address negative core beliefs (for example, "I am unlovable" or "I will always be alone"). Self-esteem and self-compassion are fostered.

- *Relapse prevention*: At the end of treatment, patients prepare to terminate formal treatment and to continue to implement learned CBT strategies.

- *Optional treatment modules* are used with patients who have relevant symptoms:
  ○ Habit reversal training is used for BDD-related skin picking or hair picking/plucking.
  ○ Depression treatment focuses on activity scheduling/behavioral activation (which may be needed early in treatment) and cognitive restructuring.
  ○ Cosmetic treatment: CBT approaches are used for patients who are seeking or receiving cosmetic treatment for BDD.
  ○ Body shape/weight concerns are addressed with CBT strategies.

Medication may be added at any time during the course of CBT.

- ○ Depression treatment
- ○ Cosmetic treatment
- ○ Body shape/weight concerns

Medication can be added to CBT at any time. It may make CBT more doable in severely ill or severely depressed patients.

Approaches that are not recommended
The following approaches are unlikely to be helpful and can even worsen BDD symptoms, depression, or suicidal ideation.

- Staring in mirrors (which reinforces the ritual of mirror checking and may potentially worsen perceptual distortions)
- Telling the patient that they are ugly (this reinforces inaccurate beliefs about appearance and is usually too distressing for patients to tolerate)
- Creating obvious "flaws," such as painting bright red spots on one's face before going out in public (this approach can cause patients to be stared at or teased, may increase referential thinking, and does not help them learn that they actually look normal)
- Flooding or excessively difficult exposures, especially early in treatment (this can be too difficult for patients to tolerate)

Session number and frequency
The duration of CBT needs to be tailored to each patient. About 6 months of weekly hour-long treatment is generally recommended,[42] although session number and frequency in published reports vary widely.[38] After formal treatment ends, patients should continue to practice CBT skills on their own.[38,42] Booster sessions with the therapist can be held as needed.[38,42]

Treatment of More Highly Suicidal and Severely Ill Patients

Although this section is not a comprehensive guide to managing highly suicidal patients with BDD, the following are some recommended approaches.[43] More highly suicidal patients need a safety plan and close monitoring for suicidality; a higher level of care should be considered. Severe comorbid conditions—especially if contributing to suicidality—as well as anxiety and insomnia should be treated in addition to BDD. It can be helpful to involve supportive family members in treatment.

For more highly suicidal and/or severely ill patients, combined treatment with medication and CBT is recommended. All such patients require treatment with an SRI, and initiation of an atypical neuroleptic (such as aripiprazole) should be considered before an adequate SRI trial is completed. More severely ill patients usually need more intensive CBT (for example, several hours a day for 5 days a week). CBT for suicidality should be considered for more highly suicidal patients.[44]

Some patients benefit from receiving dialectical behavior therapy, supportive psychotherapy, family therapy, or another type of non-CBT therapy in addition to medication plus CBT for BDD (usually provided by a different therapist than the CBT therapist). These approaches may also be helpful as adjunctive treatment for less severely ill patients. Very limited data suggest that electroconvulsive therapy does not appear effective for BDD, but it can be considered for patients with very severe depression and/or worrisome suicidality.[32,43]

Cosmetic Treatment

Many women with BDD seek and receive cosmetic treatment for BDD appearance concerns.[45] Nearly 50% of patients with BDD receive dermatologic treatment (for example, antibiotics, isotretinoin [Accutane]), and about 20% receive surgery (most commonly rhinoplasty).[45] Cosmetic dental treatment and other types of cosmetic treatment may also be received.[45] One study found that women and men were equally likely to receive cosmetic treatment for BDD concerns, but women received a greater number of treatments, which was accounted for by receiving more dermatologic treatment.[45] It is possible that, given the uptick in cosmetic procedures more generally and the widespread availability of online images of body parts (such as breasts and vulva), surgeries will become even more common among women with BDD.

Most patients with BDD are dissatisfied with the outcome of cosmetic treatment. Cosmetic treatment rarely improves overall BDD, and symptoms may worsen.[45] A 2017 Committee Opinion from the American College of Obstetricians and Gynecologists (ACOG) states "Individuals younger than 18 who request breast or labia surgery should be screened for body dysmorphic disorder. If the obstetrician–gynecologist suspects an adolescent has body dysmorphic disorder, referral to a mental health professional is appropriate."[46] Also, a 2020 ACOG Committee Opinion states "Individuals (women) should be assessed, if indicated, for body dysmorphic disorder. In women who have suspected psychological concerns, a referral for evaluation should occur before considering surgery."[47] A recent rhinoplasty practice guideline from the American Academy of Otolaryngology states that BDD symptoms and complaints may worsen following surgery and that BDD is a contraindication to elective rhinoplasty.[48]

REPRODUCTIVE ASPECTS OF BODY DYSMORPHIC DISORDER

BDD's course and clinical features across reproductive phases have scarcely been studied. However, it is known that hormonal and social changes during reproductive phases can influence other psychiatric illnesses, which may be relevant to BDD.

Body Dysmorphic Disorder in the Perinatal Period

Pregnancy rate

The pregnancy rate in women with BDD is unknown. In the authors' clinical practice, few women with BDD become pregnant. Some fear that their child will be ugly (like them), whereas some women with better insight worry that their child will be at increased risk for BDD. Some women may want to avoid the physical changes of pregnancy, and many people with BDD avoid relationships and intimacy because they do not want others to see their body.[7]

Perinatal course of body dysmorphic disorder

The sole study of perinatal BDD found that clinically significant BDD symptoms were experienced by 15% of women in the third trimester of pregnancy and by 12% at 6 to 8 weeks' postpartum (compared with a current prevalence in the general population of about 2% to 3%).[49] These rates were higher than for other obsessive-compulsive and related disorders.[49] The occurrence of postpartum BDD was associated with worse postpartum functioning.[49]

The clinical features of perinatal BDD have not been studied, but BDD may possibly have some unique clinical characteristics in the perinatal period, as does perinatal OCD (harm obsessions are more common in postpartum-onset OCD than in OCD occurring at other times).[50]

Perinatal implications of the chronicity of body dysmorphic disorder

Because BDD is often unrecognized and chronic, women with BDD may not be in remission before conception. Active antenatal psychiatric illness has a long-lasting impact on offspring[51] and also affects maternal medical and psychiatric health. People with more severe BDD are socially isolated or even housebound, which could potentially limit access to prenatal care in pregnancy and attendance at pediatrician appointments postpartum.

Risk of comorbid conditions in the perinatal period

Women with BDD have high rates of comorbid major depressive disorder, OCD, eating disorders, social anxiety disorder, and substance use disorders. These comorbid psychiatric illnesses are associated with maternal and infant morbidity during the perinatal period. Active antenatal anxiety or depressive symptoms increase risk for postpartum depression, which additionally affects child development and maternal health.[52] Maternal eating disorders can affect the health of the mother and offspring.[53] Substance use in pregnancy—including cannabis, alcohol, cigarettes, and illicit substances—affects maternal health and infant developmental outcomes.[54] **Fig. 2** shows potential perinatal risks of BDD.

Treatment considerations in the perinatal period

When selecting treatment for an illness during pregnancy or breastfeeding, treatment risks must be weighed against risks of the undertreated illness. Given BDD's severity and associated distress, impairment, and rates of suicidality, benefits of continuing high-dose SSRI treatment in the perinatal period often outweigh the risks. Antenatal relapse exposes the fetus to both active symptoms and associated risky behaviors. Psychiatric illness in pregnancy can increase obstetric risks, and high rates of suicidality in BDD can also place the mother's life at risk.[10] Postpartum BDD is also of concern owing to its impact on the mother's ability to function, and comorbid postpartum depression can adversely affect both mother and child. However, the risks and benefits of treatment options must be individually assessed for each woman.

Body Dysmorphic Disorder During Other Reproductive Phases

BDD across the menstrual cycle, at menarche, and at menopause are important topics that have not been studied. BDD most often begins at age 12 to 13 years,[17] around the

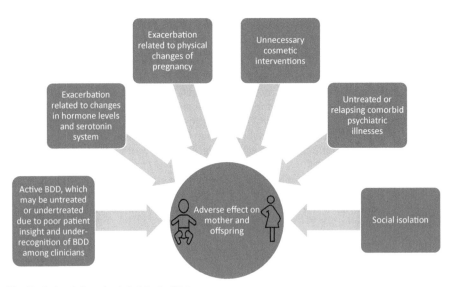

Fig. 2. Potential perinatal risks in BDD.

age of menarche, but studies have not simultaneously recorded age of menarche and onset of BDD or whether clinical features of women with onset around menarche differ from those whose symptoms develop at other times.

Clinically, the authors encounter women with premenstrual exacerbation of BDD, and BDD is more common in women with PMDD than in women without PMDD.[55] Women with premenstrual worsening of OCD have a higher frequency of suicidal ideation and suicide attempts[56]; it is not known whether this is the case for BDD. In the authors' clinical experience, SRI treatment for BDD often improves symptoms of co-morbid PMDD.

SUMMARY

BDD is common yet underrecognized and is more common in women than in men. BDD usually significantly interferes with functioning, and suicidality is common. Although many patients receive cosmetic treatment for BDD, it is virtually never effective and can worsen symptoms. SRIs, often at high doses, and CBT that is tailored to BDD's unique clinical features are first-line treatments. Certain medication augmentation strategies may be helpful. Reproductive aspects of BDD have scarcely been studied; research on this important topic is needed, as is research on other aspects of BDD that are relevant to women.

CLINICS CARE POINTS

- Body dysmorphic disorder is common yet underrecognized.
- Body dysmorphic disorder has more similarities than differences in girls and women and boys and men, but certain characteristics are more common in girls and women.
- Reproductive transitions, such as the perinatal period and menarche, may be periods of high risk for women who are susceptible to body dysmorphic disorder. Further research is warranted.
- The chronicity and severity of body dysmorphic disorder may negatively impact maternal, fetal, and infant health. Treatment is of particular importance in the perinatal period.
- Unless clinicians specifically ask patients about body dysmorphic disorder symptoms, it is likely to be undetected.
- Diagnosing body dysmorphic disorder is usually straightforward and can be made by asking questions such as those in **Box 1**.
- Clues that a patient may have body dysmorphic disorder include observation of repetitive body dysmorphic disorder behaviors (such as mirror checking) or camouflaging as well as receipt of cosmetic procedures (especially if the patient is dissatisfied with the treatment outcome).
- Cosmetic treatment, especially rhinoplasty and other surgeries, is not recommended for body dysmorphic disorder. It is virtually never helpful and can make body dysmorphic disorder symptoms worse.
- Serotonin-reuptake inhibitors are the first-line medication treatment for body dysmorphic disorder.
- High serotonin-reuptake inhibitor doses are usually needed.
- Certain medications (such as atypical neuroleptics and buspirone) may be helpful as serotonin-reuptake inhibitor augmenters.
- If one serotonin-reuptake inhibitor is not adequately helpful, another one may be.
- Cognitive-behavioral therapy is the first-line therapy for body dysmorphic disorder.

- Cognitive-behavioral therapy must be tailored to body dysmorphic disorder's unique clinical features.
- Frequency of cognitive-behavioral therapy sessions must be tailored to the individual patient; more severely ill patients need more intensive cognitive-behavioral therapy.
- Combined treatment (serotonin-reuptake inhibitors plus cognitive-behavioral therapy) is recommended for more severely ill patients.
- Patients should be monitored for suicidality.
- More highly suicidal patients may need additional treatment approaches, such as a safety plan and cognitive-behavioral therapy for suicidality.

DISCLOSURE

K.A. Phillips (past year): Oxford University Press (author, royalties), International Creative Management, Inc (author, royalties), UpToDate/Wolter's Kluwer (author, royalties), Guilford Publications (author, royalties), American Psychiatric Association Publishing (author, royalties), Merck Manual (author, honorarium), OCD Scales (scale development, honorarium), L'Oreal (presentation for Medscape, honorarium), Fabday LLC (presentation for providers of aesthetic treatment, honorarium), CeraVe/RBC Consultants (advisory board meetings, honorarium), academic institutions (speaker, honorarium). No funding supported the writing of this article. L. Susser: No disclosures.

REFERENCES

1. American Psychiatric Association. Diagnostic and statistical manual of mental disorders. Fifth Edition. Arlington VA: APA; 2013.
2. Phillips KA, Kelly MM. Body dysmorphic disorder: Clinical overview and relationship to obsessive compulsive disorder. FOCUS 2021;19:413–9.
3. Phillips KA, Menard W, Fay C, et al. Demographic characteristics, phenomenology, comorbidity, and family history in 200 individuals with body dysmorphic disorder. Psychosomatics 2005;46:317–32.
4. Simmons R, Phillips KA. Core clinical features of body dysmorphic disorder: appearance preoccupations, negative emotions, core beliefs, and repetitive and avoidance behaviors. In: Phillips KA, editor. Body dysmorphic disorder: Advances in research and clinical practice. New York, NY: Oxford University Press; 2017. p. 61–80.
5. Gazzarrini D, Perugi G. Gender and body dysmorphic disorder. In: Phillips KA, editor. Body dysmorphic disorder: Advances in research and clinical practice. New York, NY: Oxford University Press; 2017. p. 187–94.
6. Phillips KA, Pinto A, Hart AS, et al. A comparison of insight in body dysmorphic disorder and obsessive-compulsive disorder. J Psychiatr Res 2012;46:1293–9.
7. Phillips KA, Menard W, Fay C, et al. Psychosocial functioning and quality of life in body dysmorphic disorder. Compr Psychiatry 2005;46:254–60.
8. Grant JE, Kim SW, Crow SJ. Prevalence and clinical features of body dysmorphic disorder in adolescent and adult psychiatric inpatients. J Clin Psychiatry 2001;62:517–22.
9. Phillips KA, Quinn G, Stout RL. Functional impairment in body dysmorphic disorder: A prospective, follow-up study. J Psychiatr Res 2008;42:701–7.
10. Phillips KA. Suicidality and aggressive behavior in body dysmorphic disorder. In: Phillips KA, editor. Body dysmorphic disorder: Advances in research and clinical practice. New York, NY: Oxford University Press; 2017. p. 155–72.

11. Kelly MM, Zhang J, Phillips KA. The prevalence of body dysmorphic disorder and its clinical correlates in a VA primary care behavioral health clinic. Psychiatr Res 2015;228:162–5.

12. Angelakis I, Gooding P, Panagioti M. Suicidality in body dysmorphic disorder (BDD): A systematic review with meta-analysis. Clin Psychol Rev 2016;49:55–66.

13. Snorrason I, Beard C, Christensena K, et al. Body dysmorphic disorder and major depressive episode have comorbidity independent associations with suicidality in an acute psychiatric setting. J Affect Disord 2019;259:266–70.

14. Grant JE, Kim SW, Eckert ED. Body dysmorphic disorder in patients with anorexia nervosa: prevalence, clinical features, and delusionality of body image. Int J Eat Disord 2002;32:291–300.

15. Hartmann AS, Buhlmann U. Prevalence and underrecognition of body dysmorphic disorder. In: Phillips KA, editor. Body dysmorphic disorder: Advances in research and clinical practice. New York, NY: Oxford University Press; 2017. p. 49–60.

16. Veale D, Gledhill LJ, Christodoulou P, et al. Body dysmorphic disorder in different settings: A systematic review and estimated weighted prevalence. Body Image 2016;18:168–88.

17. Bjornsson AS, Didie ER, Grant JE, et al. Age at onset and clinical correlates in body dysmorphic disorder. Compr Psychiatry 2013;54:893–903.

18. Phillips KA, Menard W, Quinn E, et al. A 4-year prospective observational follow-up study of course and predictors of course in body dysmorphic disorder. Psychol Med 2013;43:1109–17.

19. Gunstad J, Phillips KA. Axis I comorbidity in body dysmorphic disorder. Compr Psychiatry 2003;44:270–6.

20. Grant JE, Menard W, Pagano ME, et al. Substance use disorders in individuals with body dysmorphic disorder. J Clin Psychiatry 2005;66:309–11.

21. Enander J, Ivanov VZ, Mataix-Cols D, et al. Prevalence and heritability of body dysmorphic symptoms in adolescents and young adults: a population-based nationwide twin study. Psychol Med 2018;48:2740–7.

22. Monzani B, Rijsdijk F, Harris J, et al. The structure of genetic and environmental risk factors for dimensional representations of DSM-5 obsessive-compulsive spectrum disorders. JAMA Psychiatr 2014;71:182–9.

23. Bienvenu OJ, Samuels JF, Wuyek LA, et al. Is obsessive-compulsive disorder an anxiety disorder, and what, if any, are spectrum conditions? A family study perspective. Psychol Med 2012;42:1–13.

24. Feusner JD, Townsend J, Bystritsky A, et al. Visual information processing of faces in body dysmorphic disorder. Arch Gen Psychiatry 2007;64:1417–25.

25. Feusner JD, Hembacher E, Moller H. Abnormalities of object visual processing in body dysmorphic disorder. Psychol Med 2011;41:2385–97.

26. McCurdy-McKinnon D, Feusner JD. Neurobiology of body dysmorphic disorder: Heritability/genetics, brain circuitry, and visual processing. In: Phillips KA, editor. Body dysmorphic disorder: Advances in research and clinical practice. New York, NY: Oxford University Press; 2017. p. 253–76.

27. Wong WW, Rangaprakash D, Moody TD, et al. Dynamic effective connectivity patterns during rapid face stimuli presentation in body dysmorphic disorder. Front Neurosci 2022;16:890424.

28. Buhlmann U, Hartmann AS. Cognitive and emotional processing in body dysmorphic Disorder. In: Phillips KA, editor. Body dysmorphic disorder: Advances in research and clinical practice. New York, NY: Oxford University Press; 2017. p. 285–98.

29. Neziroglu F, Barile N. Environmental factors in body dysmorphic disorder. In: Phillips KA, editor. Body dysmorphic disorder: Advances in research and clinical practice. New York, NY: Oxford University Press; 2017. p. 277–84.

30. Kelly Y, Zilanawala A, Booker C, et al. Social media use and adolescent mental health: Findings from the UK millennium cohort study. EClinMed 2018;6:5968.

31. Alsaidan MS, Altayar NS, Alshmmari SH, et al. The prevalence and determinants of body dysmorphic disorder among young social media users: A cross-sectional study. Dermatol Rep 2020;12:8774.

32. Phillips KA. Pharmacotherapy and other somatic treatments for body dysmorphic Disorder. In: Phillips KA, editor. Body dysmorphic disorder: Advances in research and clinical practice. New York, NY: Oxford University Press; 2017. p. 333–56.

33. Castle D, Beilharz F, Phillips KA, et al. Body dysmorphic disorder: a treatment synthesis and consensus on behalf of the International College of Obsessive-Compulsive Spectrum Disorders (ICOCS) and the Obsessive Compulsive and Related Disorders Network (OCRN) of the European College of Neuropsycho-pharmacology (ECNP). Int Clin Psychopharmacol 2021;36:61–75.

34. Curtiss JE, Bernstein EE, Wilhelm S, et al. Predictors of pharmacotherapy outcomes for body dysmorphic disorder: A machine learning approach. Psychol Med 2022;1–11.

35. Koran LM, Hanna GL, Hollander E, et al. Practice guideline for the treatment of patients with obsessive-compulsive disorder. Am J Psychiatry 2007;164(7 Suppl):5–53.

36. Pittenger C, Brennan BP, Koran L, et al. Specialty knowledge and competency standards for pharmacotherapy of adult obsessive-compulsive disorder. Psychiatr Res 2021;300:113853.

37. Phillips KA, Keshaviah A, Dougherty DD, et al. Pharmacotherapy relapse prevention in body dysmorphic disorder: A double-blind placebo-controlled trial. Am J Psychiatry 2016;173:887–95.

38. Rasmussen J, Gómez AF, Wilhelm S. Cognitive-behavioral therapy for body dysmorphic Disorder. In: Phillips KA, editor. Body dysmorphic disorder: Advances in research and clinical practice. New York, NY: Oxford University Press; 2017. p. 357–78.

39. Wilhelm S, Phillips KA, Greenberg JL, et al. Efficacy and posttreatment effects of therapist-delivered cognitive behavioral therapy vs supportive psychotherapy for adults with body dysmorphic disorder: A randomized clinical trial. JAMA Psychiatr 2019;76:363–73.

40. Phillips KA, Greenberg JL, Hoeppner SS, et al. Predictors and moderators of symptom change during cognitive-behavioral therapy or supportive psychotherapy for body dysmorphic disorder. J Affect Disord 2021;287:34–40.

41. Veale D, Neziroglu F. Body dysmorphic disorder: a treatment manual. West Sussex, UK: Wiley-Blackwell; 2010.

42. Wilhelm S, Phillips KA, Steketee G. Cognitive-behavioral therapy for body dysmorphic disorder: a treatment manual. New York, NY: Guilford Press; 2013.

43. Veale D, Phillips KA, Neziroglu F. Challenges in assessing and treating patients with body dysmorphic disorder and recommended approaches. In: Phillips KA, editor. Body dysmorphic disorder: Advances in research and clinical practice. New York, NY: Oxford University Press; 2017. p. 313–32.

44. Wenzel A, Brown GK, Beck AT. Cognitive therapy for suicidal patients: scientific and clinical Applications. Washington, DC: American Psychological Association; 2009.

45. Phillips KA, Grant J, Siniscalchi J, et al. Surgical and nonpsychiatric medical treatment of patients with body dysmorphic disorder. Psychosomatics 2001;42: 504–10.
46. American College of Obstetricians and Gynecologists. ACOG Committee Opinion: Breast and labial surgery in adolescents. ACOG 2017.
47. American College of Obstetricians and Gynecologists. ACOG Committee Opinion: Elective female genital cosmetic surgery. AGOG 2020.
48. Ishii LE, Tollefson TT, Basura GJ, et al. Clinical practice guideline: improving nasal form and function after rhinoplasty (supplement). Otolaryngol Head Neck Surg 2017;156:S1–30.
49. Miller M, Roche A, Lemon E, et al. Obsessive-compulsive and related disorder symptoms in the perinatal period: Prevalence and associations with postpartum functioning. Arch Wom Ment Health 2022;25:771–80.
50. Uguz F, Akman C, Kaya N, et al. Postpartum-onset obsessive-compulsive disorder: Incidence, clinical features, and related factors. J Clin Psychiatry 2007;68: 132–8.
51. Plant D, Pawlby S, Sharp D, et al. Prenatal maternal depression is associated with offspring inflammation at 25 years: A prospective longitudinal cohort study. Transl Psychiatry 2016;6:e936.
52. Pearlstein T, Howard M, Salisbury A, et al. Postpartum depression. AJOG 2009; 200:357–64.
53. Ante Z, Luu T, Healy-Profitos J, et al. Pregnancy outcomes in women with anorexia nervosa. Int J Eat Disord 2020;53:673–82.
54. Substance use in women research report: Substance use while pregnant and breastfeeding. National Institute on Drug Abuse https://nida.nih.gov/publications/research-reports/substance-use-in-women/substance-use-while-pregnant-breastfeeding. Accessed 10/18/22.
55. Fornaro M, Perugi G. The impact of premenstrual dysphoric disorder among 92 bipolar patients. Europ Psychiatr 2010;25:450–4.
56. Moreira L, Bins H, Toressan R, et al. An exploratory dimensional approach to premenstrual manifestation of obsessive-compulsive disorder symptoms: A multicenter study. J Psychosom Res 2013;4:313–9.

Sleep and Women's Mental Health

Meredith E. Rumble, PhD[a],*, Paul Okoyeh, MD[b],
Ruth M. Benca, MD, PhD[b]

KEYWORDS

- Women • Sleep • Mental health • Insomnia • Restless legs syndrome
- Obstructive sleep apnea • Depression • Alzheimer disease

KEY POINTS

- Sleep disturbances and mental health concerns are common among women.
- Women are more likely to experience insomnia and restless legs syndrome (RLS), and, as women age, sex differences in obstructive sleep apnea (OSA) decrease.
- Hormonal transitions are of importance when considering sleep disorders in women (onset of menses, pregnancy, and menopause for insomnia; heavy menstrual bleeding and pregnancy for RLS; pregnancy and menopause for OSA).
- Insomnia, OSA, and RLS are related to increased risk of depression.
- Insomnia and sleep-disordered breathing are related to increased risk of Alzheimer disease.

INTRODUCTION

Starting as early as adolescence and persisting across women's remaining lifetimes, both sleep disturbance and mental health concerns disproportionally affect women over men. Although the importance of sleep in relation to physical health has long been accepted, it has only been more recently that the complex, bidirectional, and critical relationship between sleep and mental health has been recognized. Given that women have higher risks for both sleep disturbances and psychiatric disorder, in this article, the authors consider the crucial relationship between sleep and women's mental health.

This article starts by first providing an overview of sleep, normative age-related changes in sleep, and sex-specific differences in sleep. Then, the article considers common sleep disorders in women as well as the relationships between sleep disturbances and mental health more broadly. Finally, the authors discuss the relationships

[a] Department of Psychiatry, University of Wisconsin, 6001 Research Park Boulevard, Madison, WI 53719, USA; [b] Department of Psychiatry and Behavioral Medicine, Wake Forest School of Medicine, 791 Jonestown Road, Winston-Salem, NC 27103, USA
* Corresponding author.
E-mail address: rumble@wisc.edu

Psychiatr Clin N Am 46 (2023) 527–537
https://doi.org/10.1016/j.psc.2023.04.008
0193-953X/23/© 2023 Elsevier Inc. All rights reserved.

psych.theclinics.com

between sleep disturbance and depression, schizophrenia, and Alzheimer disease (AD) in women.

OVERVIEW OF SLEEP

Sleep is divided into 2 categories: rapid eye movement (REM) and non–rapid eye movement (NREM) sleep, with NREM further divided into 3 stages based on electro-encephalographic (EEG) patterns.[1,2] Stage N1 consists of theta activity (4–7 Hz) and vertex sharp waves, with decreased muscle activity and slow, rolling eye movements. The following stage is N2, which is characterized by the appearance of sleep spindles (11–16 Hz). Other prominent features in N2 include K-complexes, which are negative, high-amplitude waves, followed by positive slow waves. Eye movements are absent. In stage N3, slow-wave patterns become much more frequent, occupying at least 20% of each 30-second epoch of sleep. Finally, REM sleep features an activated EEG pattern compared with stages N1–N3, including a return of theta activity as well as a characteristic sawtooth wave pattern (2–6 Hz). As the name suggests, this stage also features rapid, irregular eye movements along with tonic muscle atonia and superimposed muscle twitches. REM is the stage most often associated with dreaming, although dreaming can occur in NREM sleep as well.

A typical night of sleep consists of alternating between NREM and REM sleep, with each NREM/REM cycle lasting roughly 90 minutes. Stage N3/slow-wave sleep is most prominent during the first part of the night, as it represents the homeostatic response to wakefulness, whereas REM sleep episodes are longer and more intense in the latter part of the night.[1,2] Sleep structure and timing are determined by a two-part process, the circadian rhythm (ie, the physiologic process related to the timing and pattern of sleep and wakefulness and other essential functions like heart rate and temperature) and the homeostatic mechanism (ie, the body's pressure for sleep related to the amount wakefulness).[3]

Normative Age-Related Changes in Sleep

There are significant changes in sleep and circadian rhythm patterns roughly associated with stages of development. In infants, sleep occupies most of the day (up to 20 hours), with no clear diurnal pattern.[4] In addition, a significant portion of time asleep, up to 50%, is spent in REM or "active" sleep.[5] From birth to age 2, overall sleep duration and daytime sleep (napping) also decrease.[4] Across childhood, slow-wave sleep amounts are high, but slow-wave sleep amounts start to decrease during adolescence owing to synaptic pruning.[6] Total sleep amounts gradually decrease across childhood and adolescence as well.[7] In adolescence, there are significant changes in circadian rhythms, with teenagers tending to go to sleep later in the night and wake up later in the morning.[8] At the same time, during waking hours, sleep pressure increases at a slower rate, permitting later bedtimes. However, the rate at which sleep pressure decreases with sleep does not change, demonstrating the continued need for sleep in adolescence.[8]

A meta-analysis of quantitative sleep measures in 3577 individuals from ages 5 to 102 years old has shown large age-related effects for decreased total sleep time, sleep efficiency (the percentage of time spent asleep during the period set aside for sleep), and N3/slow-wave sleep and increased wake time after sleep onset.[7] A majority of these changes were found to occur between the ages of 18 to 60 years old, with about a 10-minute decrease in total sleep time, 2% decrease in slow-wave sleep, and 10-minute increase in wake time after sleep onset per decade. The exception was decreased sleep efficiency, which was present from age 40 onward with about a

3% decrease per decade.[7] In contrast to the delay in circadian rhythms seen during adolescence, the circadian rhythm shows a phase advance with increasing age (ie, going to sleep and waking up earlier).[9]

Sex Differences in Sleep

Across stages of development, there are significant differences between women and men. First, sex differences emerge in the timing and magnitude of the adolescent circadian phase delay. Female adolescents tend to experience an earlier onset and peak of this delay compared with male adolescents, which is theorized to be associated with the earlier onset of puberty in women.[10] Furthermore, male adolescents experience a greater magnitude of phase delay (ie, going to sleep and waking up later) during adolescence than female adolescents.[10] In adulthood, this sex difference in chronotype persists, although generally there is phase advancement throughout adulthood, with women tending to go to bed earlier than men.[9,10]

Although both men and women exhibit broadly similar changes in sleep over the lifespan (eg, decreased total sleep time, increased sleep fragmentation), sex differences have been documented in objective sleep as measured by polysomnography. A meta-analysis found that women fall asleep more quickly and have more total sleep time compared with men.[7] On the other hand, in this same meta-analysis, women demonstrated greater amounts of time awake after sleep onset in comparison to men.[7] Similar findings were demonstrated in a study of 69,650 adults aged 19 to 67 years old using data from wearable activity tracking devices, in that women had more total sleep time in comparison to men, but women also demonstrated more nighttime awakenings than men.[11] Sleep EEG oscillations (slow-wave sleep and spindles) start to decrease starting in adolescence, but there is evidence to suggest that women go through this decline at least 1 year earlier than men.[6,12] Overall, from adolescence through adulthood, women exhibit greater slow-wave and spindle activity (especially spindle density) as compared with men.[13]

Women also experience unique periods of hormonal and physiologic changes that impact sleep architecture, namely menstruation, pregnancy, and menopause. In regards to self-report, women tend to report sleep disturbances during the late luteal and early follicular phases of the menstrual cycle (ie, last few premenstrual days through the first few days of menstruation), corresponding with low levels of circulating progesterone and estradiol.[14] In regard to objective measurement of sleep, one notable change on EEG during the menstrual cycle is a significant increase in sleep spindle duration and density during the luteal phase compared with the follicular phase, a change which becomes less pronounced in older women with insomnia.[14] Links between specific sleep disorders and onset of menstruation, pregnancy, and menopause are discussed in the next section, outlining common sleep disorders in women.

COMMON SLEEP DISORDERS IN WOMEN
Insomnia

Insomnia symptoms, including difficulty falling asleep, difficulty staying asleep, and waking up earlier than desired, are common, with about one-third of the population reporting at least one insomnia symptom.[15] Insomnia disorder is defined as having at least one insomnia symptom along with daytime consequences occurring at least 3 times per week for 3 months or more, while having sufficient opportunity for sleep.[16] About 6% to 10% of the adult population meet criteria for insomnia disorder.[15]

Women are about 1.4 times as likely as men to meet criteria for insomnia disorder.[17] These sex differences have been shown to emerge at the onset of menses, with one study demonstrating a 2.75-fold increase in risk of insomnia in women versus men at the same level of maturation, but with no differences between women and men before the onset of menses.[18] Furthermore, a meta-analysis found that clinically significant insomnia symptoms occurred at a higher rate within pregnancy in the third trimester versus the first and second trimester (approximately 40% vs 25 or 27%, respectively).[19] Insomnia symptoms have also been found to be more prevalent in postmenopausal women (approximately 60%) in comparison to reproductive women (approximately 48%) cross-sectionally.[20] In a longitudinal analysis, women experienced increased insomnia symptoms in the 2 years before and after the menopausal transition.[20] Thus, hormonal transitions are an important factor contributing to insomnia in women.

Obstructive Sleep Apnea

Obstructive sleep apnea (OSA) is characterized by complete (apnea) or partial (hypopnea) decrements in breathing during sleep, in which there is oropharyngeal collapse for 10 seconds or more, resulting in drops in blood oxygenation and sleep fragmentation.[21] OSA symptoms include loud snoring, witnessed apneas, gasping or choking during sleep, daytime sleepiness, and fatigue. OSA severity is classified by the apnea-hypopnea index (AHI), the number of respiratory events per hour of sleep: mild, ≥ 5 to <15 events/h; moderate, ≥ 15 to <30 events/h; and severe, ≥ 30 events/h. In the general adult population, studies have estimated an overall prevalence of OSA between 9% and 38%.[22]

Men are more likely to have OSA than women, with an estimated prevalence between 13% and 33% for men and 6% and 19% for women. On the other hand, studies have demonstrated smaller differences in OSA prevalence related to sex with age.[22] In addition, women with OSA may present with somewhat different symptoms than men with OSA. One study found that women with mild OSA were more likely to report insomnia symptoms and excessive sleepiness in comparison to men with mild OSA.[23] Hormonal transitions also impact OSA prevalence. Pregnancy is associated with increased prevalence of OSA, with a meta-analysis demonstrating a pooled prevalence of about 15%, with greater pooled prevalence in the Western Pacific and Region of Americas (17% and 20%) versus the European Region (5%).[24] In addition, during menopause, one study found that AHI increased by 4% with each additional year in menopause for women, and these relationships were independent of other known common OSA risk factors, such as age and body mass index.[25]

Restless Legs Syndrome

Diagnostic criteria for restless legs syndrome (RLS) include (1) recurrent, unpleasant sensations in the legs while sitting or lying down; (2) urges to move the legs while sitting or lying down; (3) symptoms temporarily relieved by movement; and (4) symptoms greater in the evening or at night.[26] In a population-based study of 15,391 respondents, about 7% of respondents endorsed all RLS diagnostic symptoms.[27] Notably, women were more likely to report all RLS symptoms than men (9.0 vs 5.4%, respectively).[27] The higher prevalence of RLS in women has been shown to be related to parity, with each additional pregnancy a woman experiences increasing the odds of developing RLS in a dose-response fashion.[28] Iron deficiency is also a risk factor for RLS,[21] and reproductive-age women are at particular risk for iron deficiency owing to increased iron demands during pregnancy and heavy menstrual bleeding.[29] Finally, the relationship of higher prevalence of RLS with aging has also been demonstrated, so older women are also at higher risk.[28,30]

RELATIONSHIP OF SLEEP DISTURBANCE TO GENERAL MENTAL HEALTH

In general, there is a collective understanding that sleep is important for health, but it is only within the last few decades that we have begun to truly understand the key role that sleep plays in mental health. A 1992 meta-analysis incorporating 171 studies with over 7000 subjects demonstrated associations between changes in aspects of sleep architecture (eg, total sleep time, sleep efficiency, slow-wave activity) with various psychiatric disorders, including mood disorders, alcohol use disorder, psychosis, and certain personality disorders.[31] Although the relationship between sleep and mental health started to become better acknowledged with such evidence, sleep disturbance was often only considered a secondary symptom of mental health concerns. For example, insomnia was seen as a symptom of depression, so depression was the focus for assessment and treatment, resulting in sleep disturbance often being ignored in both assessment and treatment.

Continued longitudinal research has demonstrated a more complex and bidirectional relationship between sleep disturbance and mental health. These findings underscored the importance of assessing and treating sleep disturbance in a comorbid model. The most studied relationship between sleep and mental health has been with insomnia and depression. More specifically, one meta-analysis of 21 studies detailed the predictive nature of insomnia symptoms with depression, finding that those with insomnia alone at baseline were about twice as likely to develop depression in comparison to those without insomnia symptoms at baseline.[32] Another meta-analysis of 13 studies that required at least a 12-month follow-up has broadened these findings, showing how those with insomnia at baseline were not only about twice as likely to report future depression (10 studies), but also were about 3 times as likely to endorse future anxiety (6 studies) and about 1.5 times more likely to report future alcohol abuse (2 studies) and psychosis (1 study).[33] By examining broader definitions of sleep disturbance (eg, shorter sleep duration, sleep quality, and nightmares), a recent meta-analysis of 6 studies demonstrated bidirectional relationships between sleep disturbance and posttraumatic stress disorder (PTSD).[34] More specifically, shorter sleep duration and poorer sleep quality predicted next-day PTSD symptoms, and conversely, higher levels of PTSD symptoms predicted nightmares and poorer sleep quality that night.[34] Sleep disturbance is an important and common comorbidity for psychiatric disorders that demands consideration in research and clinical care.

Relationship of Sleep Disturbance to Depression for Women

Major depressive disorder (MDD) is a common mental health concern associated with significant impairment.[35] Moreover, women are twice as likely to be classified as having MDD compared with men.[35] Through a variety of assessment approaches, sex differences in sleep disturbance have been demonstrated in those experiencing depression. For example, the higher prevalence of insomnia symptoms in women in the general population has also been replicated in individuals with depression. In a sample of 55,000 individuals from the United Kingdom, health record and self-report data demonstrated a higher prevalence of insomnia symptoms in women across the sample in comparison to men, whether they were classified as individuals with probable MDD, harmful alcohol use, a combination of MDD and harmful alcohol use, or controls.[36] Using accelerometer data in a population-based sample of 418 adults, another study demonstrated that the relationship between sleep and rest-activity indices and depressive symptoms was moderated by sex[37]; women with greater depressive symptoms took longer to fall asleep and had less total sleep time than women with fewer depressive symptoms, whereas men with more depressive symptoms had lower mean activity level and amplitude than men with lower depressive symptoms. Using high-density EEG measurement of sleep in a well-defined clinical sample of 30 young, middle-aged individuals with unipolar MDD, slow-wave activity and sleep spindle density, amplitude, and duration were increased in women with MDD versus healthy female controls, whereas there were no differences in slow-waves or sleep spindles detected between men with MDD and controls.[38,39] Taken together, sex differences present more broadly in sleep in healthy individuals also seem to be present in individuals experiencing major depression (ie, greater self-reported sleep disturbance, greater sleep spindle, and slow-wave power in women). In addition, there is some evidence of greater sleep disturbance as measured by actigraphy in women with higher versus lower levels of depressive symptoms.

Relationships between specific sleep disorders and depression in women have also been reported. As noted above, several meta-analyses have confirmed the longitudinal relationship between baseline insomnia and future depression, so insomnia is an established and significant risk factor for depression, and women were well represented in these studies.[32,33] OSA and RLS have also been found to be associated with depression. In a nationally representative population of 9714 adults, women with physician-diagnosed sleep apnea were more likely to endorse probable depression (OR = 5.3) versus men (OR = 2.4).[40] A longitudinal study of 1428 women found that those with definite RLS were at significantly higher risk of depressive symptoms during pregnancy (17 and 32 weeks) and postdelivery (6 weeks) versus those without RLS, even when adjusting for parity, prepregnancy smoking status, and psychiatric history.[41] Outside of pregnancy, in a prospective study of 56,399 women without depression at baseline, those with physician-diagnosed RLS at baseline were at a higher age-adjusted relative risk of subsequent clinical depression versus women without RLS.[42] Thus, a variety of sleep disorders are related to increased risk of depressive symptoms in women.

Relationship of Sleep Disturbance to Schizophrenia for Women

Schizophrenia has a well-documented association with sleep disturbance, and acute psychosis is associated with the most severe disruptions of sleep.[31] Schizophrenia also has been associated with circadian rhythm disruption,[43] and, as discussed earlier in this article, insomnia is known to be a significant predictor for a variety of mental health disorders, including psychosis.[33] In terms of sleep EEG, one of the most consistent differences between those with schizophrenia and those without the disease is the level of sleep spindle activity during sleep. People with schizophrenia demonstrate significantly reduced spindle activity compared with healthy controls, including early in the course of the illness.[43,44] This reduction in spindle activity has also been reported in unaffected first-degree relatives of those with schizophrenia, which is significant considering that schizophrenia often has a strong genetic component.[43,45]

However, the role of sex in mediating the relationship between sleep and schizophrenia is less clear. It is well-known that the incidence of schizophrenia is significantly higher in men, and that male sex is associated with worse outcomes.[46,47] It is also established, as previously mentioned, that women exhibit greater sleep spindle activity compared with men, starting in adolescence.[13] Taken together, this raises an interesting question as to whether greater spindle activity in women confers a protective effect against the development in schizophrenia. However, more work is needed to establish firm genetic and physiologic differences between men and women in the interplay between sleep and schizophrenia.

Relationship of Sleep Disturbance to Alzheimer Disease for Women

As of 2021, AD is the seventh-leading cause of death in the United States and the fifth-leading cause of death among Americans aged 65 and older.[48] It is also one of the few major chronic diseases in which the number of deaths has steadily increased over the past 2 decades, in contrast with overall mortality in other diseases, such as cardiovascular disease, HIV, and cancer.[48] Briefly, AD pathologic condition is linked to the buildup of 2 proteins in the brain: extracellular plaques of amyloid beta (Aβ) protein and intracellular tangles of tau protein. Sleep disturbance is an important aspect of AD pathologic condition, and Aβ has been of particular interest because it is well-established that it is cleared from the brain during sleep, particularly stage N3.[49] Insomnia and sleep-disordered breathing are known to be predictive risk factors for AD,[50] and sleep deprivation is associated with greater deposition of amyloid protein in the adult brain, regardless of level of cognitive impairment.[51]

This relationship between AD and sleep disturbances becomes even more pronounced when accounting for sex differences, particularly in women. Among the more than 6 million people in the United States suffering from AD, roughly two-thirds of them are women.[48] In addition, insomnia, a risk factor for AD, is a more common complaint in women, especially in the perimenopausal and postmenopausal period.[20] There seems to be some genetic evidence for the sex-specific nature of sleep disturbances and AD pathologic condition as well. APOE4, a gene that confers an increased risk of developing AD, is associated with shorter sleep duration,[52] and women with APOE4 are more likely to develop AD as compared with men,[53] which may suggest APOE4 as a mediating factor between insomnia and increased risk of AD in women. Another proposed mediating factor between sleep disruption and AD is neuroinflammation. Studies have shown that chronic inflammation is a contributing factor to the development of AD, with sleep loss and fragmentation promoting an increase in neuroinflammation.[54,55] Of note, women tend to have higher levels of neuroinflammation compared with men,[56] suggesting that increased rates of insomnia in women may lead to neuroinflammation and the subsequent development of AD.

SUMMARY

In contrast to men, women have increased risks for sleep disturbances and psychiatric symptoms beginning in adolescence with the onset of menstruation and continuing for the remainder of their lives. In terms of specific sleep disorders, women are more likely to have insomnia disorder and RLS in comparison to men. Although men have an overall higher prevalence of OSA, sex differences in OSA prevalence decrease with age. Hormonal transitions are one important consideration for sleep disturbance in women, as increased risk of insomnia has been demonstrated with the onset of menses, during pregnancy, and during menopause; increased risk of RLS is associated with heavy menstrual bleeding and pregnancy, and OSA risk increases during pregnancy and menopause.

It is important to acknowledge the complexity and bidirectionality in the relationship between sleep and mental health. Not only is sleep disturbance a consequence of psychiatric disorders but also sleep disturbances and disorders confer increased risk for future onset and/or exacerbation of psychiatric disorders. For example, as discussed in this article, insomnia, OSA, and RLS are all related to increased risk of depression for women, and insomnia and sleep-disordered breathing are related to increased risk of AD for women. These findings underscore the importance of assessment and treatment of sleep and mental health concerns in women. Continued research examining the relationship between sleep and mental health, particularly in women, given their distinct and greater vulnerability, is also necessary to expand the understanding and improve clinical care for women.

CLINICS CARE POINTS

- Regular assessment and treatment of sleep and mental health in women is essential, given the high prevalence of sleep disturbance and mental health issues for this population.
- Common sleep concerns for women include insomnia, RLS, and OSA.
- Refer women with significant sleep disorders to appropriate sleep specialists as needed.
- When considering assessment and treatment options, keep in mind the following
  - There is strong evidence for a complex and bidirectional relationship between sleep and mental health (e.g., insomnia, RLS, and OSA are related to increased risk of depression; insomnia and sleep-disordered breathing are related to increased risk of Alzheimer disease; psychiatric disorders can worsen sleep disturbances and disorders).
  - Hormonal transitions can present greater vulnerability to sleep disturbances (onset of menses, pregnancy, and menopause for insomnia; heavy menstrual bleeding and pregnancy for RLS; and pregnancy and menopause for OSA).

DISCLOSURES

Dr M.E. Rumble has received grant support from Merck. Dr P. Okoyeh has no disclosures. Dr R.M. Benca has served as a consultant to Eisai, Idorsia, Merck, Jazz, and Sage and has received grant support from Merck, United States and Eisai, Japan.

REFERENCES

1. American Academy of Sleep Medicine. The ASSM manual for the scoring of sleep and associated events: rules, terminology and technical specification. Westchester, IL: American Academy of Sleep Medicine; 2007.
2. Rechtschaffen A, Kales A. A manual of standardized terminology, techniques, and scoring system for sleep stages of human subjects. Washington, DC: Brain Information Service/Brain Research Institute; 1968.
3. Borbely AA. A two process model of sleep regulation. Hum Neurobiol 1982;1(3): 195–204.
4. Paavonen EJ, Saarenpää-Heikkilä O, Morales-Munoz I, et al. Normal sleep development in infants: findings from two large birth cohorts. Sleep Med 2020;69: 145–54.
5. Knoop MS, de Groot ER, Dudink J. Current ideas about the roles of rapid eye movement and non-rapid eye movement sleep in brain development. Acta Paediatr 2021;110(1):36–44.
6. Franco P, Putois B, Guyon A, et al. Sleep during development: Sex and gender differences. Sleep Med Rev 2020;51:101276.
7. Ohayon MM, Carskadon MA, Guilleminault C, et al. Meta-analysis of quantitative sleep parameters from childhood to old age in healthy individuals: developing normative sleep values across the human lifespan. Sleep 2004;27(7):1255–73.
8. Crowley SJ, Wolfson AR, Tarokh L, et al. An update on adolescent sleep: New evidence informing the perfect storm model. J Adolesc 2018;67:55–65.
9. Duffy JF, Zitting KM, Chinoy ED. Aging and Circadian Rhythms. Sleep Med Clin 2015;10(4):423–34.

10. Bailey M, Silver R. Sex differences in circadian timing systems: implications for disease. Front Neuroendocrinol 2014;35(1):111–39.
11. Jonasdottir SS, Minor K, Lehmann S. Gender differences in nighttime sleep patterns and variability across the adult lifespan: a global-scale wearables study. Sleep 2021;44(2). https://doi.org/10.1093/sleep/zsaa169.
12. Zhang ZY, Campbell IG, Dhayagude P, et al. Longitudinal Analysis of Sleep Spindle Maturation from Childhood through Late Adolescence. J Neurosci 2021; 41(19):4253–61.
13. Markovic A, Kaess M, Tarokh L. Gender differences in adolescent sleep neurophysiology: a high-density sleep EEG study. Sci Rep 2020;10(1):15935.
14. Baker FC, Lee KA. Menstrual Cycle Effects on Sleep. Sleep Med Clin 2018;13(3): 283–94.
15. Ohayon MM. Epidemiology of insomnia: what we know and what we still need to learn. Sleep Med Rev 2002;6(2):97–111.
16. American Psychiatric Association. Diagnostic and statistical manual of mental disorders. 5th edition. Arlington, VA: American Psychiatric Association; 2013.
17. Zhang B, Wing YK. Sex differences in insomnia: a meta-analysis. Sleep 2006; 29(1):85–93.
18. Johnson EO, Roth T, Schultz L, et al. Epidemiology of DSM-IV insomnia in adolescence: lifetime prevalence, chronicity, and an emergent gender difference. Pediatrics 2006;117(2):e247–56.
19. Sedov ID, Anderson NJ, Dhillon AK, et al. Insomnia symptoms during pregnancy: A meta-analysis. J Sleep Res 2021;30(1):e13207.
20. Ballot O, Ivers H, Ji X, et al. Sleep Disturbances During the Menopausal Transition: The Role of Sleep Reactivity and Arousal Predisposition. Behav Sleep Med 2022;20(4):500–12.
21. Benca REM. Sleep disorders: the clinician's guide to diagnosis and management. New York, NY: Oxford University Press; 2012.
22. Senaratna CV, Perret JL, Lodge CJ, et al. Prevalence of obstructive sleep apnea in the general population: A systematic review. Sleep Med Rev 2017;34:70–81.
23. Morris JL, Mazzotti DR, Gottlieb DJ, et al. Sex differences within symptom subtypes of mild obstructive sleep apnea. Sleep Med 2021;84:253–8.
24. Liu L, Su G, Wang S, et al. The prevalence of obstructive sleep apnea and its association with pregnancy-related health outcomes: a systematic review and meta-analysis. Sleep Breath 2019;23(2):399–412.
25. Mirer AG, Young T, Palta M, et al. Sleep-disordered breathing and the menopausal transition among participants in the Sleep in Midlife Women Study. Menopause 2017;24(2):157–62.
26. American Academy of Sleep Medicine. International classification of sleep disorders. 3rd edition. Darien, IL: American Academy of Sleep Medicine; 2014.
27. Allen RP, Walters AS, Montplaisir J, et al. Restless legs syndrome prevalence and impact: REST general population study. Arch Intern Med 2005;165(11):1286–92.
28. Berger K, Luedemann J, Trenkwalder C, et al. Sex and the risk of restless legs syndrome in the general population. Arch Intern Med 2004;164(2):196–202.
29. Moisidis-Tesch CM, Shulman LP. Iron Deficiency in Women's Health: New Insights into Diagnosis and Treatment. Adv Ther 2022;39(6):2438–51.
30. Wesstrom J, Nilsson S, Sundstrom-Poromaa I, et al. Restless legs syndrome among women: prevalence, co-morbidity and possible relationship to menopause. Climacteric 2008;11(5):422–8.
31. Benca RM, Obermeyer WH, Thisted RA, et al. Sleep and psychiatric disorders. A meta-analysis. Arch Gen Psychiatry 1992;49(8):651–68, discussion 669-70.

32. Baglioni C, Battagliese G, Feige B, et al. Insomnia as a predictor of depression: a meta-analytic evaluation of longitudinal epidemiological studies. J Affect Disord 2011;135(1–3):10–9.
33. Hertenstein E, Feige B, Gmeiner T, et al. Insomnia as a predictor of mental disorders: A systematic review and meta-analysis. Sleep Med Rev 2019;43:96–105.
34. Slavish DC, Briggs M, Fentem A, et al. Bidirectional associations between daily PTSD symptoms and sleep disturbances: A systematic review. Sleep Med Rev 2022;63:101623.
35. Bromet E, Andrade LH, Hwang I, et al. Cross-national epidemiology of DSM-IV major depressive episode. BMC Med 2011;9:90.
36. Kolla BP, Biernacka JM, Mansukhani MP, et al. Prevalence of insomnia symptoms and associated risk factors in UK Biobank participants with hazardous alcohol use and major depression. Drug Alcohol Depend 2021;229(Pt A):109128.
37. White KH, Rumble ME, Benca RM. Sex Differences in the Relationship Between Depressive Symptoms and Actigraphic Assessments of Sleep and Rest-Activity Rhythms in a Population-Based Sample. Psychosom Med 2017;79(4):479–84.
38. Plante DT, Landsness EC, Peterson MJ, et al. Sex-related differences in sleep slow wave activity in major depressive disorder: a high-density EEG investigation. BMC Psychiatr 2012;12:146.
39. Plante DT, Goldstein MR, Landsness EC, et al. Topographic and sex-related differences in sleep spindles in major depressive disorder: a high-density EEG investigation. J Affect Disord 2013;146(1):120–5.
40. Wheaton AG, Perry GS, Chapman DP, et al. Sleep disordered breathing and depression among U.S. adults: National Health and Nutrition Examination Survey, 2005-2008. Sleep 2012;35(4):461–7.
41. Wesström J, Skalkidou A, Manconi M, et al. Pre-pregnancy restless legs syndrome (Willis-Ekbom Disease) is associated with perinatal depression. J Clin Sleep Med 2014;10(5):527–33.
42. Li Y, Mirzaei F, O'Reilly EJ, et al. Prospective study of restless legs syndrome and risk of depression in women. Am J Epidemiol 2012;176(4):279–88.
43. Ferrarelli F. Sleep Abnormalities in Schizophrenia: State of the Art and Next Steps. Am J Psychiatry 2021;178(10):903–13.
44. Ferrarelli F. Sleep disturbances in schizophrenia and psychosis. Schizophr Res 2020;221:1–3.
45. Zhang Y, Quiñones GM, Ferrarelli F. Sleep spindle and slow wave abnormalities in schizophrenia and other psychotic disorders: Recent findings and future directions. Schizophr Res 2020;221:29–36.
46. Santos S, Ferreira H, Martins J, et al. Male sex bias in early and late onset neurodevelopmental disorders: Shared aspects and differences in Autism Spectrum Disorder, Attention Deficit/hyperactivity Disorder, and Schizophrenia. Neurosci Biobehav Rev 2022;135:104577.
47. Gogos A, Ney LJ, Seymour N, et al. Sex differences in schizophrenia, bipolar disorder, and post-traumatic stress disorder: Are gonadal hormones the link? Br J Pharmacol 2019;176(21):4119–35.
48. 2022 Alzheimer's disease facts and figures. Alzheimers Dement 2022;18(4):700–89.
49. Ngo HV, Claassen J, Dresler M. Sleep: Slow Wave Activity Predicts Amyloid-β Accumulation. Curr Biol 2020;30(22):R1371–3.
50. Shi L, Chen SJ, Ma MY, et al. Sleep disturbances increase the risk of dementia: A systematic review and meta-analysis. Sleep Med Rev 2018;40:4–16.

51. Sprecher KE, Koscik RL, Carlsson CM, et al. Poor sleep is associated with CSF biomarkers of amyloid pathology in cognitively normal adults. Neurology 2017; 89(5):445–53.

52. Spira AP, An Y, Peng Y, et al. APOE Genotype and Nonrespiratory Sleep Parameters in Cognitively Intact Older Adults. Sleep 2017;40(8). https://doi.org/10.1093/sleep/zsx076.

53. Zhu D, Montagne A, Zhao Z. Alzheimer's pathogenic mechanisms and underlying sex difference. Cell Mol Life Sci 2021;78(11):4907–20.

54. Irwin MR, Vitiello MV. Implications of sleep disturbance and inflammation for Alzheimer's disease dementia. Lancet Neurol 2019;18(3):296–306.

55. Ozben T, Ozben S. Neuro-inflammation and anti-inflammatory treatment options for Alzheimer's disease. Clin Biochem 2019;72:87–9.

56. Contreras JA, Aslanyan V, Albrecht DS, et al, (ADNI) AsDNI. Higher baseline levels of CSF inflammation increase risk of incident mild cognitive impairment and Alzheimer's disease dementia. Alzheimers Dement (Amst) 2022;14(1): e12346.

Examining Associations Between Women's Mental Health and Obesity

Jennifer V.A. Kemp, MSc[a,b,1], Vivek Kumar, MBBS, MPH[a,b,1],
April Saleem, BSc[c], Gabrielle Hashman, MSc[a,b,d],
Mashael Hussain, MBBS[a,b], Valerie H. Taylor, MD, PhD[a,*]

KEYWORDS

- Women's mental health • Mental illness • Obesity • Weight gain • Quality of life
- Self-esteem • Vulnerable

KEY POINTS

- Mental illness and obesity form a vicious cycle, each impacting the onset and management outcomes of the other. This article looks at the existing literature that provides links between women's mental health and obesity. The biological and psychological factors that modulate such associations are reviewed.
- Studies have shown that individuals with a higher body mass index score significantly lower on the quality-of-life metrics and that there is a higher predispositio in women.
- Self-esteem and cultural beliefs play an important role in manifesting mental illnesses, especially during the vulnerable periods of the female life span. Further research is warranted to better understand these relationships and to assist in improving well-being.

ABSTRACT

Obesity is a common comorbidity associated with mental illness. Women seem disproportionally impacted by the weight gain side effects of medications, and issues such as weight gain are more likely to impact symptoms of mental illness, impacting self-esteem. Women are also overrepresented in illnesses such as binge eating

[a] Department of Psychiatry, University of Calgary, Foothills Campus, Calgary, Alberta, Canada; [b] Matheson Centre for Mental Health Research & Education, University of Calgary, Foothills Campus, 3280 Hospital Drive Northwest, 1D-57, Calgary, Alberta T2N 4Z6, Canada; [c] Department of Pathology and Molecular Medicine, Gastrointestinal Disease Research Unit, Queen's University, 76 Stuart Street, Sheth Lab (Floor 3), Kingston, Ontario K7L 2V7, Canada; [d] Medical School for International Health, Faculty of Health Sciences, Ben-Gurion University of the Negev, Beer Sheva, Israel
[1] Co-first authors.
* Corresponding author. AW259B, Special Services Building Foothills Medical Centre, 1403 29 Street Northwest, Calgary, Alberta T2N 2T9, Canada.
E-mail address: Valerie.taylor@ucalgary.ca

Psychiatr Clin N Am 46 (2023) 539–549
https://doi.org/10.1016/j.psc.2023.04.009
0193-953X/23/© 2023 Elsevier Inc. All rights reserved.

disorder, major depressive disorder, and attention-deficit/hyperactivity disorder, which can have weight gain symptoms. The hormonal impacts of various life stages, menarche, pregnancy and the postpartum, and perimenopause/menopause periods, can also impact weight gain.

Aim: To summarize the existing literature on the associations between women's mental health and obesity. Methods: For literature searching and screening: The search strategy was developed in consultation with a health sciences librarian. Six databases were searched including MEDLINE, Embase, Web of Science, PsycInfo, CINAHL, and CENTRAL. The authors also searched the reference list of key papers and older systematic reviews for additional papers. Screening was done in duplicate, and conflicts resolved by a third author.

Conclusion: It is important to understand the many ways weight gain and obesity can impact the cause and course of mental illness in women, with a special focus on vulnerable life stages. Understanding this association will lead to better health outcomes.

BACKGROUND

The obesity epidemic is of major public health concern. According to the World Health Organization, more than 1 billion people worldwide are obese, and it is estimated that by 2025, approximately 167 million people will have their health negatively impacted due to being overweight or having obesity.[1] The worldwide prevalence of obesity has approximately tripled since 1975 and is significantly higher in women when compared with men, in all age groups.[2]

Obesity is a risk factor for several medical conditions, including but not limited to glucose intolerance, hypertension, dyslipidemia, cardiovascular disease, sleep apnea, endocrine disorders such as polycystic ovarian syndrome, various cancers, reflux, nonalcoholic fatty liver, and ultimately, increased mortality.[3] Obesity is also a risk factor for worsening mental health issues.[3] In a review by Hjorthøj and colleagues,[4] there was an estimated 14.5 years of potential life lost among individuals with schizophrenia (SCZ) and psychosis when compared with the general population, and the mortality gap has increased with cardiometabolic risk factors as the major contributors.[5–7] These associated comorbidities have, as a consequence, led to increased health care costs causing tremendous economic burden[3]; for example, the 2019 annual medical care costs related to obesity in the United States were estimated to be nearly $173 billion.[8] Considering comorbid mental health conditions, both obesity and severe mental illness together lead to a magnified increase in adverse health outcomes due to increased disability, morbidity, and mortality.[9]

The reasons for rising rates of obesity are complex, with biological, cultural, socioeconomic, and gender-related disparities all contributing. For many people, obesity is ultimately a consequence of an imbalance between caloric intake and energy expenditure, such as a carbohydrate- and fat-rich diet along with a sedentary lifestyle.[10] The factors leading to this imbalance are often quite complex; however, a myriad of variables contribute to the cause of this illness.[11] Lifetime stress, especially in women, is associated with a higher risk for obesity,[12] and sex hormones also have a major role to play on both metabolism and patterns of fat distribution.[10] For example, men exhibit visceral fat accumulation, whereas in women fat usually accumulates subcutaneously[10]; this is significant because visceral adiposity is much more metabolically active and is linked to increased morbidity and mortality.[13] Other contributing factors include a genetic risk, along with epigenetic modifications.[11]

The bidirectional[14] associations between mental health and obesity in children, adolescents,[15] and adults[16] are well-documented. Vittengl[17] reported that people with major depressive disorder (MDD) have a 58% chance of developing obesity and people with obesity have a 55% likelihood of developing MDD. Mood disorders are characterized by alterations to appetite, sleep, energy levels, and motivation,[18] all of which are factors that also impact weight gain. The risks are not equal across sex and gender; however, it is becoming increasingly evident that women, in particular, are at elevated risk for developing comorbid MDD and obesity.[18–21]

This review looks at various factors that may be involved in the pathophysiological processes linking obesity and women's mental health, as well as is an overview of the current management of obesity, with a focus on sex and gender.

Mental Illnesses Linked to Obesity from a Female Lens

Several biological and psychosocial factors are potential mediators or moderators of the association between mental illness and obesity in women. These factors include hypothalamic-pituitary-adrenal (HPA) axis dysregulation,[22] body image perturbations,[20] socioeconomic status (SES),[23] and cyclical hormones.[16,19,21]

Mental illnesses such as MDD, bipolar disorder, and SCZ are often marked by increased levels of stress and subsequent increases in peripheral cortisol.[22,24] Cortisol is a glucocorticoid that is released when the body's stress response system (the HPA axis) is activated by exogenous stressors. It is well documented that excessive cortisol levels confer increased risk for obesity, hypertension, diabetes, and cardiovascular disease.[25] Although cortisol levels in people with mental illnesses do not reach levels associated with hypercortisolemic disorders such as Addison disease, they can still drive the conversion of preadipocytes to mature adipocytes,[26] which in turn promotes deposition of adipose tissue in central regions of the body.[27] Likewise, sustained increases in cortisol levels can impair the negative feedback mechanism responsible for shutting down the HPA axis. This impairment may alter one's ability to process and respond appropriately to new environmental stressors and can perpetuate depressionlike symptoms seen in various mood disorders.[28] As such, HPA axis dysregulation is associated with mood disorders[22,24] and obesity[26] and may serve to mediate the association between mental illness and obesity.

Women in particular show higher incidence of mental illness and obesity compared with their male counterparts.[16,29] From a body image perspective, the Social Comparison Theory[30] posits that women are more likely to be affected by thin body image ideals that social media perpetuates, and these ideals, in turn, are associated with negative mood.[20,31] In addition, previous literature has noted associations between comorbid obesity and mood disorders and SES, although the direction of effect seems to differ between studies (ie, some studies report lower SES is associated with a higher incidence of MDD and obesity in women, whereas other studies report higher SES is associated with a higher incidence of MDD and obesity in women).[23,32,33] Social ideals and SES may serve as exogenous stressors for women and interact negatively with the HPA axis to perpetuate negative emotions, although the exact relationship between these variables requires further exploration.[34]

A specific biological factor conferring increased risk for mental illness and comorbid obesity in females is cyclical hormones. Women are at elevated risk for MDD during periods of their life marked by significant hormonal fluctuations; these periods are menarche, pregnancy, postpartum, and menopause.[35] Estrogen in particular is highly associated with MDD because it interacts with the serotonergic system, which plays a large role in mood regulation.[16,35] Decreased levels of estrogen as seen during menopause or the postpartum period are associated with reduced brain-derived neurotrophic factor (BDNF).[16] BDNF is responsible for promoting serotonin neurons, and a reduction of BDNF may result in reduced serotonin expression, which is an antecedent to the development of mood disorders.[36] Furthermore, decreased estrogen is also associated with altered adipocyte metabolism[37] and may confer risk for obesity during menopause.[38] As such, during times when estrogen levels are lower, women may be at elevated risk both for mood dysregulation and obesity.

Role of Medication

Women are at higher risk for several mental illnesses and thus receive more pharmacologic treatments.[39] From a bioavailability perspective, factors such as gastrointestinal transit time (slower in women), stomach pH (lower in men), and mucosal enzymes and transporters, which are influenced by gonadal hormones and, as a consequence, differ in men and women indicate a sex influence that is difficult to predict and is drug dependent.[40,41] Increased typical subcutaneous fat distribution seen in women with obesity results in poorer perfusion and slower absorption, impacting the rate of absorption from intramuscular injections.[42] When discussing psychotropic medications, women are more likely to report disturbing side effects.[43] Weight gain is a side effect repeatedly reported as more prevalent in women than in men, with further risk during the postpartum period.[44–46]

Weight and Quality of Life

Obesity and weight gain have a significant impact on an individual's physical and psychosocial well-being, consequently affecting all aspects of daily functioning and overall quality of life (QoL).[47] QoL is a subjective and broad evaluation of an individual's lived experiences based on values, expectations, abilities, beliefs, and needs.[48] Principal domains encompass standard of living such as quality of housing and community, SES contributors such as financial stability and job satisfaction, social support such as family relationships, perceived self-esteem and self-worth, and other social determinants of health.[49–51] Focusing on factors contributing to the QoL considerably influences treatment efficacy, in addition to weight loss, providing a patient-centered approach when addressing the multifactorial cause, severity, and chronicity of obesity.[48]

Recent studies have shown a negative association between patients with obesity and QoL, with those with obesity scoring significantly lower on health-related quality of life (HRQoL) scale metrics across physical, health perceptions, and vitality measures, when compared with nonoverweight patients.[50] This association is further pronounced in women who are overweight compared with men and nonoverweight women.[52–55] For example, Stephenson and colleagues[52] compared the HRQoL scores of adults residing in England (n = 64,631, $n_{females}$ = 40,668) across body mass index (BMI) levels and found that an increase in BMI was associated with a reduced HRQoL score in participants reporting 3 or more mental or physical health conditions compared with those reporting fewer conditions. Kurscheid and colleagues[53] provided app-controlled feedback devices (eg, bioimpedance scale, blood pressure monitor, and activity tracking bracelet) to adults with obesity living in Germany (n = 89, $n_{females}$ = 54) undergoing a 12-week weight reduction modified diet program. The results showed women benefiting from the app-controlled feedback devices and achieved an increase in HRQoL while reducing their BMI compared with baseline and those who did not receive the feedback devices.[53] Arikawa and colleagues[54] conducted a parallel group randomized controlled trial assessing HRQoL in overweight and obese postmenopausal breast cancer survivors (n = 20) undergoing either a three-month calorie deficit diet and exercise intervention or a weight management counseling intervention in the United States. Although both intervention groups experienced significant weight loss and improvement in HRQoL, the calorie deficit diet and exercise cohort reported a decrease in sleep quality.[54] Busutil and colleagues[55] investigated the impact of obese BMI on HRQoL of a Spanish adult population (n = 18,682) primarily with BMI greater than 35 kg/m^2. Individuals with BMI greater than 35 reported reduced HRQoL scores even without chronic disease symptoms; women and individuals aged 65 years and older reported significantly worse HRQoL than the average.[55] Ul-Haq and colleagues[56] analyzed data from a Scottish cross-sectional study collected since 1995 (n = 5608, n$_{female}$ = 3077) specifically looking at the impact of overweight BMI, metabolic comorbidity, and HRQoL. Obese individuals reported significantly reduced HRQoL, and those with metabolic comorbidity reported poorer HRQoL regardless of BMI.[56]

Similar associations have been found in various studies, highlighting a reduction in HRQoL scores as BMI increases, suggesting a linear reduction of HRQoL with an increase in BMI. The negative association appears to greatly affect women, individuals older than 65 years, and those with comorbid conditions,[50–52] warranting further research and analysis to better understand the relationships between weight gain, self-esteem, and QoL.

Impact on Self-Esteem

The associations between women's mental health, obesity, and self-esteem have been increasingly explored over the last several years. Recent literature on the topic of female self-esteem and weight refers to the objectification theory[57] as the foundational framework for understanding the implications that body-related self-conscious emotions have on women's mental health.[58–60] The objectification theory highlights the impact of sociocultural norms and beliefs on body surveillance and negative self-conscious emotions such as shame and guilt,[57] postulating that women who perceive themselves as not being what they view as a BMI in the range to confer a diagnosis of obesity are significantly more likely to develop depressive symptoms compared with their male counterparts with similar BMI.[61]

Body weight contingent on self-worth (CSW) is a concept closely associated with self-esteem and mental health. Recent studies have shown that in adult and adolescent women, body weight CSW is significantly associated with unstable self-esteem and depressive symptoms.[58,62] It is suggested that body weight CSW is a risk factor for individuals developing depressive symptoms, in part, because their self-esteem is particularly impacted by stressful life events and external feedback.[58] Of note, Ching and colleagues[58] found that prior levels of unstable self-esteem were a predictor for depressive symptoms over time, whereas prior levels of depressive symptoms did not significantly predict higher instability of self-esteem. These findings align with a meta-analysis conducted by Sowislo and Orth[63], which concluded that self-esteem had a 2-fold impact on depression, when compared with the effects of depression on self-esteem.

Brunet and colleagues (2019) found that young adults with low self-esteem had a significant positive correlation between body-related guilt and depressive symptoms, but no significant relationship was seen with the same factors in participants with high self-esteem. This finding highlights the possible protective effect that elevated self-esteem can have on depressive symptoms in young adults experiencing body-related guilt. A 3-year prospective study also found that self-esteem acted as a resilience factor against the development of attention problems, anxiety, and depression in a clinical sample of adolescents being treated for mental health problems.[64] This finding underscores the significance of addressing self-esteem in a clinical setting as a potential moderator of longer-term outcomes of depressive symptoms.[64] Additional research has found that the impact of body-related shame on depressive symptoms in women can be significantly moderated by high levels of self-compassion, which is thought to compensate as a protective mechanism when self-esteem falls short.[60]

It is also important to consider the role culture plays in the internalization of weight bias and thus, the subsequent impact of weight gain on self-esteem. Multiple studies have shown the variable impact of cultural norms, beliefs, and values on one's weight-based self-esteem,[65–67] with cultural differences in body image ideals being a critical underlying factor. Rakhkovskaya and Warren[67] found ethnic identity to be protective against body dissatisfaction in African American women but not in European Americans. Similarly, Dijkstra and colleagues[65] found that women in the Caribbean Island Curacao showed more resistance to negative effects on self-esteem from imagined weight gain than women in The Netherlands.

Role of Vulnerable Periods Through the Female Life Span

According to the women's health across the nation study, before menopause, the mean annual rise in fat mass was 0.25 kg, which increased to 0.45 kg during the menopausal transition.[68] In addition, during the premenopausal period, increasing fat mass and declining proportional lean mass was apparent, accelerating by 2- to 4-folds during the menopausal transition.[68] Obesity during menopause often presents centrally, distributed from the gynoid to the abdomen due to relative hyperandrogenemia, rapid hypoestrogenism, and low sex hormone-binding globulin level.[69] Furthermore, the transitional period marked by menopause is highly associated with depressive symptoms.[70] Current treatment of menopause hormones and physical changes are often traditional antidepressants (eg, selective serotonin reuptake inhibitors and serotonin and norepinephrine reuptake inhibitors) and hormonal treatments, which, as discussed earlier, have been shown to increase weight.[71] As such, the menopausal period is marked by both considerable weight gain and an elevated risk for depressive and anxiety symptoms.

Menarche is also associated with a fast and significant increase in body weight[72,73] and a high prevalence of later-life mental illness, suggesting that pubertal timing is directly related to mental health.[74] The links between obesity and menarche can start during early childhood, because increases in obesity before menarche can result in earlier onset of puberty[75]; this is because a variety of hormonal changes such as leptin activation of the hypothalamic-pituitary axis, combined with insulin resistance, and increased adiposity, may result in the higher estrogen levels that are linked to breast development.[76,77] Young adolescents also experience a sharp decline in their level of physical activity, worsening nutritional habits, and other important psychosocial and developmental risk factors that may contribute to obesity.[78] Weight gain associated with menarche typically occurs 7 to 12 months after menarche onset and can perpetuate binge eating, purging, concerns regarding body image, and the risk of the onset of eating disorders and other mental health disorders.[73]

Pregnancy is a natural and biological reason for cyclical weight fluctuations,[79] but there is also documentation of elevated risk for obesity during the antepartum, intrapartum, and postpartum periods.[80] This elevated risk can result in an increased risk for gestational diabetes, pregnancy-induced hypertension, preeclampsia, labor induction, elective and emergency cesarean delivery, and thromboembolic complications.[81] Gestational weight gain above the Institute of Medicine recommendation can cause short-term and long-term (21-year period) postpartum weight retention.[82] This retention is relevant to mental health as women with pre-existing obesity who had weight gain during pregnancy had a higher prevalence of MDD when compared with nonobese women.[83]

SUMMARY

Mental illness and obesity represent two of the most significant contributions to morbidity and mortality globally. Each individually can impact the onset, treatment, and outcome of the other, and as such it is important that clinicians be aware of the association. This fact is especially important when considering the care of women. As described earlier, the mental illness-obesity dyad is especially complex in women, and it needs to be considered to ensure best practices and optimal outcomes.

CLINICS CARE POINTS

- Worldwide prevalence of obesity is significantly higher in women than men.
- Obesity is a risk factor for worsening mental health condition leading to increased morbidity and mortality. The bidirectional association between mental health and obesity is well-documented.
- Lifetime stress and sex hormones have a major role in metabolism and patterns of fat distribution amongst men and women, thereby causing gender-based differences, along with genetic risk and epigenetic modifications.
- Significant hormonal fluctuations in women during menarche, pregnancy, postpartum, and menopause place women at a higher risk for mental illnesses. Estrogen is highly associated with MDD as it interacts with the serotonergic system that is a major mood regulator.
- Women are more likely affected by thin body image ideals, which in turn, is associated with negative mood. In adult and adolescent women, body weight contingent on self-worth is significantly associated with unstable self-esteem and depressive symptoms. Cultural norms, beliefs, and values on one's weight-based self-esteem are critical underlying factors.
- Weight gain is a medication side-effect reported more in women than men along with other disturbing side effects. Increased subcutaneous fat deposition in women impacts rate of absorption of intramuscular injections.
- A negative association has been seen between patients with obesity and quality of life, with those with obesity scoring significantly lower on health-related quality of life scale metrics across physical, health perceptions, and vitality measures, when compared with non-overweight patients. These associations appear to greatly affect women, individuals older than 65 years, and those with comorbid conditions.

DISCLOSURE

The authors have nothing to disclose.

REFERENCES

1. World Health Organization. World Obesity Day 2022- Accelerating action to stop obesity. 2022. https://www.who.int/news/item/04-03-2022-world-obesity-day-2022-accelerating-action-to-stop-obesity#. Accessed 21 November, 2022.
2. Boutari Chrysoula, Mantozoros CA. 2022 update on the epidemiology of obesity and a call to action: as its twin COVID-19 pandemic appears to be receding, the obesity and dysmetabolism pandemic continues to rage on. Metabolism 2022; 133:155217.
3. Okunogbe Adeyemi, Nugent Rachel, Spencer Garrison, et al. Economic impacts of overweight and obesity: current and future estimates for eight countries. BMJ Glob Heal 2021;6:e006351.

4. Hjorthøj C, Stürup AE, McGrath JJ, et al. Years of potential life lost and life expectancy in schizophrenia: a systematic review and meta-analysis. Lancet Psychiatr 2017;4(4):295–301.

5. Laursen TM, Nordentoft M, Mortensen P. Excess early mortality in schizophrenia. Annu Rev Clin Psychol 2014;10(1):425–48.

6. Correll CU, Solmi M, Veronese N, et al. Prevalence, incidence and mortality from cardiovascular disease in patients with pooled and specific severe mental illness: a large-scale meta-analysis of 3,211,768 patients and 113,383,368 controls. World Psychiatr 2017;16(2):163–80.

7. Oakley P, Kisely S, Baxter A, et al. Increased mortality among people with schizophrenia and other non-affective psychotic disorders in the community: a systematic review and meta-analysis. J Psychiatr Res 2018;102(Jul):245–53.

8. Centers for Disease Control and Prevention. Consequences of Obesity. 2022. Available at: https://www.cdc.gov/obesity/basics/consequences.html. Accessed 21 November, 2022.

9. Avila Christian, Holloway Alison, Hahn Margaret K, et al. An Overview of Links Between Obesity and Mental Health. Curr Obes Rep 2015;4(3):303–10.

10. Agrawal M, Kern PA, Nikolajczyk B. The immune system in obesity: Developing paradigms amidst inconvenient truths. Curr Diab Rep 2017;17:87.

11. Sehgal Kanika, Khanna S. Gut microbiota: a target for intervention in obesity. Expert Rev Gastroenterol Hepatol 2021;15(10):1169–79.

12. Chen Yue, Qian L. Association between lifetime stress and obesity in Canadians. Prev Med 2012;55(5):464–7.

13. Bergman RN, Kim SP, Isabel C, et al. Why Visceral Fat is Bad: Mechanisms of the Metabolic Syndrome. Obesity 2006;14(Supplement):16S–9S.

14. Luppino F, de Wit L, Bouvy P, et al. Overweight, Obesity, and Depression. Arch Gen Psychiatry 2010;67(3):220–9.

15. Small L, Aplasca A. Child Obesity and Mental Health. A Complex Interaction. Child Adolesc Psychiatr Clin N Am 2016;25(2):269–82.

16. Pereira-Miranda E, Costa PRF, Queiroz VAO, et al. Overweight and Obesity Associated with Higher Depression Prevalence in Adults: A Systematic Review and Meta-Analysis. J Am Coll Nutr 2017;36(3):223–33.

17. Vittengl JR. Mediation of the bidirectional relations between obesity and depression among women. Psychiatry Res 2018;264(July 2017):254–9.

18. Taylor VH, McIntyre RS, Remington G, et al. Beyond pharmacotherapy: Understanding the links between obesity and chronic mental illness. Can J Psychiatry 2012;57(1):5–12.

19. Rajewska J, Rybakowski JK. Depression in premenopausal women: Gonadal hormones and serotonergic system assessed by D-fenfluramine challenge test. Prog Neuro-Psychopharmacology Biol Psychiatry 2003;27(4):705–9.

20. Fardouly J, Diedrichs PC, Vartanian LR, et al. Social comparisons on social media: THE impact of Facebook on young women's body image concerns and mood. Body Image 2015;13:38–45.

21. Deecher D, Andree TH, Sloan D, et al. From menarche to menopause: Exploring the underlying biology of depression in women experiencing hormonal changes. Psychoneuroendocrinology 2008;33(1):3–17.

22. Sachar EJ. Cortisol Production in Depressive Illness. Arch Gen Psychiatry 1970; 23(4):289.

23. Stunkard AJ, Faith MS, Allison KC. Depression and obesity. Biol Psychiatry 2003; 54(3):330–7.

24. Girshkin L, Matheson SL, Shepherd AM, et al. Morning cortisol levels in schizo-phrenia and bipolar disorder: A meta-analysis. Psychoneuroendocrinology 2014;49(1):187–206.
25. Pivonello R, Faggiano A, Lombardi G, et al. The metabolic syndrome and cardio-vascular risk in Cushing's syndrome. Endocrinol Metab Clin North Am 2005;34(2): 327–39.
26. Incollingo Rodriguez AC, Epel ES, White ML, et al. Hypothalamic-pituitary-adre-nal axis dysregulation and cortisol activity in obesity: A systematic review. Psy-choneuroendocrinology 2015;62:301–18.
27. Brown ES, Varghese FP, McEwen BS. Association of depression with medical illness: Does cortisol play a role? Biol Psychiatry 2004;55(1):1–9.
28. Watson S, Mackin P. HPA axis function in mood disorders. Psychiatry 2006;5(5): 166–70.
29. Carey M, Small H, Yoong SL, et al. Prevalence of comorbid depression and obesity in general practice: a cross-sectional survey. Br J Gen Pract 2014; 64(620):e122–7.
30. Festinger L., A Theory of Social Comparison Processes. *Hum Relat,* 7 (2), 1954, 115-256.
31. Myers TA, Crowther JH. Social Comparison as a Predictor of Body Dissatisfac-tion: A Meta-Analytic Review. J Abnorm Psychol 2009;118(4):683–98.
32. Chae WR, Schienkiewitz A, Du Y, et al. Comorbid depression and obesity among adults in Germany: Effects of age, sex, and socioeconomic status. J Affect Disord 2022;299:383–92.
33. Moore ME, Stunkard A, Srole L. Obesity, Social Class, and Mental Illness. JAMA 1962;181(11):962–6.
34. Milas G, Klarić IM, Malnar A, et al. Socioeconomic status, social-cultural values, life stress, and health behaviors in a national sample of adolescents. Stress Heal 2019;35(2):217–24.
35. Lokuge S, Frey BN, Foster JA, et al. Depression in Women: Windows of Vulnera-bility and New Insights Into the Link Between Estrogen and Serotonin. J Clin Psy-chiatry 2011;72(11):1563–9.
36. Martinowich K, Lu B. Interaction between BDNF and Serotonin: Role in Mood Dis-orders. Neuropsychopharmacol 2007;33(1):73–83.
37. Heine PA, Taylor JA, Iwamoto GA, et al. Increased adipose tissue in male and fe-male estrogen receptor-α knockout mice. Proc Natl Acad Sci 2000;97(23): 12729–34.
38. Lizcano F, Guzmán G. Estrogen deficiency and the origin of obesity during meno-pause. BioMed Res Int 2014;2014. https://doi.org/10.1155/2014/757461.
39. Seeman MV. Are there gender differences in the response to antipsychotic drugs. Neuropharmacology 2019;23:8.
40. Freire AC, Basit AW, Choudhary R, et al. Does sex matter? the influence of gender on gastrointestinal physiology and drug delivery. Int J Pharm 2011;415(1–2): 15–28.
41. Marazziti D, Baroni S, Picchetti M, et al. Pharmacokinetics and pharmacody-namics of psychotropic drugs: effect of sex. CNS Spectr 2001;18:118–27.
42. Brunton LL, Chabner BKBC. The pharmacological basis of therapeutics. New York: McGraw-Hill; 2011. Published online.
43. Haack S, Seeringer A, Thürmann PA, et al. Sex-specific differences in side effects of psychotropic drugs: genes or gender? Pharmacogenomics 2009;10(9): 1511–26.
44. Seeman M. Exercise and Antipsychotic Drugs. J Patient care 2016;2:114.

45. Seeman MV. Secondary Effects of Antipsychotics: Women at Greater Risk Than Men. Schizophr Bull 2009;35(5):937–48.
46. Seeman MV. Clinical interventions for women with schizophrenia: Pregnancy. Acta Psychiatr Scand 2012;127(1):12–22.
47. Taylor VH, Forhan M, Vigod SN, et al. The impact of obesity on quality of life. Best Pr Res Clin Endocrinol Metab 2013;27(2):139–46.
48. Kushner RF, Foster G. Obesity and quality of life. Nutrition 2000;16(10):947–52.
49. WHO. The World Health Organization quality of life assessment (WHOQOL): Development and general psychometric properties. Soc Sci Med 1998;46(12): 1569–85.
50. Wilkinson R. and Marmot M., World Health Organization. Social determinants of health: the solid facts, World Health Organization, 2nd ed, 2003, Regional Office for Europe https://apps.who.int/iris/handle/10665/326568.
51. Testa MA, Simonson DC. Assessment of quality-of-life outcomes. N Engl J Med 1996;334(13):835–40.
52. Stephenson J, Smith CM, Kearns B, et al. The association between obesity and quality of life: a retrospective analysis of a large-scale population-based cohort study. BMC Publ Health 2021;21(1):1990.
53. Kurscheid T, Redaelli M, Heinen A, et al. App-controlled feedback devices can support sustainability of weight loss. Multicentre QUANT-study shows additional weight loss and gain of QoL via multiple feedback-devices in OPTIFAST(R)52-program. Z Psychosom Med Psychother 2019;65(3):224–38.
54. Arikawa AY, Kaufman BC, Raatz SK, et al. Effects of a parallel-arm randomized controlled weight loss pilot study on biological and psychosocial parameters of overweight and obese breast cancer survivors. Pilot Feasibility Stud 2018;4:17.
55. Busutil R, Espallardo O, Torres A, et al. The impact of obesity on health-related quality of life in Spain. Heal Qual Life Outcomes 2017;15(1):197.
56. Ul-Haq Z, Mackay DF, Fenwick E, et al. Impact of metabolic comorbidity on the association between body mass index and health-related quality of life: a Scotland-wide cross-sectional study of 5,608 participants. BMC Publ Health 2012;12:143.
57. Fredrickson BL, Roberts TA, 'barr A, et al. Objectification theory. Psychol Women Q 1997;21:173–206.
58. Ching BHH, Wu HX, Chen TT. Body weight contingent self-worth predicts depression in adolescent girls: The roles of self-esteem instability and interpersonal sexual objectification. Body Image 2021;36:74–83.
59. Frederick DA, Schaefer LM, Hazzard VM, et al. Racial identity differences in pathways from sociocultural and objectification constructs to body satisfaction: The U.S. Body Project I. Body Image 2022;41:140–55.
60. Sick K, Pila E, Nesbitt A, et al. Does self-compassion buffer the detrimental effect of body shame on depressive symptoms? Body Image 2020;34:175–83.
61. Darimont T, Karavasiloglou N, Hysaj O, et al. Body weight and self-perception are associated with depression: Results from the National Health and Nutrition Examination Survey (NHANES) 2005–2016. J Affect Disord 2020;274:929–34.
62. Clabaugh A, Karpinski A, Griffin K. Body weight contingency of self-worth. Self Ident 2008. https://doi.org/10.1080/15298860701665032. Published online.
63. Sowislo J, Orth U. Does low self-esteem predict depression and anxiety? A meta-analysis of longitudinal studies. Psychol Bull 2013;139(1):213–40.
64. Henriksen IO, Ranøyen I, Indredavik MS, et al. The role of self-esteem in the development of psychiatric problems: A three-year prospective study in a clinical sample of adolescents. Child Adolesc Psychiatry Ment Health 2017;11(1):1–9.

65. Dijkstra P, Barelds DPH, Van Brummen-Girigori O. Weight-Influenced Self-Esteem, Body Comparisons and Body Satisfaction: Findings among Women from The Netherlands and Curacao. Sex Roles 2015;73:355–69.

66. Kessler RC, Berglund PA, Chiu WT, et al. The Prevalence and Correlates of Binge Eating Disorder in the World Health Organization World Mental Health Surveys. Biol Psychiatry 2013;73(9):904–14.

67. Rakhkovskaya LM, Warren CS. Sociocultural and identity predictors of body dissatisfaction in ethnically diverse college women. Body Image 2016;16:32–40.

68. Greendale GA, Sternfeld B, Huang M, et al. Changes in body composition and weight during the menopause transition. JCI Insight 2019;4(5):e124865.

69. Kozakowski J, Gietka-Czernel M, Leszczynska D, et al. Obesity in menopause – our negligence or an unfortunate inevitability? Menopause Rev Menopauzalny 2017;16(2):61–5.

70. Freeman EW, Sammel MD, Liu L, et al. Hormones and Menopausal Status as Predictors of Depression in Women in Transition to Menopause. Arch Gen Psychiatry 2004;61(1):62–70.

71. Serretti A, Mandelli L. Antidepressants and Body Weight: A Comprehensive Review and Meta-Analysis. J Clin Psychiatry 2010;71:10.

72. O'Dea J, Abraham S. Should body-mass index be used in young adolescents? Lancet (London, England) 1995;345(8950):657.

73. Abraham S, Boyd C, Lal M, et al. Time since menarche, weight gain and body image awareness among adolescent girls: onset of eating disorders? J Psychosom Obstet Gynaecol 2009;30(2):89–94.

74. Mendle J, Ryan RM, McKone KMP. Age at menarche, depression, and antisocial behavior in adulthood. Pediatrics 2018;141(1). https://doi.org/10.1542/PEDS.2017-1703/37687.

75. Li W, Liu Q, Deng X, et al. Association between Obesity and Puberty Timing: A Systematic Review and Meta-Analysis. Int J Env Res Public Heal 2017;14(10):1266.

76. Shimizu H, Oh S, Okada S, et al. Leptin resistance and obesity. Endocrinol J 2007;54:17–26.

77. Holly JM, Smith CP, Dunger DB, et al. Relationship between the pubertal fall in sex hormone binding globulin and insulin-like growth factor binding protein-I. A synchronized approach to pubertal development? Clin Endocrinol 1989;31:277–84.

78. Jasik CB, Lustig RH. Adolescent obesity and puberty: The "perfect storm. Ann N Y Acad Sci 2008;1135:265–79.

79. Gunderson EP, Murtaugh MA, Lewis CE, et al. PAPER Excess gains in weight and waist circumference associated with childbearing: The Coronary Artery Risk Development in Young Adults Study (CARDIA). Int J Obes 2004;28:525–35.

80. Arnolds DE, Scavone BM. Obesity in pregnancy. Int Anesthesiol Clin 2021;59(3):8–14.

81. Guelinckx I, Devlieger R, Beckers K, et al. Maternal obesity: pregnancy complications, gestational weight gain and nutrition. Obes Rev 2008;9(2):140–50.

82. Mannan M, Doi SA, Mamun AA. Association between weight gain during pregnancy and postpartum weight retention and obesity: A bias-adjusted meta-analysis. Nutr Rev 2013;71(6):343–52.

83. Bodnar LM, Wisner KL, Moses-Kolko E, et al. Prepregnancy Body Mass Index, Gestational Weight Gain, and the Likelihood of Major Depressive Disorder During Pregnancy. J Clin Psychiatry 2009;70(9):1290–6.

Psychological Aspects of Breast Cancer

Jennifer Kim Penberthy, PhD[a],*, Anne Louise Stewart, MD[a],
Caroline F. Centeno, BS[a], David R. Penberthy, MD, MBA[b]

KEYWORDS

- Breast cancer • Distress • Depression • Anxiety • Psychotherapy

KEY POINTS

- Anxiety, depression, cognitive impairment, adjustment disorders, sleep disturbance and associated fatigue, posttraumatic stress, body image issues, and sexual dysfunction are the most frequently described psychological symptoms and disorders in women with breast cancer.
- Distress screening and psychological assessment is used to identify patients with breast cancer requiring therapeutic support and intervention throughout the treatment course.
- Psychotherapeutic approaches have proved effective in managing psychological symptoms and disorders in patients diagnosed with breast cancer.
- Addressing psychological symptoms can help improve compliance with treatment, outcomes, psychological symptoms, and quality of life.
- Patients diagnosed with breast cancer should be supported with these techniques during the entire oncological trajectory.

INTRODUCTION

Prevalence of Breast Cancer

Breast cancer is a complex and heterogeneous group of diseases in terms of occurrence, impact, therapeutic response, and clinical outcomes. It is the most commonly occurring cancer in women and the most common cancer overall. More than 2.26 million new cases of breast cancer were reported in women globally in 2020 alone. At the end of that same year, there were 7.8 million women alive diagnosed with breast cancer in the past 5 years. In the United States, breast cancer is the most common malignancy diagnosed in women, with an estimated 290,560 cases diagnosed in

[a] Department of Psychiatry & Neurobehavioral Sciences, UVA Cancer Center, University of Virginia School of Medicine & Health System, PO Box 800623, Charlottesville, VA 22908, USA;
[b] Department of Radiation Oncology, Penn State Cancer Institute, Penn State Health Milton S. Hershey College of Medicine, Hershey, PA, USA
* Corresponding author.
E-mail address: jkp2n@UVAHealth.org

Psychiatr Clin N Am 46 (2023) 551–570
https://doi.org/10.1016/j.psc.2023.04.010
0193-953X/23/© 2023 Elsevier Inc. All rights reserved.

2022 and 43,780 deaths from the disease in the same year.[1] One in eight women will develop breast cancer in her lifetime.

Breast cancer occurs worldwide and can occur at any age after puberty and with increasing rates in later life.[2] Breast cancer represents the number two oncological cause of death and 25% of all new cancer diagnoses in women, with the highest incidence in the age range from 55 to 64 years.[2] Breast cancer is a rare malignancy in men, accounting for less than 1% of all cases of cancer.[3] Rates of breast cancer in the United States vary by race and ethnicity. Non-Hispanic white women (137.6 per 100,000) and non-Hispanic Black women (129.6 per 100,000) have the highest incidence of breast cancer (rate of new breast cancer cases) overall. Hispanic women have the lowest incidence (99.9 per 100,000). Incidence rates for non-Hispanic Asian and Pacific Islanders and non-Hispanic American Indian/Alaska Natives are in the middle at 106.9 and 111.3 per 100,000 cases, respectively.[4]

Despite the growing and aging global population, and the increasing number of new breast cancer diagnoses, survival rates have improved due to advancements in early detection and treatment.[5] Women with a history of breast cancer are the largest group of cancer survivors in high-income countries, and as of January 2022, there were more than 3.8 million women with a history of breast cancer in the United States, which include women currently being treated and women who have finished treatment.[6] Thus, this growing population of women warrants our attention and our efforts to better understand their stressors and mental health needs.

Most women diagnosed with breast cancer experience at least some psychosocial distress during the course of their breast cancer diagnosis and treatment. The level of distress varies from woman to woman and over the course of diagnosis and treatment. Cancer-related distress can be expected to dissipate with time for most of the women diagnosed with cancer. For others, however, such distress may interfere substantially with their psychological well-being, quality of life, physical comfort, and the ability to make appropriate treatment decisions and adhere to treatment.[7] Psychosocial distress can be related to physical problems such as illness or disability, psychological problems, family issues, and social concerns such as those related to employment, insurance, and supportive care access. In this chapter, the authors focus on the *psychological impact* of the diagnosis and treatment of breast cancer in women specifically, including psychological symptoms and disorders. They also explore research regarding effective treatments.

Definitions

Breast cancer arises in the lining cells of the ducts or lobules in the glandular tissue of the breast. Initially, the cancerous growth is confined to the duct or lobule ("in situ") where it generally causes no symptoms and has minimal potential for spread. Over time, these in situ cancers may progress and invade the surrounding breast tissue, spreading to the nearby lymph nodes or other organs in the body. If a woman dies of breast cancer, it is typically because of widespread metastasis.[8]

Breast cancer is not a transmissible or infectious disease. Unlike some cancers that have infection-related causes, such as human papillomavirus infection and cervical cancer, there are no known viral or bacterial infections linked to the development of breast cancer. In fact, about half of breast cancers develop in women who have no identifiable breast cancer risk factor other than gender (female) and age (over 40 years). Certain factors increase the risk of breast cancer, including increasing age, obesity, harmful use of alcohol, family history of breast cancer, history of radiation exposure, reproductive history (such as age that menstrual periods began and age at first pregnancy), tobacco use, and unopposed estrogen over time, including postmenopausal hormone therapy.[9] Pregnancy may lower risk due to the interruption of the stimulatory effects of estrogen. Patients with breast cancer who know that they are at increased risk of having hereditary breast cancer may experience heightened levels of psychological distress.[10]

Modern breast cancer treatments are varied and highly effective, especially when the disease is identified early and the patient is adherent to treatment. Typical treatment of breast cancer consists of a combination of surgical removal, radiation therapy, and medication such as hormonal therapy, chemotherapy, or targeted biological therapy. These treatments target the microscopic cancer that has spread from the breast tumor through the blood. The combination of treatments prevents cancer growth and saves lives and can be physically and psychologically stressful to endure. Psychological and physical symptoms can interfere with well-being and treatment compliance[11] and are therefore very important to address.

BACKGROUND
Psychological Impact

Breast cancer diagnosis and treatments are often associated with significant psychological distress. This distress negatively affects psychosocial adjustment to the disease process and health outcomes.[12] Importantly, increased distress in patients with breast cancer has been associated with poorer physical and mental health during treatment.[11]

Being given the diagnosis of breast cancer is often overwhelmingly distressing in and of itself and can create an enormous stress for the patient who now has to deal with new and challenging issues of treatment choices.[13] Undergoing testing, receiving the diagnosis, understanding the prognosis, undergoing treatments, handling side effects, managing possible relapses, and facing an uncertain future are all stages of a stressful process that can cause psychological distress and negatively affect psychological health and well-being, including quality of life, treatment compliance, and outcome.

This heightened stress can lead to or worsen existing anxiety, depression, or other psychological symptoms. Many patients experience multiple concurrent psychological issues during their cancer care trajectory. The most prevalent psychological symptoms in patients with breast cancer include anxiety, depression, impaired cognitive function, as well as physical symptoms such as pain, sleep disturbances, sexual dysfunction, and fatigue, which can trigger fear of death or recurrence, altered body image, and diminished well-being.[14–18]

Patients who receive the diagnosis of breast cancer may progress through stages of coping with the news. These stages include difficulty accepting the diagnosis, failing to acknowledge the seriousness of the situation, and feeling angry or becoming tearful and distraught. Eventually these phases of shock, denial, and emotional reaction typically give way to efforts to adjust, a desire to seek treatment, and hope for health. It is important for providers to understand these stages in their patients and not assume that a patient's emotional response is fixed or even necessarily unhealthy. Allowing time for the patient to process the news of their diagnosis and evaluate treatment options is an important and ongoing part of effective treatment and support.[18]

Different psychological issues arise in different phases of treatment. These phases coincide with aspects of the clinical course of the illness and related treatments. Studies show highest distress at transition points in treatment: at the time of diagnosis, awaiting treatment, during and on completion of treatment, at follow-up visits, at time of recurrence, and at time of treatment failure.[19] In addition, multiple variables affect distress over the course of diagnosis and treatment. These variables include age, sex, personality, and variables related to the impact of treatment such as side effects, social support, and socioeconomic status.[19] Overall, approximately 30% of women show significant distress at some point during the illness, and the number is greater in women with recurrent disease whose family members are also distressed.[20]

Cancer treatment approach can affect symptom presentation. In patients who undergo surgical procedures for breast cancer, the rate of significant psychological dysfunction ranges from 30% to 47%, without any significant difference between those who undergo breast-conserving surgery versus a modified radical mastectomy. Significantly, 20% to 45% continue to meet criteria for their psychiatric disorder 1 year postsurgery, and 10% endorse ongoing disorders 6 years after their operation.[21] Research indicates that 40% of patients with breast cancer report anxiety while undergoing radiotherapy, and this percentage remains stable throughout the course of radiation.[22] Chemotherapy is one of the most stressful aspects of a breast cancer diagnosis, with up to 90% of patients reporting some level of distress during their course of chemotherapy.[23] Chemotherapies can lead to poor functioning, fatigue, depression, anger, and mood disturbance posttreatment.[24] Much of the distress surrounding chemotherapy stems from the anticipation and experiences of unpleasant physical side effects,[25] which are related to specific chemotherapy agents used.

Why Identifying Psychological Symptoms Is Important

The link between psychological and physical health in patients with breast cancer is well documented. Anxiety can manifest as physical symptoms such as muscle tension or sleep disturbance, which may increase the risk of depression.[26] For patients with breast cancer diagnosed with depressive symptoms, mortality rates were found to be nearly 26 times higher and 39 times higher in patients diagnosed with major depression. Importantly, a decrease in depression symptoms was associated with longer survival.[27,28] Diagnosis and treatment of psychological symptoms and disorders improves patients' adherence to therapy and quality of life.[29] Adherence to treatment is important because the effectiveness of breast cancer therapies depends on receiving the full course of treatment. Partial treatment is less likely to lead to a positive outcome.[30]

Distress Screening and Psychological Assessment

It is important to identify psychological stressors in order to plan a proper treatment approach. A full discussion of all psychological assessment tools is beyond the scope of this chapter. A comprehensive literature review published in *Seminars in Oncology Nursing* concluded that psychological health in patients with cancer was determined by a balance between the stress and burden posed by the cancer experience and the resources available for coping.[31] For all of these reasons, screening, assessing, and treating psychological symptoms and disorders is of utmost importance in this patient population.

The Institute of Medicine's 2008 report, Cancer Care for the Whole Patient: Meeting Psychosocial Health Needs, called attention to the importance of addressing the psychological problems associated with cancer and noted that leaving these needs unmet could result in decreased well-being and reduced treatment adherence and threaten patients' return to health.[32] Recognizing this, the National Comprehensive Cancer Network issued a consensus statement recommending distress screening and management as a standard of care within oncology health services delivery. In 2012, the American College of Surgeons Commission on Cancer (CoC) added distress screening to its accreditation standards for cancer programs; this requires development and implementation of a process to integrate and monitor on-site psychosocial distress screening and referral for the provision of psychosocial care.[32]

Distress, defined as the overburden or the inability to cope with negative affect–eliciting events, exists along a continuum, ranging from feelings of vulnerability, sadness, and fears to problems that can become disabling. Distress may be experienced as a reaction to the disease and its treatment and also as a result of the consequences of the disease on social functioning.[33] Many of the instruments used to assess patients with breast cancer attempt to measure what is referred to as health-related quality of life (HRQOL).[34,35] HRQOL assessments are self-rated subjective evaluations of health and well-being generally in at least 4 areas: psychological functioning, physical functioning, social functioning, and symptoms and side effects. In this chapter the authors focus on the areas of psychological functioning.

An instrument commonly used to assess psychological distress is the Distress Thermometer and Problem List from the National Comprehensive Cancer Network. The Distress Thermometer itself is a one-item, 11-point Likert scale represented on a visual graphic of a thermometer that ranges from 0 (no distress) to 10 (extreme distress), with which patients indicate their level of distress over the course of the prior week.[36] Specific problems encountered can also be endorsed.

Specific symptoms can be assessed by more specialized assessments including the Hospital Anxiety and Depression scale,[37] the Short Form-36 of the Medical Outcomes Study,[38] Brief Symptom Inventory,[39] Cancer Rehabilitation Evaluation System tool,[40] the Functional Assessment of Cancer Therapy-Breast,[41] and the Quality of Life Breast Cancer Instrument.[42] Distress screening followed by targeted assessment of relevant symptoms with standardized, valid, and reliable psychological assessment tools is recommended in order to create an appropriate and effective treatment intervention.

Inconsistency in research methodology, including use of various assessment tools, some of which are not validated or reliable, has led to differing reports of symptoms and their impact. Distress and psychological assessment in patients with breast cancer has made progress, but caution is recommended in evaluating the research.[43]

DISCUSSION
Common Psychological Symptoms

Although research demonstrates common psychological symptoms that occur in patients with breast cancer, it is important to remember the wide variability across individual women. The psychosocial impact of breast cancer must be understood in the context of multiple issues that affect women's coping, quality of life, and well-being, including socioeconomic and cultural factors, social support, access to health care, and the presence of other chronic illness or life crises. In addition, there are differing psychological challenges that coincide with clinical course of the illness and related treatments. With these caveats in mind, the authors briefly review the research regarding common psychological symptoms (**Table 1**).

Adjustment Disorders

Problems in adjusting to a breast cancer diagnosis or treatment may lead to significant distress beyond what is normally seen in response to such stressor and lead to functional impairment, resulting in a diagnosis of adjustment disorder. Adjustment disorders can be defined as with depression or anxiety or both. Recent research found that 38.6% of patients with breast cancer met criteria for adjustment disorder with depression.[44] Another 2020 study found that 37.5% of patients with breast cancer met criteria for

Table 1
Common psychological symptoms and estimates of prevalence in breast cancer

Symptom	Prevalence (%)
PTSD	0–32
Anxiety	10–30
Depression	10–30
Cognitive impairment	12–82
Sexual dysfunction	43–83
Sleep disturbances	50–90
Body image disturbances	75–92

adjustment disorder symptoms during the course of treatment and up to 5 years post-treatment.[45] Onset of an adjustment disorder can occur at any time during the cancer continuum but is most likely, as are many symptoms, to present during transition points, where new stressors ensue. Making a diagnosis of adjustment disorder can be challenging, as it is can seem similar to other depressive and anxiety disorders.

Anxiety and Depression

Research shows that about one-third of patients with breast cancer display symptoms of anxiety and depression,[46] and these numbers were found to be even higher during COVID, with one study reporting more than half of patients with breast cancer suffered from depression (51.2%), anxiety (62.8%), sleep problems (51.2%), and posttraumatic stress disorder (PTSD) symptoms (35.3%).[47] Clinically relevant symptoms of anxiety and depression are common at the initial diagnosis and during active treatment, when treatment side effects may have more of a negative impact.[48] High prevalence of depressive symptoms and anxiety have also been observed in survivorship,[49] with one study finding depressive symptoms persisting for at least 2 years after diagnosis in 20% of women.[50]

Anxiety is common in patients with breast cancer,[13] with rates ranging from 10% to 30%. Anxiety may be related to anticipation of negative outcomes and the uncertainty about the future. Anxiety is also frequently related to concern over recurrence and the worry of treatment side effects during and after treatments.[51] Recent findings suggest that anxiety is more prevalent than depression, although other studies report comparable rates of between 10% and 30%.[46]

The rate of depression in patients with breast cancer is estimated to be between 10% and 30%, depending on the study population, study design, and choice of depression measure.[13] Depressive symptoms have been shown to negatively affect compliance with treatment regime, reduce patient quality of life and self-care, and decrease immunity and chances of survival.[52] Diagnosing depression can be challenging in patients with cancer because symptoms of depression overlap with physical symptoms related to treatment. Chronic fatigue and decreased social interactions are also common responses to breast cancer that can affect depressive symptoms.[53] Research indicates that women with a primary breast cancer diagnosis remain vulnerable to psychological disorders for many years,[54] highlighting the significant psychological impact of this medical condition.

Cancer-Related Cognitive Impairment

Cognitive difficulties in patients with breast cancer began to appear in the literature in the 1990s,[55] associated with the increasing use of postoperative adjuvant chemotherapy. Because symptoms were more frequently reported in women who received very high-dose chemotherapy, the concern was that cognitive impairment might become a dose-limiting treatment toxicity. Fortunately, over the past 20 years, there has been a deescalation of both the intensity and generalized use of adjuvant chemotherapy in patients with breast cancer. Because of this initial association of cognitive impairment with chemotherapy treatment, early research focused on what was referred to as "chemobrain."

The reported prevalence of cognitive impairment following treatment of breast cancer is somewhat variable. There was preliminary evidence of measurable neurocognitive effects among patients with breast cancer who were exposed to chemotherapy. Subsequent studies have documented cognitive changes before any cancer-directed therapies, as well as in association with other common breast cancer treatments (eg, radiation, endocrine therapy). According to one survey, 77% of patients who received chemotherapy with and without endocrine therapy and 45% who received only endocrine therapy reported cognitive symptoms during or soon after treatment.[56]

A commonly cited range suggests that 12% to 82% of women will experience cognitive impairment as a result of their cancer treatment.[57] This variability may be attributable to a range of patient factors such as age, menopausal status, and education level.[58] Research also demonstrates that cognitive impairment is often present before the start of chemotherapy,[59] potentially arising as a result of cancer itself. The evolving body of research has led to a renaming of the condition as *cancer-related cognitive impairment*. Although symptoms are most commonly reported in close proximity to initial breast cancer treatments, for some patients, symptoms of cognitive impairment can persist for years after treatment completion.[60]

Sleep Disturbances

Similar to other symptoms, the incidence of sleep disturbance, including insomnia, varies across studies depending on the study design and assessment methods, but most studies report that 60% to 90% of patients with breast cancer endorse significant sleep disturbances.[61] This is much higher than in the healthy population. The prevalence of sleep disorders is higher among patients with breast cancer compared with other cancers, possibly due to the impact of menopausal symptoms triggered by this therapy.[62] Insomnia in patients with breast cancer can be associated with various factors such as psychological distress arising from the cancer diagnosis or adverse effects of cancer therapy. Patients who receive adjuvant endocrine therapy remain at increased risk for insomnia because of the occurrence of menopause.[63] Research exploring the prevalence of patients with breast cancer meeting criteria for an insomnia syndrome report rates of 18.6% to 19%.[64]

Body Image Disturbances and Sexual Dysfunction

A woman's body image is conceptualized as the mental representation of her social and psychological experiences and is shaped by her impression and sense of her physical appearance.[65] Breast cancer treatments typically involve significant changes to a woman's body, potentially including disfiguring surgeries, hair loss, and the emotional and physical impact of hormonal changes resulting from the treatments. A recent study reports that 92% of patients with breast cancer after modified radical mastectomy endorsed body image disturbances.[66] Another study examining patients with breast cancer posttreatment reported a prevalence of body image dissatisfaction of 74.8% confidence interval (CI) (65%–82%).[67]

Psychologically, body image disturbance has demonstrated a direct relationship with low self-confidence, weak social relationships, depression, and problems in sexual functioning.[68,69] Sexual dysfunction in patients with breast cancer is commonly reported, with prevalence rates across the globe between 43% and 75%, and average prevalence rates of 66% to 68%, depending on age.[70] These symptoms have been found to exist during treatment and after treatment. Recent research on young women breast cancer survivors showed an incidence rate as high as 83%.[71] Other recent studies showed that 50% to 75% of breast cancer survivors reported persistent sexual dysfunction.[72] In patients with breast cancer with body image disturbance, 73.4% endorse sexual dysfunctions, suggesting that these women constitute a high-risk group.[73] Body image disturbance and sexual dysfunction are a significant problem for most of the patients with breast cancer and must be addressed in order to facilitate improved quality of life.

Acute Stress Disorder and Posttraumatic Stress Disorder

Acute stress disorder (ASD) and PTSD occur in response to a perceived life-threatening trauma and subsequent related symptoms including recurrent and intrusive thoughts of the experiences associated with cancer, feelings of detachment and emotional numbness, increased arousal, sudden outbursts of anger, avoidance of cancer and treatment-related stimuli, and an exaggerated startle response. These symptoms frequently occur in patients with breast cancer, especially posttreatment. Patients may describe constant concerns, nightmares about the treatment, and worries about recurrence of cancer. Acute stress is differentiated from PTSD by the duration of symptoms, which are limited to 1 month. Most of the research conducted are on PTSD.

Subthreshold symptoms are different than meeting full diagnostic criteria for ASD or PTSD, and some of the challenges in the research literature result from a lack of clarity in assessment, treatment phase, and diagnosis of symptoms or disorder. For example, a 2019 study found that greater than 90% of patients with breast cancer experienced posttraumatic stress symptoms after diagnosis, with no significant improvement until 2 years after hospital discharge.[74] However, in a study that examined full criteria for PTSD, researchers found only 2% of patients breast cancer met criteria 1 year after diagnosis.[75] Another study[76] found the prevalence of breast cancer–related PTSD diagnosis to be 8.1%, and a 2016 meta-analysis reported 9.6% of patients with breast cancer in their sample diagnosed with PTSD.[77] In a recent meta-analysis researchers reported PTSD in 10% of women and endorsed that depending on the methods and inclusion criteria of the studies, the incidence of a PTSD diagnosis after the diagnosis of breast cancer varied widely, with some studies reporting up to 32.3%.[78] Additional research report clinically significant levels of PTSD symptoms from 7.3% to 13.8% depending on the assessment and scoring criteria used.[79] In a study from 2013 on a diverse breast cancer population, researchers found that 23% reported symptoms consistent with a diagnosis of PTSD at baseline, 16.5% at first follow-up, and 12.6% at the second follow-up. Persistent PTSD was observed among 12.1% participants. Among participants without PTSD at baseline, 6.6% developed PTSD at the first follow-up interview. Younger age at diagnosis, being black, and being Asian were associated with PTSD.[80]

PSYCHOTHERAPEUTIC APPROACHES

Increased psychological screening and assessment has heightened the need for effective psychological intervention in patients with breast cancer. Women may present with multiple psychological symptoms that can be addressed at the same time. Some specialized interventions have also been developed and studied to address specific symptoms. It is important to recognize that treating one symptom, such as insomnia, may positively affect other symptoms, such as depression or anxiety. Thus, even targeted treatment approaches may impact other symptoms. Ideally, treatment is provided in an integrated system of care. Supportive services are crucial in a comprehensive cancer center and help ensure care is patient-centered and holistic.

With the growing number and types of interventions for breast cancer survivors, it can be difficult to determine which interventions are appropriate for patients. Rather than using diagnostic or medical treatment status as a guide for psychosocial treatment selection, practitioners can be guided by the patient's psychological needs, such as addressing anxiety or coping with adjusting to their bodily changes. These psychological needs can then be mapped onto relevant evidence-based psychological treatments. Interventions can be offered at any point during the course of diagnosis, treatment, and survivorship. The authors briefly review commonly used empirically based psychotherapeutic interventions with recommendations for use when appropriate (**Table 2**).

Psychoeducation

Psychological and emotional support is often given in conjunction with providing education about breast cancer, its diagnosis, treatment, and other aspects of the cancer experience. This support provides comfort, instills confidence, and reduces the stress of illness and of having to think through and decide on treatment options.[81] Given the complexity of breast cancer care, physicians often do not have the time to extensively discuss treatment options and concerns regarding those options. Psychologists and other mental health care professionals can provide additional information, directly address psychosocial concerns, and aid in the shared decision-making process. Psychoeducation is also often a component in supportive and cognitive–behavioral interventions.

Psychoeducational therapy (PET) is an interdisciplinary approach, including an educational program and a psychological intervention.[82] Research supports the efficacy of psychoeducation in improving adaptive coping strategies and quality of life, reducing depression and anxiety, and increasing treatment compliance and self-efficacy in women with breast cancer.[83]

Table 2	
Psychological interventions used in patient populations with breast cancer	
Psychological Intervention	**Definition**
Psychoeducational	Focus on providing information about illness in a social and supportive interaction
Cognitive behavioral psychotherapy	Focus on self-monitoring, behavior change, and cognitive restructuring of maladaptive thoughts and beliefs
Mindfulness-based therapy	Focus on self-regulation, present moment awareness, and acceptance of experience without judgment
Supportive-expressive therapy	Focus on social support, especially in the context of encouraging expression of emotion
Meaning-centered psychotherapy	Focus on sense of self and meaning making
Acceptance and commitment therapy	Focus on increasing psychological flexibility and acceptance

Cognitive Behavioral Therapy

Cognitive behavioral therapy (CBT) is a widely used evidence-based practice and is focused on improving coping skills and affect. It is based on a combination of the basic principles of behavioral and cognitive psychology and typically has 3 components: self-monitoring, behavior change, and cognitive restructuring of maladaptive thoughts and beliefs.

In a 2016 review, CBT approaches were shown to be effective for treatment of mood, anxiety, sleep, disorders, PTSD, sexual dysfunction and adjustment disorders, as well as treatment-related side effects in patients with breast cancer.[84] In a more recent meta-analyses, CBT was found to be effective in restructuring negative automatic cognitive schemas,[85] and increasing optimism and positive thought, which help to improve the quality of life of patients with breast cancer.[86]

CBT has been found to be effective in managing anxiety and depression,[87] insomnia,[88] fatigue,[89] and menopausal symptoms[90] and improve quality of life and self-esteem.[91] CBT has been also shown to be effective in managing physical symptoms such as pain, headache, irritable bowel syndrome, nausea, and vomiting[92] and thus may help patients with breast cancer suffering from treatment side effects.

Cognitive and Behavioral Cancer Stress Management (CBCSM) is a structured intervention focused on cancer-related stress management that has demonstrated mixed results in outcome studies with patients with breast cancer. In a recent meta-analysis, CBCSM was found to significantly increase relaxation scores, positive affect, decrease serum cortisol, anxiety, depression, thought avoidance, thought intrusion, and negative mood. However, there was no significant impact on reducing stress or mood disturbances.[93]

Mindfulness-Based Therapy

Mindfulness-based approaches focus on helping patients achieve self-regulation, present moment awareness, and acceptance of experience without judgment. These approaches are particularly appropriate for coping with loss of control, general loss, and grief. Research on such interventions shows benefits including decreased distress, improved sleep, reduced fatigue, improved mood, and reduced anxiety.[94,95] Compared with usual care, mindfulness approaches were found superior in decreasing depression and anxiety in patients with breast cancer.[96]

Mindfulness-based cancer recovery (MBCR) is a cancer-specific modification of mindfulness-based stress reduction.[97] Several MBCR clinical trials have shown efficacy in improving mood, quality of life, and reducing stress.[98,99] Recent meta-analyses provide further support for the effectiveness of mindfulness-based interventions in cancer with moderate to large effect sizes. The investigators reported significant reductions in anxiety and depression in patients receiving mindfulness-based therapy versus control treatment.[100]

Supportive-Expressive Therapy

Supportive-expressive therapy (SET) promotes social support among peers and encourages patients to express disease-related emotions and existential concerns, with a focus on facing and grieving losses.[101] The goals of the therapy include increasing support, enhancing openness and emotional expressiveness, integrating a changed self and body image into the view of self, improving coping skills and interpersonal relationships, and detoxifying feelings around death and dying. SET is based on the idea that participants learn to better cope with their cancer and feel less distressed by expressing emotions and increasing the experience of social support.

Clinical trials have examined the effects of SET on potential working mechanisms, finding a decrease in suppression of negative affect and improvements in social functioning. SET has been shown to reduce stress symptoms and improve quality of life in patients with breast cancer.[102]

Meaning-Centered Psychotherapy

Meaning-centered psychotherapy (MCP) emerged from SET and is tailored to patients with advanced cancer. Components include exploring the patient's cancer story, eliciting sense of self, impact of cancer, and exploring sources of meaning. MCP targets psychological, existential, and spiritual distress of patients with breast cancer, with demonstrated significant beneficial effects on quality of life, depression, and hopelessness.[103]

Acceptance and Commitment Therapy

Acceptance and commitment therapy (ACT) has fairly recently been studied in patients with breast cancer. It includes strategies to modify a patient's relationship with their thoughts and feelings so that they can experience them without being dominated by them. Basic ACT strategies include value clarification, commitment to engaging in value-consistent activities, and use of acceptance strategies to cope. These strategies are used to increase psychological flexibility and adaptability, which may increase acceptance of relapse and reduce fears related to breast cancer. In a 2021 study, patients with breast cancer showed significant improvement in subjective cognitive impairment, depression, anxiety, and psychological inflexibility after the ACT intervention.[104] In a recent review and meta-analysis, ACT was found to have significantly improved anxiety, depression, stress, and increased hope in patients with breast cancer.[105]

Diversity Considerations

Although evidence suggests that psychosocial interventions are beneficial for patients with breast cancer at all phases of treatment, historically, most studies have lacked diversity; thus less is known about the effectiveness in these underrepresented populations. Certain populations face unique stressors such as lack of health information, poor patient–provider communication, fearful perceptions of treatment, and distrust of the health care system. Black women are more likely to report lack of social support, greater cancer-related stigma, and poorer breast cancer–related quality of life than White women.[106] Significantly, Black women are 41% more likely to die from breast cancer than White women[106] despite a lower incidence rate. Limited research demonstrates that Black women's coping skills are improved through cognitive reframing and increased knowledge.[107] In addition, a CBT decision-making intervention showed significantly improved self-efficacy, thus enabling Black women to more comfortably engage with their health care team on treatment decisions such as chemotherapy.[107] Overall, effective interventions for diverse populations may have the greatest success when they are culturally informed, but more research is needed.

Psychopharmacologic Drugs and Breast Cancer

Psychiatric treatment holds an important place in the treatment of psychological symptoms in patients with breast cancer. Medications are commonly prescribed in the oncology setting to treat psychiatric disorders frequently exacerbated by cancer. Psychiatric disorders are serious medical conditions that can alter the course and treatment of cancer and often require psychopharmacologic interventions. These medications can also be a useful tool in treating psychiatric symptoms secondary

Table 3
Psychopharmacologic interventions used in patient populations with breast cancer[a]

Pharmacologic Drug	Targeted Symptoms
Mirtazapine	Insomnia, low appetite, nausea[b,c]
Olanzapine	Nausea/vomiting[d]
Lorazepam	Specific procedures or phobias[e]
Bupropion	Fatigue,[f] smoking cessation[g]
Duloxetine	Neuropathic pain[h]
Venlafaxine	Hot flashes[i]
Stimulants	Fatigue[j]

[a] Adapted from Elsevier.[108]
[b] Adapted from Investigational New Drugs.[109]
[c] Adapted from Psychiatry Clin Neurosci.[110]
[d] Adapted from Cochrane Database of Syst Rev.[111]
[e] Adapted from Journal of Clinical Oncology.[112]
[f] Adapted from BMC Cancer.[113]
[g] Adapted from Cancer Causes & Control.[114]
[h] Adapted from Clin J Pain.[115]
[i] Adapted from Breast Cancer Research and Treatment.[116]
[j] Adapted from Cochrane Database Syst Rev.[117]

to the cancer itself and secondary to the cancer treatment. Psychiatrists trained to prescribe to the oncology patient are preferred, as they can tailor medications to the patient, the cancer, and any current or future cancer treatments to avoid drug-drug interactions. A detailed description of appropriate medications is beyond the scope of this chapter, but in addition to treatment of any underlying psychiatric illness, some general thoughts specific to pharmacologic treatment in oncology patients are provided in **Table 3**.

SUMMARY

Breast cancer is the most common cancer in women, with about 1 in 8 women developing breast cancer in their lifetime. Many women diagnosed with breast cancer will experience some distress during their diagnosis or course of treatment or in survival. Cancer-related distress can be expected to dissipate with time for most of the women diagnosed, but in others distress may lead to significant symptoms that interfere with their psychological well-being. Such symptoms include anxiety, depression, sleep and sex disturbances, as well as cognitive disruptions and post-traumatic symptoms. Left untreated, these symptoms can lead to poor quality of life and negatively affect treatment compliance and ultimately, treatment outcome. Thus, distress and related psychological symptoms must be routinely assessed in patients with breast cancer and used to inform care. Various psychotherapeutic interventions have been demonstrated to be effective in addressing symptoms of patients with breast cancer. It is recommended that the patient's psychological needs are used to guide treatment, with specific issues or symptoms mapped onto relevant evidence-based treatments. Psychoeducation and CBT may be most helpful for reducing stress, depression, and anxiety and improving overall coping skills. Mindfulness-based therapies are particularly helpful in coping with loss of control, loss, and grief and can also reduce symptoms of depression and anxiety and improve cognitive functioning. Supportive emotional therapies and meaning-centered therapy focus on connecting with others and enhancing openness and may be most effective for improving social functioning, reducing negative affect, improving quality of life, and reducing hopelessness. ACT focuses on increasing psychological flexibility and acceptance and has promise in reducing stress, anxiety, fears, and depression. Less research has been conducted on patients of color who face unique stressors. Limited research supports the need to implement tailored culturally informed assessments and treatments to these populations. Psychiatric medications also play an important role in addressing the symptoms of this patient population and should be used in conjunction with psychosocial interactions as appropriate.

CLINICS CARE POINTS

- Patients diagnosed with breast cancer have an increased risk for depression, anxiety, cognitive impairments, sleep disruptions, and sexual dysfunction.

- Patients may go through stages of adjusting to the breast cancer diagnosis and treatments. It is important to understand that patients may display a range of emotions and behaviors over time. Do not assume that a patient's emotional response is fixed or even necessarily unhealthy.

- Transition times during diagnosis and treatment (such as diagnosis, treatment implementation, survivorship) are periods of higher risk for patients with breast cancer to experience psychological symptoms.

- Research demonstrates that addressing psychology symptoms can improve compliance with treatment and improve psychological symptoms and quality of life.

- Effective psychotherapeutic interventions are best used to match the patient's presenting symptoms and can be varied over time to address patient needs.

- Psychotropic medications are frequently helpful in addressing symptoms not helped by psychotherapy and are an important aspect of treatment.

DISCLOSURE

The authors have no financial disclosures to make and have no funding sources that supported writing this chapter.

REFERENCES

1. Siegel RL, Miller KD, Fuchs HE, et al. Cancer statistics, 2022. CA Cancer J Clin 2022;72(1):7–33.
2. Stewart BW, Wild CP, Weiderpass E, editors. World cancer report: cancer research for cancer prevention. Lyon: IARC Press; 2020. Available at: https://www.iccp-portal.org/system/files/resources/IARC%20World%20Cancer%20Report%202020.pdf.
3. Rojas K, Stuckey A. Breast cancer epidemiology and risk factors. Clin Obstet Gynecol 2016;59(4):651–72.
4. Cancer stat facts: Female breast cancer. SEER. Available at: https://seer.cancer.gov/statfacts/html/breast.html. Accessed 8 November, 2022.
5. DeSantis C, Ma J, Bryan L, et al. Breast cancer statistics, 2013. CA Cancer J Clin 2014;64(1):52–62.
6. Miller KD, Nogueira L, Devasia T, et al. Cancer treatment and survivorship statistics, 2022. CA Cancer J Clin 2022;72(5):409–36.

7. Zaker MR, Safaripour A, Sabegh SRZ, et al. Supportive intervention challenges for patients with breast cancer: A systematic review. Asian Pacific Journal of Environment and Cancer 2021;4(1). https://doi.org/10.31557/APJEC.2021.4.1. 19-24.

8. Mutebi M, Anderson BO, Duggan C, et al. Breast cancer treatment: A phased approach to implementation. Cancer 2020;126(Suppl 10):2365–78.

9. Feng Y, Spezia M, Huang S, et al. Breast cancer development and progression: Risk factors, cancer stem cells, signaling pathways, genomics, and molecular pathogenesis. Genes Dis 2018;5(2):77–106.

10. Chiriac VF, Baban A, Dumitrascu DL. Psychological stress and breast cancer incidence: a systematic review. Clujul Med 2018;91(1):18–26.

11. Dinapoli L, Colloca G, Di Capua B, et al. Psychological aspects to consider in breast cancer diagnosis and treatment. Curr Oncol Rep 2021;23(3):1–7.

12. Montgomery M, McCrone SH. Psychological distress associated with the diagnostic phase for suspected breast cancer: systematic review. J Adv Nurs 2010; 66(11):2372–90.

13. Ng CG, Mohamed S, Kaur K, et al. Perceived distress and its association with depression and anxiety in breast cancer patients. PLoS One 2017;12(3): e0172975.

14. Bower JE. Cancer-related fatigue: mechanisms, risk factors, and treatments. Nat Rev Clin Oncol 2014;11(10):597–609.

15. Nowicki A, Krzemkowska E, Rhone P. Acceptance of illness after surgery in patients with breast cancer in the early postoperative period. Pol Przegl Chir 2015; 87(11):539–50.

16. Hall DL, Antoni MH, Lattie EG, et al. Perceived fatigue interference and depressed mood: comparison of chronic fatigue syndrome/Myalgic encephalomyelitis patients with fatigued breast cancer survivors. Fatigue 2015;3(3): 142–55.

17. Schmid-Büchi S, Halfens RJG, Dassen T, et al. A review of psychosocial needs of breast-cancer patients and their relatives. J Clin Nurs 2008;17:2895–909.

18. Ganz PA. Psychological and social aspects of breast cancer. Oncology (Williston Park) 2008;22(6):642–53.

19. Andrykowski MA, Manne SL. Are psychological interventions effective and accepted by cancer patients? I. Standards and levels of evidence. Ann Behav Med 2006;32(2):93–7.

20. Institute of Medicine (US) and National Research Council (US) National Cancer Policy Board. In: Hewitt M, Herdman R, Holland J, editors. Meeting psychosocial needs of women with breast cancer. Washington (DC): National Academies Press (US); 2004.

21. Moyer A. Psychosocial outcomes of breast-conserving surgery versus mastectomy: a meta-analytic review [published correction appears in Health Psychol 1997 Sep;16(5):442]. Health Psychol 1997;16(3):284–98.

22. Izawa H, Karasawa K, Kawase E, et al. The assessment of anxiety about radiotherapy in patient with early breast cancer receiving breast irradiation. Int J Radiat Oncol Biol Phys 2007;69(3):S589–90.

23. Costanzo ES, Lutgendorf SK, Mattes ML, et al. Adjusting to life after treatment: distress and quality of life following treatment for breast cancer. Br J Cancer 2007;97(12):1625–31.

24. Hack TF, Pickles T, Ruether JD, et al. Predictors of distress and quality of life in patients undergoing cancer therapy: impact of treatment type and decisional role. Psycho Oncol 2010;19(6):606–16.

25. Gibbons A, Groarke A. Coping with chemotherapy for breast cancer: Asking women what works. Eur J Oncol Nurs 2018;35:85–91.

26. Smith HR. Depression in cancer patients: Pathogenesis, implications and treatment (Review). Oncol Lett 2015;9(4):1509–14.

27. Satin JR, Linden W, Phillips MJ. Depression as a predictor of disease progression and mortality in cancer patients: a meta-analysis. Cancer 2009;115(22): 5349–61.

28. Giese-Davis J, Collie K, Rancourt KM, et al. Decrease in depression symptoms is associated with longer survival in patients with metastatic breast cancer: a secondary analysis. J Clin Oncol 2011;29(4):413–20.

29. Hardman A, Maguire P, Crowther D. The recognition of psychiatric morbidity on a medical oncology ward. J Psychosom Res 1989;33(2):235–9.

30. Blaschke TF, Osterberg L, Vrijens B, et al. Adherence to medications: insights arising from studies on the unreliable link between prescribed and actual drug dosing histories. Annu Rev Pharmacol Toxicol 2012;52:275–301.

31. Andrykowski MA, Lykins E, Floyd A. Psychological health in cancer survivors. Semin Oncol Nurs 2008;24(3):193–201.

32. Adler NE, Page AEK, Institute of Medicine (US), Committee on Psychosocial Services to Cancer Patients/Families in a Community Setting. Cancer care for the Whole patient: meeting psychosocial health needs. Washington (DC): National Academies Press (US); 2008.

33. McEvoy MD, McCorkle R. Quality of life issues in patients with disseminated breast cancer. Cancer 1990;66(6 Suppl):1416–21.

34. Cella DF, Bonomi AE, Lloyd SR, et al. Reliability and validity of the Functional Assessment of Cancer Therapy-Lung (FACT-L) quality of life instrument. Lung Cancer 1995;12(3):199–220.

35. Mandelblatt JS, Eisenberg JM. Historical and methodological perspectives on cancer outcomes research. Oncology (Williston Park) 1995;9(11 Suppl):23–32.

36. Ownby KK. Use of the distress thermometer in clinical practice. J Adv Pract Oncol 2019;10(2):175–9.

37. Stern AF. The hospital anxiety and depression scale. Occup Med (Lond) 2014; 64(5):393–4.

38. Zhou K, Li M, Wang W, et al. Reliability, validity, and sensitivity of the Chinese Short-Form 36 Health Survey version 2 (SF-36v2) in women with breast cancer. J Eval Clin Pract 2019;25(5):864–72.

39. Calderon C, Ferrando PJ, Lorenzo-Seva U, et al. Factor structure and measurement invariance of the Brief Symptom Inventory (BSI-18) in cancer patients. Int J Clin Health Psychol 2020;20(1):71–80.

40. Schag CA, Ganz PA, Heinrich RL. CAncer Rehabilitation Evaluation System–short form (CARES-SF). A cancer specific rehabilitation and quality of life instrument. Cancer 1991;68(6):1406–13.

41. Brady MJ, Cella DF, Mo F, et al. Reliability and validity of the Functional Assessment of Cancer Therapy-Breast quality-of-life instrument. J Clin Oncol 1997; 15(3):974–86.

42. Levine MN, Guyatt GH, Gent M, et al. Quality of life in stage II breast cancer: an instrument for clinical trials. J Clin Oncol 1988;6(12):1798–810.

43. Adeyemi OJ, Gill TL, Paul R, et al. Evaluating the association of self-reported psychological distress and self-rated health on survival times among women with breast cancer in the U.S. PLoS One 2021;16(12):e0260481.

44. Tang HY, Xiong HH, Deng LC, et al. Adjustment Disorder in Female Breast Cancer Patients: Prevalence and Its Accessory Symptoms. Curr Med Sci 2020; 40(3):510–7.

45. Wijnhoven LMA, Custers JAE, Kwakkenbos L, et al. Trajectories of adjustment disorder symptoms in post-treatment breast cancer survivors. Support Care Cancer 2022;30(4):3521–30.

46. Saboonchi F, Petersson LM, Wennman-Larsen A, et al. Changes in caseness of anxiety and depression in breast cancer patients during the first year following surgery: patterns of transiency and severity of the distress response. Eur J Oncol Nurs 2014;18(6):598–604.

47. Cui Q, Cai Z, Li J, et al. The Psychological Pressures of Breast Cancer Patients During the COVID-19 Outbreak in China-A Comparison With Frontline Female Nurses. Front Psychiatry 2020;11:559701.

48. Burgess C, Cornelius V, Love S, et al. Depression and anxiety in women with early breast cancer: five year observational cohort study. BMJ 2005; 330(7493):702.

49. Maass SW, Roorda C, Berendsen AJ, et al. The prevalence of long-term symptoms of depression and anxiety after breast cancer treatment: A systematic review. Maturitas 2015;82(1):100–8.

50. Avis NE, Levine BJ, Case LD, et al. Trajectories of depressive symptoms following breast cancer diagnosis. Cancer Epidemiol Biomarkers Prev 2015; 24(11):1789–95.

51. Walker LG, Heys SD, Walker MB, et al. Psychological factors can predict the response to primary chemotherapy in patients with locally advanced breast cancer. Eur J Cancer 1999;35(13):1783–8.

52. Boing L, Pereira GS, Araújo CDCR, et al. Factors associated with depression symptoms in women after breast cancer. Rev Saude Publica 2019;53:30.

53. Denieffe S, Gooney M. A meta-synthesis of women's symptoms experience and breast cancer. Eur J Cancer Care 2011;20(4):424–35.

54. Cohee AA, Adams RN, Fife BL, et al. Relationship Between Depressive Symptoms and Social Cognitive Processing in Partners of Long-Term Breast Cancer Survivors. Oncol Nurs Forum 2017;44(1):44–51.

55. Van Dyk K, Ganz PA. Cancer-Related Cognitive Impairment in Patients With a History of Breast Cancer. JAMA 2021;326(17):1736–7.

56. Buchanan ND, Dasari S, Rodriguez JL, et al. Post-treatment Neurocognition and Psychosocial Care Among Breast Cancer Survivors. Am J Prev Med 2015;49(6 Suppl 5):S498–508.

57. Janelsins MC, Heckler CE, Peppone LJ, et al. Cognitive complaints in survivors of breast cancer after chemotherapy compared with age-matched controls: An analysis from a nationwide, multicenter, prospective longitudinal study. J Clin Oncol 2017;35(5):506–14.

58. Vardy J. Cognitive function in breast cancer survivors. Cancer Treat Res 2009; 151:387–419.

59. Lange M, Giffard B, Noal S, et al. Baseline cognitive functions among elderly patients with localised breast cancer. Eur J Cancer 2014;50(13):2181–9.

60. Hurria A, Somlo G, Ahles T. Renaming "chemobrain. Cancer Invest 2007;25(6): 373–7.

61. Weng YP, Hong RM, Chen VC, et al. Sleep quality and related factors in patients with breast cancer: A cross-sectional study in Taiwan. Cancer Manag Res 2021; 13:4725–33.

62. Simeit R, Deck R, Conta-Marx B. Sleep management training for cancer patients with insomnia. Support Care Cancer 2004;12(3):176–83.
63. Bardwell WA, Profant J, Casden DR, et al. The relative importance of specific risk factors for insomnia in women treated for early-stage breast cancer. Psycho Oncol 2008;17(1):9–18.
64. Savard J, Simard S, Blanchet J, et al. Prevalence, clinical characteristics, and risk factors for insomnia in the context of breast cancer. Sleep 2001;24(5):583–90.
65. Esplen MJ, Wong J, Warner E, et al. Restoring body image after cancer (ReBIC): Results of a randomized controlled trial. J Clin Oncol 2018;36(8):749–56.
66. Thakur M, Sharma R, Mishra AK, et al. Psychological distress and body image disturbances after modified radical mastectomy among breast cancer survivors: A cross-sectional study from a tertiary care centre in North India. Lancet Regional Health-Southeast Asia 2022;7(100077). https://doi.org/10.1016/j.lansea.2022.100077.
67. Guedes TSR, Dantas de Oliveira NP, Holanda AM, et al. Body image of women submitted to breast cancer treatment. Asian Pac J Cancer Prev 2018;19(6):1487–93.
68. Fobair P, Stewart SL, Chang S, et al. Body image and sexual problems in young women with breast cancer. Psycho Oncol 2006;15(7):579–94.
69. Fang SY, Lin YC, Chen TC, et al. Impact of marital coping on the relationship between body image and sexuality among breast cancer survivors. Support Care Cancer 2015;23(9):2551–9.
70. Esmat Hosseini S, Ilkhani M, Rohani C, et al. Prevalence of sexual dysfunction in women with cancer: A systematic review and meta-analysis. Int J Reprod Biomed 2022;20(1):1–12.
71. Qi A, Li Y, Sun H, et al. Incidence and risk factors of sexual dysfunction in young breast cancer survivors. Ann Palliat Med 2021;10(4):4428–34.
72. Ljungman L, Ahlgren J, Petersson LM, et al. Sexual dysfunction and reproductive concerns in young women with breast cancer: Type, prevalence, and predictors of problems. Psycho Oncol 2018;27(12):2770–7.
73. Jing L, Zhang C, Li W, et al. Incidence and severity of sexual dysfunction among women with breast cancer: a meta-analysis based on female sexual function index. Support Care Cancer 2019;27(4):1171–80.
74. Oliveri S, Arnaboldi P, Pizzoli SFM, et al. PTSD symptom clusters associated with short- and long-term adjustment in early diagnosed breast cancer patients. Ecancermedicalscience 2019;13:917.
75. Swartzman S, Booth JN, Munro A, et al. Posttraumatic stress disorder after cancer diagnosis in adults: A meta-analysis. Depress Anxiety 2017;34(4):327–39.
76. Carletto S, Porcaro C, Settanta C, et al. Neurobiological features and response to eye movement desensitization and reprocessing treatment of posttraumatic stress disorder in patients with breast cancer. Eur J Psychotraumatol 2019;10(1):1600832.
77. Wu X, Wang J, Cofie R, et al. Prevalence of posttraumatic stress disorder among breast cancer patients: A meta-analysis. Iran J Public Health 2016;45(12):1533–44.
78. Brown LC, Murphy AR, Lalonde CS, et al. Posttraumatic stress disorder and breast cancer: Risk factors and the role of inflammation and endocrine function. Cancer 2020;126(14):3181–91.
79. Bulotiene G, Matuiziene M. Posttraumatic stress in breast cancer patients. Acta Med Litu 2014;21(2):43–50.

80. Vin-Raviv N, Hillyer GC, Hershman DL, et al. Racial disparities in posttraumatic stress after diagnosis of localized breast cancer: the BQUAL study. J Natl Cancer Inst 2013;105(8):563–72.

81. Fawzy FI, Fawzy NW, Arndt LA, et al. Critical review of psychosocial interventions in cancer care. Arch Gen Psychiatry 1995;52(2):100–13.

82. Cipolletta S, Simonato C, Faccio E. The effectiveness of psychoeducational support groups for women with breast cancer and their caregivers: A mixed methods study. Front Psychol 2019;10:288.

83. Dolbeault S, Cayrou S, Brédart A, et al. The effectiveness of a psychoeducational group after early-stage breast cancer treatment: results of a randomized French study. Psycho Oncol 2009;18(6):647–56.

84. Zhang J, Xu R, Wang B, et al. Effects of mindfulness-based therapy for patients with breast cancer: A systematic review and meta-analysis. Complement Ther Med 2016;26:1–10.

85. Getu MA, Chen C, Panpan W, et al. The effect of cognitive behavioral therapy on the quality of life of breast cancer patients: a systematic review and meta-analysis of randomized controlled trials [published correction appears in Qual Life Res. 2022 Oct;31(10):3089]. Qual Life Res 2021;30(2):367–84.

86. Stagl JM, Bouchard LC, Lechner SC, et al. Long-term psychological benefits of cognitive-behavioral stress management for women with breast cancer: 11-year follow-up of a randomized controlled trial. Cancer 2015;121(11):1873–81.

87. Ren W, Qiu H, Yang Y, et al. Randomized controlled trial of cognitive behavioural therapy for depressive and anxiety symptoms in Chinese women with breast cancer. Psychiatry Res 2019;271:52–9.

88. Aricò D, Raggi A, Ferri R. Cognitive behavioral therapy for insomnia in breast cancer survivors: A review of the literature. Front Psychol 2016;7:1162.

89. Abrahams HJG, Gielissen MFM, Donders RRT, et al. The efficacy of Internet-based cognitive behavioral therapy for severely fatigued survivors of breast cancer compared with care as usual: A randomized controlled trial. Cancer 2017;123(19):3825–34.

90. Hunter MS, Coventry S, Hamed H, et al. Evaluation of a group cognitive behavioural intervention for women suffering from menopausal symptoms following breast cancer treatment. Psycho Oncol 2009;18(5):560–3.

91. Wojtyna E, Jolanta Ż, Patrycja S. The influence of cognitive-behaviour therapy on quality of life and self-esteem in women suffering from breast cancer. Rep Practical Oncol Radiother 2007;12(2):109–17.

92. Gielissen MF, Verhagen S, Witjes F, et al. Effects of cognitive behavior therapy in severely fatigued disease-free cancer patients compared with patients waiting for cognitive behavior therapy: a randomized controlled trial. J Clin Oncol 2006;24(30):4882–7.

93. Tang M, Liu X, Wu Q, et al. The effects of cognitive-behavioral stress management for breast cancer patients: A systematic review and meta-analysis of randomized controlled trials. Cancer Nurs 2020;43(3):222–37.

94. Cillessen L, Johannsen M, Speckens AEM, et al. Mindfulness-based interventions for psychological and physical health outcomes in cancer patients and survivors: A systematic review and meta-analysis of randomized controlled trials. Psycho Oncol 2019;28(12):2257–69.

95. Xunlin NG, Lau Y, Klainin-Yobas P. The effectiveness of mindfulness-based interventions among cancer patients and survivors: a systematic review and meta-analysis. Support Care Cancer 2020;28(4):1563–78.

96. Cramer H, Lauche R, Paul A, et al. Mindfulness-based stress reduction for breast cancer-a systematic review and meta-analysis. Curr Oncol 2012;19(5): e343–52.

97. Carlson LE, Speca M. Mindfulness-based cancer Recovery: a Step-by-Step MBSR approach to help you cope with treatment and reclaim your life. New Harbinger, Oakland, CA; 2010.

98. Johannsen M, O'Connor M, O'Toole MS, et al. Efficacy of mindfulness-based cognitive therapy on late post-treatment pain in women treated for primary breast cancer: A randomized controlled trial. J Clin Oncol 2016;34(28):3390–9.

99. Lengacher CA, Reich RR, Paterson CL, et al. Examination of broad symptom improvement resulting from mindfulness-based stress reduction in breast cancer survivors: A randomized controlled trial. J Clin Oncol 2016;34(24):2827–34.

100. Zhang MF, Wen YS, Liu WY, et al. Effectiveness of mindfulness-based therapy for reducing anxiety and depression in patients with cancer: A meta-analysis. Medicine (Baltim) 2015;94(45):e0897.

101. Classen CC, Kraemer HC, Blasey C, et al. Supportive-expressive group therapy for primary breast cancer patients: a randomized prospective multicenter trial. Psycho Oncol 2008;17(5):438–47.

102. Kissane DW, Grabsch B, Clarke DM, et al. Supportive-expressive group therapy for women with metastatic breast cancer: survival and psychosocial outcome from a randomized controlled trial. Psycho Oncol 2007;16(4):277–86.

103. Lichtenthal WG, Roberts KE, Pessin H, et al. Meaning-Centered Psychotherapy and cancer: Finding meaning in the face of suffering. Psychiatr Times 2020; 37(8):23–5.

104. Shari NI, Zainal NZ, Ng CG. Effects of brief acceptance and commitment therapy (ACT) on subjective cognitive impairment in breast cancer patients undergoing chemotherapy. J Psychosoc Oncol 2021;39(6):695–714.

105. Li H, Wu J, Ni Q, et al. Systematic review and meta-analysis of effectiveness of acceptance and commitment therapy in patients with breast cancer. Nurs Res 2021;70(4):E152–60.

106. Whitehead NE, Hearn LE. Psychosocial interventions addressing the needs of Black women diagnosed with breast cancer: a review of the current landscape. Psycho Oncol 2015;24(5):497–507.

107. Sheppard VB, Wallington SF, Willey SC, et al. A peer-led decision support intervention improves decision outcomes in black women with breast cancer. J Cancer Educ 2013;28(2):262–9.

108. Stern TA, Rosenbaum JF, Fricchione GL, et al. Massachusetts general hospital handbook of general hospital Psychiatry. 7th edition. Philadelphia: Elsevier; 2018.

109. Cao J, Ouyang Q, Wang S, et al. Mirtazapine, a dopamine receptor inhibitor, as a secondary prophylactic for delayed nausea and vomiting following highly emetogenic chemotherapy: An open label, randomized, Multicenter Phase III trial. Invest N Drugs 2020;38(2):507–14.

110. Kim SW, Shin IS, Kim JM, et al. Effectiveness of mirtazapine for nausea and insomnia in cancer patients with depression. Psychiatry Clin Neurosci 2008; 62(1):75–83.

111. Sutherland A, Naessens K, Plugge E, et al. Olanzapine for the prevention and treatment of cancer-related nausea and vomiting in adults. Cochrane Database Syst Rev 2018;2018(9). https://doi.org/10.1002/14651858.cd012555.pub2.

112. Traeger L, Greer JA, Fernandez-Robles C, et al. Evidence-based treatment of anxiety in patients with cancer. J Clin Oncol 2012;30(11):1197–205.

113. Salehifar E, Azimi S, Janbabai G, et al. Efficacy and safety of bupropion in cancer-related fatigue, a randomized double blind placebo controlled clinical trial. BMC Cancer 2020;20(1). https://doi.org/10.1186/s12885-020-6618-9.
114. Schnoll RA, Martinez E, Tatum KL, et al. A bupropion smoking cessation clinical trial for cancer patients. Cancer Causes & Control 2010;21(6):811–20.
115. Guan J, Tanaka S, Kawakami K. Anticonvulsants or antidepressants in combination pharmacotherapy for treatment of neuropathic pain in cancer patients: a systematic review and meta-analysis. Clin J Pain 2016;32(8):719–25.
116. Ramaswami R, Villarreal MD, Pitta DM, et al. Venlafaxine in management of hot flashes in women with breast cancer: A systematic review and meta-analysis. Breast Cancer Res Treat 2015;152(2):231237.
117. Minton O, Richardson A, Sharpe M, et al. Drug therapy for the management of cancer related fatigue. Cochrane Database Syst Rev 2010;7:CD006704.

Racial/Ethnic Disparities and Women's Mental Health

Considerations for Providing Culturally Sensitive Care

Nina Ballone, MD, Erica Richards, MD, PhD*

KEYWORDS

- Minority • Black women • Underrepresented • Ethnicity • Culturally sensitive
- Mental health

KEY POINTS

- Racial and ethnic underrepresented minority women are more likely to experience a mental health diagnosis but less likely to receive treatment.
- Mental health providers have a duty to educate themselves on how to provide culturally sensitive care to all women.
- Community resources including churches and service providers provide additional opportunities for mental health outreach.

INTRODUCTION

Women are roughly twice as likely to be diagnosed with depression compared with men. When discussing the topic of women's mental health, there are many considerations that clinicians should incorporate when attempting to provide the best care for their patients. Once gender differences are addressed, it is then necessary to consider other contributing factors, including the role of racial and ethnic disparities and how these factors influence diagnosis and treatment outcomes. Understanding these differences and actively trying to change the circumstances underlying disparities in the mental health realm should be a goal of every provider seeking to make a positive impact in their patient's lives.

Before talking about racial and ethnic disparities, it is first important to start with a basic understanding of why women are more likely to experience a mood or anxiety disorder during their lifetime. The reasons that women are more likely than men to experience depression are multifactorial. Psychosocial stressors including differences

Department of Psychiatry and Behavioral Sciences, Johns Hopkins University, 600 North Wolfe Street, Baltimore, MD 21205, USA
* Corresponding author. Sibley Memorial Hospital/Johns Hopkins Medicine, 5255 Loughboro Road, NW, Building C, Room 708, Washington, DC 20016.
E-mail address: ericha25@jhmi.edu

Psychiatr Clin N Am 46 (2023) 571–582
https://doi.org/10.1016/j.psc.2023.04.011
0193-953X/23/© 2023 Elsevier Inc. All rights reserved.

psych.theclinics.com

in socioeconomic status, education, and abuse are known contributors to elevated rates of depression in women.[1] In addition, there are biological factors that play a role in the disproportionate development of mood symptoms in women. Puberty and menopause mark the beginning and the end of the female reproductive cycle. These hormonal transitions correlate with the gender gap of increased prevalence of mood disorders seen in women compared with men.[2] Many factors likely contribute to this, including, but not limited to, endocrine and inflammatory processes during different stages of the reproductive cycle, societal and individual stresses, and individual vulnerability.[3]

Although it is important to note that biological sex differences play a significant role in the development of depression (highlighted by studies that show similar rates of depression in prepubertal sexes[4]), it is at least equally important to enhance our understanding of the influence of other contributing factors including race and ethnicity on the development and treatment of mood disorders.

Accurately defining the terms "race" and "ethnicity" is imperative before reviewing the health literature because it enhances the ability of providers to understand important discussion points. Specifically, it empowers clinicians to join the discussion about potential techniques to implement when delivering culturally competent mental health care. The social constructs of race and ethnicity are not bound to any scientific or biological meaning and have continued to evolve. Race often refers to a group of people with a connection made from common ancestral origin with associated common physical features. Ethnicity, on the other hand, is defined by a group of people with common cultural traditions, language, or religion. Associations between health outcomes and race and ethnicity are reported throughout many disciplines of medicine; however, gaining a better understanding for what drives these differences in health outcomes may help guide us as mental health professionals in providing competent and high-quality health care.[5] Within the literature reported, frameworks developed by the National Institute of Minority Health and Health Disparities (NIMHD) describes the complexities of health disparities defined as a difference in health that negatively effects what is determined to be a racial or ethnic minority populations including Blacks/African Americans, Hispanics/Latinos, Asians, American Indians/Alaska Natives, and Native Hawaiians or other Pacific Islanders.[6]

This article seeks to provide insight into the effects of racial and ethnic disparities on women's mental health including statistics regarding how likely women are to be affected by a mental health disorder and new considerations for providers interested in continuing their education related to treating diverse patient populations. It does not provide a "one-size-fits-all" approach to caring for women of color. Instead, it continues a conversation that is, finally, starting to gain momentum in the field and contributes additional thoughts for mental health professionals who seek to enhance their ability to provide culturally sensitive care. To provide a fuller picture of the life of racial and ethnic minorities, this discussion will start at the "beginning," looking at factors that might negatively affect mental health during infancy and pediatric years. Traveling through the reproductive life cycle of a woman will highlight additional factors, some hormonal and others related to the effects of race and culture that also warrant consideration. Finally, aging also presents its own unique issues related to the mental health of women of color.

PART I: PEDIATRIC CONSIDERATIONS

Rates of new-onset mental health diagnoses are the same for both sexes before puberty. Nevertheless, it is important to examine other factors that predispose women of color to poor outcomes, even if they predate the influence of biological hormonal influences. As recently as 2020, studies showed that infant mortality rates were nearly twice as high in Black babies compared with white babies. Reasons for this disparity are multifactorial, including access to care, location of services, and race of physician caring for the newborn.[7] Babies born to women of color are more likely to have low birth weight, be preterm, and have higher rates of infant mortality.[8] Outcomes of those that require care in the neonatal intensive care unit are also influenced by unequal access to care.[9] This impaired access to appropriate care predates mental health concerns but disparities in mental health care for the infant but not for the parents worried about the health of their newborn, contributing to additional psychosocial stressors in environmental influences.

Disproportionate access to care is often seen in early childhood, with untreated mental health concerns resulting in worsening social functioning and integration. Surveys have assessed that minority groups, specifically African American and Latino youth, have lower rates of mental health utilization compared with non-Latino white youths. Even when access to care is more readily available, minority youth are undertreated.[10] Most concerning regarding these missed opportunities to treat these populations is the fact that suicide is the second leading cause of death for youths between ages 12 and 19 years. Suicide attempts between 1991 and 2019 have increased by 22.5% in adolescents with a disproportionate increase seen among Black adolescents relative to other racial and ethnic groups. Black and American Indian/Alaska Native women showed an increase in prevalence of suicidal ideation during that same age range compared with other female groups that showed overall decreasing rates.[11] Although more adolescent boys die by suicide, in the United States, adolescent girls are almost twice as likely to report suicidal ideation. Suicidal thoughts and behaviors increase significantly during the onset of puberty, with adolescent girls reporting more thoughts compared with boys.[12] Differences seen in adolescent girls have raised the possibility for hormone sensitivity during puberty development and the menstrual cycle, predisposing some girls to experience emotional, physical, and behavioral symptoms including increased suicidal thoughts. Some identified risk factors for girls who experience increased suicidal thoughts and behaviors during the premenstrual period include earlier age of menarche and early adverse life events.[13]

In addition to identifying youths who are at risk of mental health diagnoses and suicide, adolescence is an ideal opportunity to introduce and educate about sexual health care to include contraception, sexually transmitted disease prevention, and the discussion of family planning.[14] Unplanned pregnancy occurs most often in African American and Hispanic women compared with non-Hispanic white women in the United States and has been associated with delayed prenatal care, low birth weight, and prematurity.[15] Access to reproductive health care and education has been less reported and less available in nonwhite youths, with some factors including structural barriers, family influence such as religious beliefs against contraception, distrust in providers, and implicit bias among providers themselves.[14] With this known discrepancy in the number of unintended pregnancy and barriers for accessing contraception care, the recent overturning of *Roe v. Wade* puts these already at-risk women at a higher risk of negative maternal health outcomes and adds another level of barriers for reproductive health care.[16]

Discussions related to challenges with conception have historically been taboo in communities of color; this too has been associated with stigma, often leading to mood symptoms and social isolation for women facing these obstacles. Although options such as adoption, fertility assistance, and surrogacy have been around for decades, women of color have been slower to pursue these options. Now, they are more readily talking about assisted reproductive technology including oocyte cryopreservation (egg freezing) and in vitro fertilization (IVF). However, Black women have lower live birth rates following IVF compared with white women, which creates additional mental health needs for this population.[17,18] Not every woman of color wants to be a mother but that too can be met with stigma. The mental health issues surrounding very personal reproductive decisions for women of color remain pertinent to consider when efforts are made to develop effective therapeutic interventions designed to enhance delivery of culturally competent care.

PART II: PREGNANCY AND POSTPARTUM

Nearly 30% of all pregnant women experience depressive symptoms or anxiety.[19,20] These rates are higher in women of color.[21] If left untreated, depression and anxiety throughout pregnancy have been associated with multiple adverse outcomes for both mother and baby, including, but not limited to, lack of medical care, poor nutrition, preterm birth, low birth weight, smoking, substance use, increased risk of postpartum mood or anxiety disorders, suicide, and infanticide.[22] Postpartum depression is the most common mental health diagnosis that occurs within the first 1 year after delivery, with the average prevalence close to 20%. Untreated postpartum depression may have negative consequences such as mother-baby bonding, mother's quality of life and relationships, father's mental health, and children's emotional and behavioral development.[23] In a study screening mothers for early postpartum depression symptoms at 2 weeks, 46.8% of Hispanic mothers and 43.9% of Black mothers reported symptoms consistent with postpartum depression compared with 31% of white mothers. These differences in depressive symptoms remained true after controlling for other demographics and social factors such as age, marital status, delivery type, education, parity, and history of depression.[24]

Screening mothers during their first postpartum visit is an opportunity to identify symptoms of postpartum depression and anxiety that may prompt an appropriate referral. Despite the differences in prevalence of postpartum depression and anxiety symptoms among different racial and ethnic backgrounds, minority women have been shown to be less likely to consult with a provider about mental health symptoms compared with white mothers. Understanding differences in seeking consultation in a formal medical setting is, most likely, multifactorial and unique. However, these disparities often depend on a mom's cultural background, including differences such as cultural beliefs, language barriers, distrust of providers, discrimination during prior encounters, stigma of mental health care, health literacy, insurance limitations, and the preference to seek informal supports such as that through family, friends, and other members of the community.[23]

Despite implementing standardized screening tools during prenatal care, differences remain in self-reporting of symptoms, leading to missed opportunities for referring and treating women with psychiatric diagnoses during the peripartum period. Current screening for perinatal and postpartum mood and anxiety disorders typically uses the Edinburgh Postnatal Depression Scale (EPDS); however, self-reporting of symptoms across different backgrounds has shown some differences, likely at least partially based on racial and ethnic differences. In a large sample of postpartum mothers, Hispanic women, compared with non-Hispanic or African American subgroups, reported a different cluster of symptoms including general distress and feeling overwhelmed that may not be represented fully on the EPDS with limited items that specifically address postpartum anxiety. The occurrence of perinatal and postpartum mood and anxiety disorders is not equally distributed across different backgrounds. Mothers who are younger in age, have a trauma background, and who have a lower socioeconomic status have higher rates of postpartum mood and anxiety disorders. In addition, non-Hispanic white mothers are reported to have a lower prevalence of postpartum depression.[25]

Implicit bias developed through early life experiences through reinforcement of stereotypes and structural discrimination is an unconscious thought or belief that may influence attitudes, understanding, and actions toward others. Data suggest that implicit bias negatively affects the quality of care for patients by influencing medical decision-making and patient-provider communication. Within maternal health care, the rates of cesarean section deliveries are higher among Hispanic and African American women known to be associated with increased risks of adverse health outcomes for both mom and baby. Another example of implicit bias in maternal health care is the false belief regarding differences in African American mothers and increased pain tolerance causing patients to be undertreated for pain. Providers with a high implicit bias often demonstrate a condescending tone, higher verbal dominance, and unsatisfactory care for mothers who are Hispanic and African American compared with white mothers. Negative consequences of differences seen with medical decision-making and communication are associated with higher rates of traumatic births or mistreatment seen in 30% of Hispanic and African American women compared with 21% of white women. The increased rates of preeclampsia and hypertension associated with poor birth outcomes in nonwhite populations of women is partly thought to be related to feeling dismissed, resulting in minimizing symptoms and delaying interventions.[26] These factors have the potential to contribute to mental health issues in women of color during their reproductive years.

Despite increased rates of perinatal depression and anxiety in nonwhite pregnant women, studies have demonstrated that African American, Hispanic, and other non-Hispanic nonwhite women are significantly less likely to receive treatment of peripartum mental health symptoms, including medication management. Taking prescription medications for mental health treatment is often regarded as unacceptable based on cultural values but, provider bias may also exist, resulting in undertreatment of racial/ethnic minority pregnant patients (also presenting the possibility that white pregnant patients are overtreated in some instances).[27] Becoming better versed in implicit biases and how potential rates of illness differ based on racial and cultural considerations will empower providers to better meet the needs of all patients.

PART III: MENOPAUSE TRANSITIONS

The average age of menopause is 52 years, providing another unique cohort of patients to consider for mental health outreach. Similar to other generations, minority geriatric populations are less likely to seek mental health care.[28] When discussing menopause, African American women report more positive attitudes toward this change in life when compared with Hispanic, white, Japanese, or Chinese women.[29] There may be differences between menopause symptoms among different racial and ethnic backgrounds, which prompt these attitudes toward menopause such as vasomotor, urogenital, affective, and somatic symptoms. African American women have as high as an 8-fold increase of earlier onset of menopause compared with other races and ethnicities when controlling for women with irregular menstrual cycles. They are also 1.5 times more likely to experience vasomotor symptoms associated with menopause. Across all populations, risk factors that predispose some women to depressive symptoms during the menopause transition include a preexisting history of depression, premenstrual mood changes, poor sleep, hot flashes, and elevated follicle-stimulating hormone levels. Even after controlling for these known risk factors, African American women are twice as likely to experience depression symptoms during the transition to menopause compared with non-Hispanic white women. Another survey found that Hispanic women reported a higher prevalence of mood changes, low energy, cognitive changes, vaginal dryness, and palpitations compared with non-Hispanic postmenopausal white women.

Understanding differences in individual symptoms during menopause may help to guide symptomatic treatment considerations including medications, creams, and patches. Despite higher rates of mood symptoms during the menopause transition, African American and Hispanic women are less likely to use hormone replacement therapy compared with non-Hispanic white women and are more often interested in complementary and alternative options.[30] Some themes identified in the personalized choice to take a medication during the menopause transition include seeking formal versus informal advice, viewing medication as either the first choice versus the last resort, targeting specific symptoms versus a holistic approach, and the idea of optimizing nutrition therapy. Non-Hispanic white women were more likely to seek advice in formal settings from physicians, take prescription medications to alleviate specific symptoms, and avoid trigger foods compared with other racial and ethnic populations who more often preferred to seek guidance from family and friends, viewed medications as a last resort, and approached managing symptoms preferably through mind-body interventions and optimizing nutrition.[31] Although each of these interventions may be appropriate for individual patients, being well versed in the options and why certain groups seek and select specific treatments is an important skillset required for providers caring for patients from diverse racial and ethnic backgrounds.

PART IV: ADDRESSING DISPARITIES AND TREATMENT CONSIDERATIONS
Identifying Stigma

Forty-six percent of adults in the United States experience at least one mental illness over their lifetime. In racial and ethnic minority groups in the United States, stigma is often one of the barriers to receiving care.[32] Stigma is often considered a discrediting aspect that may include negative beliefs and actions. It can be categorized into public stigma, self-stigma, and structural stigma, all inhibiting access to care for diverse populations. Culture may influence stigma with mental illness such that individuals may view mental illness as a detrimental quality, and the care of mental illness itself, including medication management, may be viewed as harmful. Across all racial and ethnic minority groups, public stigma was elevated compared with white Americans. Additional studies have found differences with self-stigma as being higher in Asian Americans, Latinx Americans, and Black Americans compared with white Americans. Structural stigma was identified as the result of lack of access and impaired quality of care in addressing specific cultural needs. It also includes ongoing racism, family influence of past experiences, unique values based on views pertaining to mental health treatment from cultural stereotypes, and negative outlooks on having a mental illness such that it may be perceived as a weakness and shameful.[33] One way to reduce stigma is to increase numbers of minorities trained and available to provide mental health care to women of color. Women from underrepresented racial and ethnic groups express an interest in receiving treatment from other women of color. However, within psychiatry, women and underrepresented minorities have less representation than expected based on overall numbers in the US population[34]; this has also been highlighted as an issue in aging populations where minorities are less likely to enroll in palliative care and hospice options.[35] Both stigma and access to culturally sensitive care create barriers to mental health treatment, even before actual treatment options can be discussed.

Conventional Treatments and Novel Therapeutics

When discussing treatment options, it is typical to discuss both medication management and therapy, realizing that at times both are supported to provide the best outcomes, whereas some will opt for one or the other treatment modality alone. Ethnic minorities are less likely to initiate treatment compared with their white counterparts.[36] Disparities in access to mental health care have been widely identified,[37] and for many ethnic minority groups, there is a stigma associated with seeking access to mental health.[38] For example, Black women diagnosed with depression in the peripartum period are less likely to accept recommended interventions including therapy or medications. Although there are a host of nonpharmacologic interventions available to pregnant woman,[39] it is important that a goals-of-care discussion be held between the patient and the provider to help determine which options are best in each circumstance. If medications are deemed necessary, women of color should receive a detailed discussion about options including side-effect profiles. Although medication management options have not changed much over the last few decades, it is also important to acknowledge that we still do not know a lot about efficacy and side effects from a race/cultural perspective, as inclusion of people of color in research studies continues to fall behind their white counterparts; this remains true for novel therapeutics such as the recently Food and Drug Administration–approved brexanolone, a 60-hour infusion targeting treatment of postpartum depression and esketamine, an intranasally administered medication used in patients with treatment-resistant depression. Although inclusion of people of color has increased over time, they remain underrepresented in demographics of subjects included in these studies. Transcranial magnetic stimulation (TMS) has also been shown to be an effective treatment of patients with major depressive disorder who have not responded to antidepressant treatment or cannot tolerate side effects associated with medication management. To date, little remains known about differences in response based on gender and race.

Even more telling is an understanding of the cultural nuances to consider when offering specific services. One example is the cap used as part of the treatment of TMS. This cap is placed on the head before initiation of treatment. For women of color who have dreadlocks or braids that incorporate hair extensions, these caps can be painfully small, creating additional stress during the treatment process. Similarly, one of the most effective treatments for depression, electroconvulsive therapy requires application of gel to the head. For women of color who may have different hair-washing and styling schedules compared with women from other backgrounds, having an open discussion about hair care would help normalize this treatment as well. Although mental health providers are not expected to be experts in hair care, suggesting a discussion with a professional in that realm or simply an understanding about why this might be perceived as a barrier to care may help patients ultimately accept these types of interventions. Providing culturally sensitive care in these cases means, at a minimum, normalizing the issue and helping to find an appropriate solution with the patient. These are the small interventions that reduce barriers to care and increase the likelihood that patients will remain in treatment.

Lifestyle Interventions

A consideration for improving mental health outcomes in women who may prefer to avoid medications or conventional therapy includes targeting modifiable risk factors often associated with poorer mental health including nutrition and physical activity. Adolescence and young adulthood are an ideal time to start education and ensuring access to achieving healthy lifestyle interventions. A diet that consists of a high intake of fruits and vegetables has been associated with improving mental health outcomes.[40,41] In addition, regular physical activity in women is linked to improvements in symptoms of depression, anxiety, and overall stress.[42]

Racial and ethnic differences in reporting of consuming high-quality diets and engaging in regular physical activity are seen in minority women starting in adolescence and young adulthood. In a study of evaluating dietary patterns in young women, African American and Hispanic women tended to consume more fast food and less fruits and vegetables compared with white women of the same age range.[40] Among a population of men and women between the ages of 12 and 29 years, women across all demographics showed less physical activity with disparities seen in Black and Hispanic women. Of note, Black women were reported to have the shortest amount of physical activity particularly between the ages of 25 and 29 years.[43] Understanding these disparities requires further investigation; however, finding ways within diverse communities that are accessible and affordable may be a direction to explore in providing lifestyle interventions to improve mental health outcomes.

Faith-Based Interventions

Another potential option to enhance access to care for women of color is to partner with churches and other faith-based organizations (FBO). African Americans and non-US born Hispanics are more likely to receive FBO interventions compared with non-Hispanic whites and US-born Hispanics.[44] These organizations have been instrumental in reducing stigma and enhancing access to care in minority communities, especially when the elders of these organizations are known to support outreach efforts.[45] When considering the role of faith-based organizations in facilitating identification of people who may benefit from mental health services, programs such as the Johns Hopkins Congregational Depression and Awareness Program provide a curriculum to train members of congregations to identify and support their peers who are experiencing mental health issues. This initiative is similar to those rolled out in The Confess Project, an organization founded in 2016 that targets barbershops as potential service locations to enhance access to mental health care for Black men who also have decreased likelihood of seeking professional help for mental health issues.[46] This movement has spawned The Beyond the Shop program, which has trained more than 600 barbers to become mental health advocates. In terms of women of color, this idea has been harder to roll out for many reasons but the importance of involving the community surrounding minority women should continue to be investigated.[47]

SUMMARY

Major depression is growing in overall disease burden around the world. It is predicted to be the leading cause of disease burden by 2030 and is already the leading cause in women worldwide.[48]

Although the lived experiences of women of color are much more than can be discussed in a single article, there are a growing number of topics that still warrant further exploration including experiences of women navigating gender identity and laws changing in relation to access to appropriate contraceptive options including abortion and prevention of infertility. Recommendations aimed at improving care for minority populations are often aimed at increasing access to care and decreasing stigma but it is important to keep this discussion going. At the heart of these recommendations is the need to incorporate a multidisciplinary approach, targeting culturally sensitive components of care, whereas integrating treatment and therapy with the patient's primary care providers will all serve to decrease barriers and increase accessibility to care for women of color. Only through frequent acknowledgment of the concepts that make women similar combined with those that make them different will we be able to make significant strides in caring for women from all racial and ethnic backgrounds.

CLINICS CARE POINTS

- Women are about twice as likely to experience a lifetime major depressive episode compared to men so routine screening for mood symptoms at provider visits is important.
- Suicide screening is imperative for all age groups during provider visits.
- Nearly 30% of pregnant women experience some form of depression and/or anxiety.
- When providing care for patients for the first time, consider ways in which to provide culturally sensitive care.
- Awareness of implicit biases and how it may affect quality of care provided to patients is an important consideration for all providers.
- Consideration for treatment of mental health illness should consider a variety of approaches including medications, therapy, referral to faith-based organizations and lifestyle changes.

DISCLOSURE

The authors have no conflicts of interest to disclose.

REFERENCES

1. Rai D, Zitko P, Jones K, et al. Country- and individual-level socioeconomic determinants of depression: Multilevel cross-national comparison. Br J Psychiatry 2013;202(3).
2. Hoyt LT, Falconi AM. Puberty and perimenopause: Reproductive transitions and their implications for women's health. Soc Sci Med 2015;132.
3. Stickel S, Wagels L, Wudarczyk O, et al. Neural correlates of depression in women across the reproductive lifespan – An fMRI review. J Affect Disord 2019;246.
4. Cyranowski JM, Frank E, Young E, et al. Adolescent onset of the gender difference in lifetime rates of major depression. A theoretical model. Arch Gen Psychiatry 2000;57(1).
5. Flanagin A, Frey T, Christiansen SL. Updated Guidance on the Reporting of Race and Ethnicity in Medical and Science Journals. JAMA, J Am Med Assoc 2021;326(7).
6. Alvidrez J, Castille D, Laude-Sharp M, et al. The National Institute on Minority Health and Health Disparities Research Framework. Am J Public Health 2019; 109(S1).
7. Greenwood BN, Hardeman RR, Huang L, et al. Physician-patient racial concordance and disparities in birthing mortality for newborns. Proc Natl Acad Sci U S A 2020;117(35).
8. Braveman P. Black–White Disparities in Birth Outcomes: Is Racism-Related Stress a Missing Piece of the Puzzle?. In: Lemelle AJ, Reed W, Taylor S, editors. *Handbook of African American Health*. New York: Springer; 2011. p. 155–63.

9. Horbar JD, Edwards EM, Greenberg LT, et al. Racial Segregation and Inequality in the Neonatal Intensive Care Unit for Very Low-Birth-Weight and Very Preterm Infants. JAMA Pediatr 2019;173(5).

10. Alegria M, Vallas M, Pumariega AJ. Racial and ethnic disparities in pediatric mental health. Child Adolesc Psychiatr Clin N Am 2010;19(4).

11. Xiao Y, Cerel J, Mann JJ. Temporal trends in suicidal ideation and attempts among US adolescents by sex and race/ethnicity, 1991-2019. JAMA Netw Open 2021;4(6).

12. Nock MK, Green JG, Hwang I, et al. Prevalence, correlates, and treatment of life-time suicidal behavior among adolescents: Results from the national comorbidity survey replication adolescent supplement. JAMA Psychiatr 2013;70(3).

13. Owens SA, Eisenlohr-Moul TA, Prinstein MJ. Understanding When and Why Some Adolescent Girls Attempt Suicide: An Emerging Framework Integrating Menstrual Cycle Fluctuations in Risk. Child Dev Perspect 2020;14(2).

14. Badolato GM, Sadeghi N, Goyal MK. Racial and Ethnic Disparities in Receipt of Sexual Health Care and Education Among A Nationally Representative Sample of Adolescent Females. J Racial Ethn Health Disparities 2022;9(4).

15. Murray Horwitz ME, Ross-Degnan D, Pace LE. Contraceptive initiation among women in the United States: Timing, methods used, and pregnancy outcomes. Pediatrics 2019;143(2).

16. Coen-Sanchez K, Ebenso B, El-Mowafi IM, et al. Repercussions of overturning Roe v. Wade for women across systems and beyond borders. Reprod Health 2022;19(1).

17. McQueen DB, Schufreider A, Lee SM, et al. Racial disparities in in vitro fertiliza-tion outcomes. Fertil Steril 2015;104(2).

18. Patel A, Sharma PSVN, Kumar P. Role of mental health practitioner in infertility clinics: A review on past, present and future directions. J Hum Reprod Sci 2018;11(3).

19. Dunkel Schetter C, Tanner L. Anxiety, depression and stress in pregnancy: Impli-cations for mothers, children, research, and practice. Curr Opin Psychiatry 2012;25(2).

20. Henderson J, Redshaw M. Anxiety in the perinatal period: Antenatal and post-natal influences and women's experience of care. J Reprod Infant Psychol 2013;31(5).

21. Katz J, Crean HF, Cerulli C, et al. Material Hardship and Mental Health Symptoms Among a Predominantly Low Income Sample of Pregnant Women Seeking Prena-tal Care. Matern Child Health J 2018;22(9).

22. Kendig S, Keats JP, Camille Hoffman M, et al. Consensus bundle on maternal mental health perinatal depression and anxiety. Obstet Gynecol 2017;129(3).

23. Dagher RK, Pérez-Stable EJ, James RS. Socioeconomic and racial/ethnic dispar-ities in postpartum consultation for mental health concerns among US mothers. Arch Womens Ment Health 2021;24(5).

24. Howell EA, Mora PA, Horowitz CR, et al. Racial and ethnic differences in factors associated with early postpartum depressive symptoms. Obstet Gynecol 2005;105(6).

25. Chiu YHM, Sheffield PE, Hsu HHL, et al. Subconstructs of the Edinburgh Post-natal Depression Scale in a multi-ethnic inner-city population in the U.S. Arch Womens Ment Health 2017;20(6).

26. Saluja B, Bryant Z. How Implicit Bias Contributes to Racial Disparities in Maternal Morbidity and Mortality in the United States. J Womens Health 2021;30(2).

27. Salameh TN, Hall LA, Crawford TN, et al. Racial/ethnic differences in mental health treatment among a national sample of pregnant women with mental health and/or substance use disorders in the United States. J Psychosom Res 2019;121.

28. Jimenez DE, Cook B, Bartels SJ, et al. Disparities in mental health service use of racial and ethnic minority elderly adults. J Am Geriatr Soc 2013;61(1).

29. Pham KTC, Grisso JA, Freeman EW. Ovarian aging and hormone replacement therapy: Hormonal levels, symptoms, and attitudes of African-American and white women. J Gen Intern Med 1997;12(4).

30. Rice VM. Strategies and issues for managing menopause-related symptoms in diverse populations: Ethnic and racial diversity. Am J Med 2005;118(12).

31. Richard-Davis G, Wellons M. Racial and ethnic differences in the physiology and clinical symptoms of menopause. Semin Reprod Med 2013;31(5).

32. Ward EC, Wiltshire JC, Detry MA, et al. African American men and women's attitude toward mental illness, perceptions of stigma, and preferred coping behaviors. Nurs Res 2013;62(3).

33. Misra S, Jackson VW, Chong J, et al. Systematic Review of Cultural Aspects of Stigma and Mental Illness among Racial and Ethnic Minority Groups in the United States: Implications for Interventions. Am J Community Psychol 2021;68(3–4).

34. Wyse R, Hwang WT, Ahmed AA, et al. Diversity by Race, Ethnicity, and Sex within the US Psychiatry Physician Workforce. Acad Psychiatr 2020;44(5):523–30.

35. Bazargan M, Bazargan-Hejazi S. Disparities in Palliative and Hospice Care and Completion of Advance Care Planning and Directives Among Non-Hispanic Blacks: A Scoping Review of Recent Literature. Am J Hospice Palliat Med 2021;38(6).

36. Alegría M, Chatterji P, Wells K, et al. Disparity in depression treatment among racial and ethnic minority populations in the United States. Psychiatr Serv 2008;59(11).

37. Cook B le, Trinh NH, Li Z, et al. Trends in racial-ethnic disparities in access to mental health care, 2004-2012. Psychiatr Serv 2017;68(1).

38. Quinn DM, Chaudoir SR. Living With a Concealable Stigmatized Identity: The Impact of Anticipated Stigma, Centrality, Salience, and Cultural Stigma on Psychological Distress and Health. J Pers Soc Psychol 2009;97(4).

39. Richards EM, Payne JL. The management of mood disorders in pregnancy: Alternatives to antidepressants. CNS Spectr 2013;18(5).

40. Lee J, Seon J. Racial/ethnic differences in health behaviors and its roles on depressive symptoms among young female adults. Int J Environ Res Public Health 2020;17(19).

41. Lim E, Davis J, Chen JJ. The Association of Race/Ethnicity, Dietary Intake, and Physical Activity with Depression. J Racial Ethn Health Disparities 2021;8(2).

42. Marconcin P, Werneck AO, Peralta M, et al. The association between physical activity and mental health during the first year of the COVID-19 pandemic: a systematic review. BMC Publ Health 2022;22(1).

43. Armstrong S, Wong CA, Perrin E, et al. Association of physical activity with income, race/ethnicity, and sex among adolescents and young adults in the United States findings from the national health and nutrition examination survey, 2007-2016. JAMA Pediatr 2018;172(8).

44. Dalencour M, Wong EC, Tang L, et al. The role of faith-based organizations in the depression care of African Americans and Hispanics in Los Angeles. Psychiatr Serv 2017;68(4).

45. Codjoe L, Barber S, Ahuja S, et al. Evidence for interventions to promote mental health and reduce stigma in Black faith communities: systematic review. Soc Psychiatry Psychiatr Epidemiol 2021;56(6).

46. The Johns Hopkins University. Congregational Depression Awareness Program. 2022. Available at: https://www.hopkinsmedicine.org/about/community_health/johns-hopkins-bayview/services/healthy_community_partnership/cdap/. Accessed November 12, 2022.

47. The Confess Project of America. About. 2022. Available at: https://www.theconfessprojectofamerica.org/. Accessed November 12, 2022.

48. World Health Organization. The global burden of disease: 2004 update. 2008. Available at: https://apps.who.int/iris/handle/10665/43942. Accessed June 3, 2015.

Mental Health Disparities in Sexual Minority and Transgender Women

Implications and Considerations for Treatment

Kareen M. Matouk, PhD[a],*, Julie K. Schulman, MD[b],
Julia A.C. Case, PhD[a]

KEYWORDS

- Mental health • Minority stress • Sexual minority • Gender minority • Women
- Transgender • Lesbian • Bisexual

KEY POINTS

- Sexual minority and transgender women are at high risk of discrimination, marginalization, harassment, and violence. Minority stress theory explains the link between these experiences and increased rates of mental health disparities.
- Sexual minority women are at higher risk than heterosexual women for a wide range of mental health issues. In addition, bisexual women are at higher risk than both lesbians and heterosexual women. This higher risk is partly attributable to stigmatization of bisexual women in both the gay/lesbian and heterosexual communities. Similarly, transgender women are at higher risk compared with cisgender women.
- Family acceptance and social, school, and community support have been shown to contribute to the resiliency of sexual minority and transgender women by reducing stigma and contributing to positive coping in the face of adversity.
- Sexual minority and transgender women often avoid mental health treatment due to fear of discrimination or previous negative experiences with clinicians or treatment programs.
- Clinicians should not burden their sexual minority and transgender clients with the task of educating them; instead, they should seek out resources to develop cultural competence.

INTRODUCTION

The acronym LGBTQ refers to the lesbian, gay, bisexual, transgender, and queer community. Lesbian, gay, and bisexual are terms used to describe *sexual orientation*,

a Department of Psychiatry, Columbia University Irving Medical Center, 710 West 168th Street, 12th Floor, New York, NY 10032, USA; b Department of Psychiatry, Columbia University Irving Medical Center, 5141 Broadway, 3 River East, New York, NY 10034, USA
* Corresponding author. Department of Psychiatry, Columbia University Irving Medical Center, 710 West 168th Street, 12th Floor, New York, NY 10032.
E-mail address: kmm2264@cumc.columbia.edu

Psychiatr Clin N Am 46 (2023) 583–595
https://doi.org/10.1016/j.psc.2023.04.012
0193-953X/23/© 2023 Elsevier Inc. All rights reserved.

referring to the gender of those to whom a person is attracted, both emotionally and/or physically. *Transgender* is a term used to describe one's gender identity, which is a person's internal sense of their gender. *Cisgender* means a person's gender identity aligns with the sex they were assigned at birth, whereas *transgender* means a person's gender identity does not align with the sex they were assigned at birth. Gender identity is different from sexuality, and transgender people may also self-identify as lesbian, gay, or bisexual (LGB). *Queer* includes a variety of sexual orientations and gender identities that are anything except heterosexual and cisgender. Although shared life experiences exist between cisgender sexual minority and transgender people, these 2 communities are also distinct.

The term *sexual minority women (SMW)* is used in this article to refer to women who do not identify as heterosexual women (HW). The 3 generally accepted dimensions of sexual orientation include sexual identity (the term people use to describe themselves, such as lesbian or bisexual), sexual attraction (used to define attraction to certain characteristics, such as personality traits or physical attributes), and sexual behavior (how one may act on or express their attraction). SMW includes women who would be considered nonheterosexual in at least one of these 3 dimensions. Consequently, SMW includes those who define themselves by sexual identity (eg, lesbian, bisexual, queer, pansexual), those who identify as heterosexual but report having sexual attraction to women, and those who identify as heterosexual but report having had female sexual partners. In the following discussion, the authors endeavor to use the most specific term possible to refer to the SMW subpopulation studied. Unless otherwise specified, when the terms *lesbian or gay women (LGW)* or *bisexual women (BW)* are used, they refer to women who self-identify as such. Last, although the term SMW can refer to both cisgender and transgender women, in most research on SMW, transgender women have either been excluded entirely or have not been fully represented. Many large US surveys simply ask whether someone is male, female, transgender, or "other." Because SMW data are limited to those who identify as "female," some transgender women may be included if they self-identify as female, but others, self-identifying as "transgender," may not.

There are transgender people who identify as nonbinary and on transfeminine spectrum, and there are gender minority women who are not transgender, and may, for example, identify as *nonbinary*, *genderfluid*, or *genderqueer*. Nonbinary refers to a person whose gender identity falls outside of the gender binary (ie, identifies with neither or multiple genders). This article focuses on binary transgender women. Transgender women were assigned male at birth and identify as women. Unfortunately, many surveys have not asked questions to distinguish transgender women from transgender men. Importantly, although transgender women are often assumed to be heterosexual, only 19% of transgender women identified as heterosexual in the US Transgender Survey.[1] In this article, if no gender specifier is used after the word transgender, participants were a mixed-gender group. If no specifier is used for sexual orientation, participants identified as transgender and were a mixed-sexual orientation group.

TRAUMA AND MINORITY STRESS

Brooks[2] first developed the minority stress theory in her work with lesbian women and defined it in 1981 as "a state intervening between the sequential antecedent stressors of culturally sanctioned, categorically ascribed inferior status, resultant prejudice and discrimination, the impact of these forces on the cognitive structure of the individual, and consequent readjustment or adaptational failure." Meyer[3] expanded on this idea in 2003, linking discrimination and violence that sexual minority individuals face, as well as the "juxtaposition of minority and dominant values and the resultant conflict with the social environment," with increased rates of mental health disparities. The minority stress model has since been expanded to other populations, including transgender people.[4] Minority stress is not only chronic but also more acute compared with distress caused by life stressors that people generally face.

Research has shown BW experience the highest levels of minority stress of all SMW. At least some of this is due to the stigmatization BW face by monosexual individuals, both HW and LGW. BW experience high rates of rejection and binegative discrimination, and may be at higher risk for becoming isolated from both HW and LGW communities. BW also demonstrate significant levels of internalized binegativity that impact well-being[5]; in response to these stressors and compounded by issues such as bisexual invisibility and erasure, BW are more likely than other SMW to engage in sexual orientation or identity concealment.[6]

Transgender people also experience significant minority stress. In the 2015 US Transgender Survey, 27% of respondents reported being denied a promotion, fired, or not hired because of gender identity.[1] Furthermore, 23% reported being evicted or refused housing and 70% who stayed in a shelter reported harassment, sexual or physical assault, or expulsion due to transgender identity. A survey conducted by the Center for American Progress in 2020 corroborated these statistics and also revealed that Black and Indigenous People of Color (BIPOC) are at higher risk for discrimination and violence.[7] BIPOC transgender individuals hold multiple minority identities, and the intersection of gender and race leads to multiple minority stress[8] and greater discrimination[9,10]; this is even more so the case for BIPOC transgender women.[11]

The LGBTQ community is resilient, and there are several protective factors that contribute to coping in the face of adversity.[12] Support from parents, family, friends, and school is associated with reduced negative outcomes of victimization and stigma. Relationships with others who share the lived experience of being LGBTQ can provide additional opportunities for support.

MENTAL HEALTH DISPARITIES
Body Image and Disordered Eating

Research has shown SMW in general and LGW in particular are more likely to be overweight than HW.[13,14] Despite this, studies have repeatedly found LGW fare no worse than HW in regard to body image concerns, and often fare better.[15,16] A recent meta-analysis of studies on disordered eating behaviors in SMW suggests there may be different disordered eating patterns depending on SMW subgroups.[17] LGW are less likely to restrict food and more likely to binge than HW. Furthermore, BW are more likely than LGW or HW to restrict food, more likely than LGW to purge, and more likely than HW to engage overall in disordered eating behaviors, whereas "mostly heterosexual" women fare worse than HW on food restriction, bingeing, and purging. With regard to diagnoses, a recent analysis of data from a large, nationally-representative sample of adults in the US found sexual minorities as a whole have a higher prevalence of anorexia nervosa, bulimia nervosa, and binge-eating disorder than do heterosexual individuals.[18] However, they did not examine SMW explicitly.

It has been suggested that appearance attitudes and ideals, centered on cisnormativity, are more likely to be internalized by some transgender women to avoid discrimination and pass as cisgender. However, the concept of passing promotes unrealistic gendered beauty standards, which poses another risk. Such appearance ideals may contribute to greater body surveillance and dissatisfaction, which leads to an increase in disordered eating.[19] Body surveillance is also strongly linked to the likelihood that one will compare their appearance to others, contributing to increased body shame.[20] A review of the literature on gender dysphoria, eating disorders, and body image among transgender individuals revealed that "disordered food consumption behaviors" may be used to reduce or accentuate particular gender characteristics.[21] In addition, transphobia, stress, depression, speed and access to treatment, and loss or conflict in relationships after coming out may lead to restricting food intake or emotional eating.[22]

Eating disorders are underdiagnosed in the transgender population given the attribution of symptoms to gender dysphoria.[23] However, transgender individuals report higher incidences of fasting, laxative and diet pills use, bingeing, purging, weight concerns, dietary restraint, and rates of diagnosed eating disorders compared with cisgender counterparts.[24–27] One study found that gender-expansive BIPOC students had twice the risk of an eating disorder diagnosis than gender-expansive white students,[28] even though BIPOC people are less likely to be diagnosed with an eating disorder and receive help due to racial stereotypes and assumptions.[29]

Mood and Anxiety Disorders

Studies comparing SMW with HW have consistently found higher rates of mood and anxiety disorders in SMW than HW.[30–33] However, this research comparing mixed-orientation groups of SMW with HW tends to obscure important differences between subgroups of SMW. Recent research has demonstrated that individuals in the emerging sexual categories (ie, pansexual, demisexual, asexual, queer, and questioning) report significantly higher rates of depression and anxiety when compared with heterosexual individuals, and even significantly more than those who identify as LGB.[34]

In examining differences between subsets of SMW, BW demonstrate a higher risk of developing mood and anxiety disorders compared with HW and LGW.[30,35,36] A recent systematic review and meta-analysis conducted by Ross and colleagues[37] examined the prevalence of depression and anxiety among BW compared with HW and LGW, finding depression scores of BW were higher than those of LGW and HW. Results also showed BW demonstrated higher scores on anxiety than LGW and HW. Some studies have also examined differences in mood and anxiety between more specific subsets of SMW; for instance, a study by Lewis and colleagues[38] examined rates of anxiety and depression in women who identified as "exclusively lesbian," "mostly lesbian," and "bisexual," finding mostly lesbian and bisexual SMW reported greater severity of depression and anxiety. Given these findings, further research is needed to improve our understanding of the development of nonmonosexual identities and how stigma may impact development of mood and anxiety disorders.

Many studies on mood and anxiety symptoms in transgender women have a narrow focus on particularly vulnerable populations. Nonetheless, numerous studies have shown depression and anxiety are found at high rates in transgender communities.[39–41] One 2018 study found 57% of transgender women reported depression diagnoses and 42.1% reported anxiety diagnoses, after controlling for gender-affirming surgeries and racial identity.[42] Transgender women and nonbinary individuals assigned male at birth experience higher rates of negative health outcomes and risk factors than transgender men.[43] Nonbinary people experience higher rates of psychological distress than either transgender women or men; this is likely due to nonconformity to society's binary expectations, which increases minority stress and lack of acceptance by a society focused more on binary identities and gender norms (eg, man vs woman, gay vs straight.)[44]

Suicidality and Nonsuicidal Self-Injury

Many studies have found SMW as a whole are more likely than HW to engage in non-suicidal self-injury (NSSI).[31,45–47] Similarly, studies have consistently found higher rates of suicidal ideation (SI) and suicidal behavior in SMW as a whole than those of HW.[48,49] However, like the research on mood and anxiety disorders, some studies have suggested the rates of NSSI and SI and/or suicidal behavior in BW may be higher than in LGW, and none have found a lower risk in BW than LGW.[50] Two studies using data from the National Survey of Drug Use and Health have also shown that even though white, black, and Hispanic/Latina women differ significantly from each other in risk of suicidality, when compared with women of the same race/ethnicity, SMW are consistently more likely than HW to experience SI, make suicide plans, or make suicide attempts.[49,50]

Data on mortality rates from suicide in SMW is now increasingly available. One recent study using data from the National Violent Death Reporting System (NVDRS) showed that when controlled for demographic factors, there is little difference between SMW and HW in the method used for completed suicides.[51] Another analysis of NVDRS data revealed that when compared with HW, suicides by BW were more likely to have been preceded by family rejection, peer rejection, or bullying, whereas LGW suicide deaths were more likely to have been preceded by a romantic breakup.[52]

Recent research on suicidality has shown transgender people have a three to four times higher risk for SI and attempts than their cisgender peers.[53] According to the 2015 US Transgender Survey,[1] 81.7% of respondents reported seriously considering suicide, whereas 48.3% had done so in the past year. Suicide attempts were also high, with 40.4% lifetime suicides attempts and 7.3% attempts in the past year. Another study found 59.3% of transgender women experienced SI within the past year; SI was more prevalent among those who had lower income; identified as bisexual, pansexual, queer, or asexual; or faced stigma in regard to gender identity.[54] SI reported by transgender women has also been associated with anxiety, gender-based discrimination, sexual abuse, family verbal abuse, and stranger verbal abuse.[55]

NSSI is also present at high rates for transgender individuals, and many report engaging in NSSI as a means to reduce or distract themselves from gender dysphoria.[54] In a community sample, 53.3% of transgender participants reported prior NSSI, including 22.3% within the past year.[45] Notably, transgender women are at lower risk of NSSI compared with transgender men, and this may be because transmasculine individuals come out earlier in life than transfeminine individuals and may therefore be more susceptible to NSSI at younger ages.[45,56,57]

Substance use

Research has consistently found SMW are more likely than HW to consume alcohol, to engage in binge drinking or hazardous drinking (defined as a quantity or pattern of use increasing the risk of adverse health events[58]), experience negative consequences of drinking, or meet criteria for alcohol use disorder.[59–65] Differences in alcohol use behaviors also exist between subsets of SMW. For example, data from the 2015 to 2017 National Survey on Drug Use and Health (NSDUH) showed BW have significantly elevated odds of binge drinking and alcohol use disorder relative to LGW. Lewis and colleagues[38] also examined substance use in SMW, finding lesbian women drank the most frequently and reported the most alcohol-related consequences as well as the highest levels of hazardous drinking. Finally, there are associations between alcohol use and use of other substances; among women with a lifetime history of alcohol use disorder, SMW are more likely than HW to have a history of drug use disorders.[66]

Multiple studies have also found SMW demonstrate higher odds of substance use than HW, including tobacco use, illicit substance use, and misuse of prescription medications. In particular, SMW exhibit higher odds of experimental use of tobacco products or regular use of cigarettes, e-cigarettes, cigars, and hookah than HW, although rates are higher in BW compared with LGW.[67] Similarly, rates of lifetime marijuana use are higher in BW than LGW, and BW endorse higher rates of use for other illicit substances, including cocaine, hallucinogens, and inhalants, than LGW.[68] According to data from the 2015 NSDUH, SMW are at higher risk for the misuse of prescription medications compared with HW; however, BW are at highest risk for opioid misuse, lifetime heroin use, and lifetime injection heroin use when compared with LGW and HW.[68,69] Last, SMW exhibit higher odds of 12-month alcohol use disorder, cannabis use disorder, drug use disorder, and nicotine use disorder than HW, with BW exhibiting the highest odds for these substance use disorders, compared with LGW and HW.[70–72]

Many of the existing studies on substance use have a narrow focus on particularly vulnerable transgender women, limiting the generalizability of findings.[28] A recent meta-analysis found the prevalence of substance use disorders did not differ between transgender and cisgender people,[73] but transgender people do report higher rates of substance use than their cisgender counterparts. In particular, transgender women report significantly higher rates of alcohol (which includes moderate to high risk of alcohol use disorder), marijuana, cigarette smoking, and stimulant use.[43] There are also disproportionate rates of incarceration of transgender women, especially black transgender women, in the United States, and limited medical, social, and financial support increases the likelihood of unhealthy alcohol use in incarcerated transgender women.[74] Incarceration also positively predicts illicit drug use for transgender women, even after accounting for drug dependence at baseline.[75]

TREATMENT CONSIDERATIONS
Barriers to Care

Although most research on barriers to care has been conducted within the broader LGBTQ population, these issues are also specifically applicable to SMW. Sexual minority and transgender women commonly experience social rejection and discrimination in forms such as negative attitudes, family rejection, harassment, stigma, physical violence, economic abuse and poverty, and unemployment.[76] These issues can have a significant impact on both health outcomes and overall well-being, including the postponement of seeking care or avoiding health care altogether.[77]

LGBTQ individuals do seek health care; significant systemic barriers exist, which can further prevent them from receiving appropriate care. First, LGBTQ individuals report discrimination by health care professionals, including the refusal of necessary medication and discriminatory attitudes, at rates up to 41.8%.[78] Health care providers may refuse care to LGBTQ individuals altogether; a 2020 national survey by the Center for American Progress indicated 8% of lesbian, gay, bisexual, and queer respondents were refused care by a health care provider within the last year because of sexual orientation and 29% of transgender individuals were refused care on the basis of gender identity.[7] Other forms of discrimination by health care providers include misgendering of transgender individuals and experiences of verbal or physical abuse, and LGBTQ individuals report their providers making assumptions about their behavior based on appearance.[79] Notably, belonging to an ethnic minority group has been shown to contribute to even further discrimination by health care providers for LGBTQ individuals, with BIPOC LGBTQ individuals reporting doubled rates of discrimination by a medical professional.[78] Second, experiences in health care for members of the LGBTQ community may be impacted by providers' lack of knowledge of affirming and informed care. In a nationally representative survey conducted by the Center for American Progress, 1 in 3 transgender respondents reported having to teach their doctor about transgender people to receive appropriate care and 69% of medical students reported not having received specific training on LGBT health needs.[80] Last, LGBTQ individuals face financial challenges in accessing care, even if they have health insurance. Gender-affirming services such as hormone therapy, vocal therapy, or surgical interventions may not be covered, and the reliance of billing systems on binary identification of patients can also impact coverage of affirming procedures.[81]

It is also integral to acknowledge the history of pathologization of homosexuality and any deviation from "traditional" gender roles by medical professionals. Homosexuality was considered a mental illness by the American Psychiatric Association until 1973, and gender dysphoria is still included in the *Diagnostic and Statistical Manual of Mental Disorders (Fifth Edition, Text Revision) (DSM-V-TR)* today.[82] Although the inclusion of gender dysphoria within the *DSM* allows for insurance coverage of gender-affirming care, it also contributes to continued pathologization. In addition, attempts to change or alter an individual's sexual orientation or gender identity have ranged from use of aversive stimuli, like electric shock, to the ongoing use of "conversion [or reparative] therapy." There is an abundance of evidence that conversion therapy is both ineffective and frequently causes significant physical and mental pain and suffering with long-term harmful effects[83]; however, 21 states currently have no laws or policies prohibiting the practice of conversion therapy, and even in the 20 states that fully prohibit it, religious providers are exempt.

Providing quality care

Clinicians play essential roles in reducing the barriers to health care faced by sexual minority and transgender women. The use of affirming language by office staff and on intake forms, inclusive signs in the waiting room, and the availability of gender-neutral or gender-inclusive restrooms signal whether an environment is marginalizing or welcoming.

Respect and trust are crucial components of the client-clinician relationship, and the very first interaction with a client can help foster a sense of safety. One way clinicians can do this is by initiating introductions with name and pronouns. Clients often pay close attention to the language a clinician uses, assumptions made about the client's identities, as well as the clinician's commitment to learning. Although it is good practice to acknowledge when a clinician lacks knowledge, it is highly recommended that clinicians working with sexual and gender minority women seek out educational experiences by reading articles, attending didactics and conferences, and using online educational resources. Clients may also be attentive to the language used by clinicians outside of session, in documentation or while coordinating care with other clinicians.

Last, given that we hold privilege as clinicians, we are accountable for being advocates for our clients to improve their lives and create safer spaces. One of the many ways in which we can be advocates on a daily basis is by speaking up in workplaces or within organizations. We also have opportunities to contribute to salient issues through research, by elevating platforms of sexual and gender minorities, reaching out to other clinicians on behalf of clients (eg, calling ahead to communicate a patient's concerns about sensitivity during a physical examination), and writing letters of support for gender-affirming surgery.

CLINICS CARE POINTS

- Systemic barriers, as well as discrimination by health care providers, prevent sexual minority and transgender women from receiving appropriate care.
- Negative experiences in health care may be impacted by providers' lack of knowledge of affirming and informed care.
- Mental health professionals and clinicians play an essential role in reducing barriers to health care faced by sexual minority and transgender women.
- Clinicians should not burden their sexual minority and transgender clients with the task of educating them; instead, they should seek out resources, such as articles, research, onling educational tools, conferences, and didactics, to develop cultural competence.

DISCLOSURE

The authors do not have any commercial or financial conflicts of interest to disclose.

REFERENCES

1. James SE, Herman JL, Rankin S, et al. T*he report of the 2015 US transgender survey.* Washington, DC: National Center for Transgender Equality; 2016.
2. Brooks VR. The theory of minority stress. Minority stress and lesbian women. Lexington, MA: Lexington Books; 1981. p. 71–90.
3. Meyer IH. Prejudice, social stress, and mental health in lesbian, gay, and bisexual populations: Conceptual issues and research evidence. Psychol Bull 2003; 129(5):674–97.
4. Hendricks ML, Testa RJ. A conceptual framework for clinical work with transgender and gender nonconforming clients: An adaptation of the Minority Stress Model. Prof Psychol-Res Pr 2012;43(5):460–7.
5. Lambe J, Cerezo A, O'Shaughnessy T. Minority stress, community involvement, and mental health among bisexual women. Psychol Sex Orientat Gend Divers 2017;4:218–26.
6. Balsam KF, Mohr JJ. Adaptation to sexual orientation stigma: A comparison of bisexual and lesbian/gay adults. J Couns Psychol 2007;54:306–19.
7. Mahowald L, Gruberg S, Halpin J. The state of the LGBTQ community in 2020: a national public opinion study. Center for American Progress; 2020. Available at: https://americanprogress.org/wp-content/uploads/2020/10/LGBTQpoll-report.pdf.
8. Austin SB, Nelson LA, Birkett MA, et al. Eating disorder symptoms and obesity at the intersections of gender, ethnicity, and sexual orientation in US high school students. Am J Public Health 2013;103(2):e16–22.
9. Millar K, Brooks CV. Double jeopardy: Minority stress and the influence of transgender identity and race/ethnicity. Int J Transgend Health 2022;23(1–2):133–48.
10. Levitt HM, Ippolito MR. Being transgender: Navigating minority stressors and developing authentic self-presentation. Psychol Women Quart 2014;38(1):46–64.
11. Human Rights Campaign. A national epidemic: Fatal anti-transgender violence in the United States in 2019. 2019. Available at: https://assets2.hrc.org/files/assets/resources/Anti-TransViolenceReport2019.pdf.

12. Meyer IH. Resilience in the study of minority stress and health of sexual and gender minorities. Psychology of Sexual Orientation and Gender Diversity 2015;2(3):209–13.
13. Bowen DJ, Balsam KF, Ender SR. A review of obesity issues in sexual minority women. Obesity 2008;16(2):221–8.
14. Eliason MJ, Ingraham N, Fogel SC, et al. A systematic review of the literature on weight in sexual minority women. Wom Health Issues Mar-Apr 2015;25(2): 162–75.
15. Meneguzzo P, Collantoni E, Gallicchio D, et al. Eating disorders symptoms in sexual minority women: A systematic review. Eur Eat Disord Rev 2018;26(4):275–92.
16. Morrison MA, Morrison TG, Sager CL. Does body satisfaction differ between gay men and lesbian women and heterosexual men and women? A meta-analytic review. Body Image 2004;1(2):127–38.
17. Dotan A, Bachner-Melman R, Dahlenburg SC. Sexual orientation and disordered eating in women: a meta-analysis. Eat Weight Disord 2021;26(1):13–25.
18. Kamody RC, Grilo CM, Udo T. Disparities in DSM-5 defined eating disorders by sexual orientation among U.S. adults. Int J Eat Disord 2020;53(2):278–87. https:// doi.org/10.1002/eat.23193.
19. Brewster ME, Velez BL, Breslow AS, et al. Unpacking body image concerns and disordered eating for transgender women: The roles of sexual objectification and minority stress. J Couns Psychol 2019;66(2):131–42.
20. Strubel J, Sabik NJ, Tylka TL. Body image and depressive symptoms among transgender and cisgender adults: Examining a model integrating the tripartite influence model and objectification theory. Body Image 2020;35:53–62.
21. Milano W, Ambrosio P, Carizzone F, et al. Gender dysphoria, eating disorders and body Image: an overview. Endocr, Metab Immune Disord: Drug Targets 2020; 20(4):518–24.
22. Brewer G, Hanson L, Caswell N. Body image and eating behavior in transgender men and women: The importance of stage of gender affirmation. Bulletin of Applied Transgender Studies 2022;1:71–95.
23. Chang SC, Singh A, Dickey LM. *A clinician's guide to gender-affirming care: working with transgender and gender nonconforming clients*. Oakland, CA: New Harbinger Publications, Inc; 2018.
24. Guss CE, Williams DN, Reisner SL, et al. Disordered weight management behaviors, nonprescription steroid use, and weight perception in transgender youth. J Adolesc Health 2017;60(1):17–22.
25. Watson RJ, Veale JF, Saewyc EM. Disordered eating behaviors among transgender youth: Probability profiles from risk and protective factors. Int J Eat Disord 2017;50(5):515–22.
26. Nagata JM, Murray SB, Flentje A, et al. Eating disorder attitudes and disordered eating behaviors as measured by the Eating Disorder Examination Questionnaire (EDE-Q) among cisgender lesbian women. Body Image 2020;34:215–20.
27. Simone M, Askew A, Lust K, et al. Disparities in self-reported eating disorders and academic impairment in sexual and gender minority college students relative to their heterosexual and cisgender peers. Int J Eat Disord 2020;53(4):513–24.
28. Simone M, Hazzard VM, Askew AJ, et al. Variability in eating disorder risk and diagnosis in transgender and gender diverse college students. Ann Epidemiol 2022;70:53–60.
29. Hartman-Munick SM, Silverstein S, Guss CE, et al. Eating disorder screening and treatment experiences in transgender and gender diverse young adults. Eat Behav 2021;41:101517.

30. Bostwick WB, Boyd CJ, Hughes TL, et al. Dimensions of sexual orientation and the prevalence of mood and anxiety disorders in the United States. Am J Public Health 2010;100(3):468–75.

31. King M, Semlyen J, Tai SS, et al. A systematic review of mental disorder, suicide, and deliberate self harm in lesbian, gay and bisexual people. BMC Psychiatr 2008;8:70.

32. Cochran SD, Mays VM, Sullivan JG. Prevalence of mental disorders, psychological distress, and mental health services use among lesbian, gay, and bisexual adults in the United States. J Consult Clin Psychol 2003;71(1):53–61.

33. Gilman SE, Cochran SD, Mays VM, et al. Risk of psychiatric disorders among individuals reporting same-sex sexual partners in the national comorbidity survey. American Journal of Public Health 2001;91(6):933–9.

34. Borgogna NC, McDermott RC, Aita SL, et al. Anxiety and depression across gender and sexual minorities: Implications for transgender, gender nonconforming, pansexual, demisexual, asexual, queer, and questioning individuals. Psychology of Sexual Orientation and Gender Diversity 2019;6(1):54–63.

35. Gonzales G, Henning-Smith C. Health disparities by sexual orientation: Results and implications from the Behavioral Risk Factor Surveillance System. J Community Health 2017;42(6):1163–72.

36. Pharr JR, Kachen A, Cross C. Health disparities among sexual gender minority women in the United States: A population-based study. J Community Health 2019;44(4):721–8.

37. Ross LE, Salway T, Tarasoff LA, et al. Prevalence of depression and anxiety among bisexual people compared to gay, lesbian, and heterosexual individuals: A systematic review and meta-analysis. J Sex Res 2018/06/13 2018;55(4–5):435–56.

38. Lewis RJ, Ehlke SJ, Shappie AT, et al. Health disparities among exclusively lesbian, mostly lesbian, and bisexual young women. LGBT Health Nov/2019;6(8):400–8.

39. Valente PK, Schrimshaw EW, Dolezal C, et al. Stigmatization, resilience, and mental health among a diverse community sample of transgender and gender nonbinary individuals in the U.S. Arch Sex Behav 2020;49(7):2649–60.

40. Hanna B, Desai R, Parekh T, et al. Psychiatric disorders in the U.S. transgender population. Ann Epidemiol 2019;39:1–7 e1.

41. Downing JM, Przedworski JM. Health of transgender adults in the U.S., 2014-2016. Am J Prev Med 2018;55(3):336–44.

42. Klemmer CL, Arayasirikul S, Raymond HF. Transphobia-based violence, depression, and anxiety in transgender women: The role of body satisfaction. J Interpers Violence 2021;36(5–6):2633–55.

43. Newcomb ME, Hill R, Buehler K, et al. High burden of mental health problems, substance use, violence, and related psychosocial factors in transgender, nonbinary, and gender diverse youth and young adults. Arch Sex Behav 2020;49(2):645–59.

44. de Graaf NM, Huisman B, Cohen-Kettenis PT, et al. Psychological functioning in non-binary identifying adolescents and adults. J Sex Marital Ther 2021;47(8):773–84.

45. Jackman KB, Dolezal C, Levin B, et al. Stigma, gender dysphoria, and nonsuicidal self-injury in a community sample of transgender individuals. Psychiatry Res 2018;269:602–9.

46. Kerr DL, Santurri L, Peters P. A comparison of lesbian, bisexual, and heterosexual college undergraduate women on selected mental health issues. J Am Coll Health 2013;61(4):185–94.
47. Kidd JD, White JL, Johnson RM. Mental health service contacts among sexual minority and heterosexual girls in Boston public high schools. J Gay Lesb Ment Health 2012;16:111–23.
48. Dorrell K, Berona J, Hipwell AE, et al. Longitudinal associations between peer factors and suicidal thoughts and behaviors among sexual minority women. J Psychiatr Res 2021;141:111–5.
49. Kelly LM, Shepherd BF, Becker SJ. Elevated risk of substance use disorder and suicidal ideation among Black and Hispanic lesbian, gay, and bisexual adults. Drug Alcohol Depend 2021;226:108848.
50. Ramchand R, Schuler MS, Schoenbaum M, et al. Suicidality among sexual minority adults: Gender, age, and race/ethnicity differences. Am J Prev Med 2022; 62(2):193–202.
51. Clark KA, Mays VM, Arah OA, et al. Sexual orientation differences in lethal methods used in suicide: Findings from the National Violent Death Reporting System. Arch Suicide Res Apr-Jun 2022;26(2):548–64.
52. Ream GL. An investigation of the LGBTQ + youth suicide disparity using national violent death reporting system narrative data. J Adolesc Health 2020;66:470–7.
53. Hershner S, Jansen EC, Gavidia R, et al. Associations between transgender identity, sleep, mental health and suicidality among a North American cohort of college students. Nat Sci Sleep 2021;13:383–98.
54. Maksut JL, Sanchez TH, Wiginton JM, et al. Gender identity and sexual behavior stigmas, severe psychological distress, and suicidality in an online sample of transgender women in the United States. Ann Epidemiol 2020;52:15–22.
55. Kota KK, Salazar LF, Culbreth RE, et al. Psychosocial mediators of perceived stigma and suicidal ideation among transgender women. BMC Publ Health 2020;20(1):125.
56. Bockting WO, Miner MH, Swinburne Romine RE, et al. Stigma, mental health, and resilience in an online sample of the US transgender population. Am J Public Health 2013;103(5):943–51.
57. Kuper LE, Nussbaum R, Mustanski B. Exploring the diversity of gender and sexual orientation identities in an online sample of transgender individuals. J Sex Res 2012;49(2–3):244–54.
58. Edwards G, Arif A, Hadgson R. Nomenclature and classification of drug- and alcohol-related problems: a WHO Memorandum. Bull World Health Organ 1981;59(2):225–42.
59. Drabble L, Midanik LT, Trocki K. Reports of alcohol consumption and alcohol-related problems among homosexual, bisexual and heterosexual respondents: results from the 2000 National Alcohol Survey. J Stud Alcohol 2005;66(1):111–20.
60. McCabe SE, Hughes TL, West BT, et al. DSM-5 alcohol use disorder severity as a function of sexual orientation discrimination: A national study. Alcohol Clin Exp Res 2019;43(3):497–508.
61. Paschen-Wolff MM, Kelvin E, Wells BE, et al. Changing trends in substance use and sexual risk disparities among sexual minority women as a function of sexual identity, behavior, and attraction: Findings from the National Survey of Family Growth, 2002-2015. Arch Sex Behav 2019;48(4):1137–58.
62. Hughes TL, Veldhuis CB, Drabble LA, et al. Research on alcohol and other drug (AOD) use among sexual minority women: A global scoping review. PLoS One 2020;15(3):e0229869.

63. Kidd JD, Paschen-Wolff MM, Mericle AA, et al. A scoping review of alcohol, tobacco, and other drug use treatment interventions for sexual and gender minority populations. J Subst Abuse Treat 2022;133:108539.
64. Salomaa AC, Matsick JL, Exten C, et al. Different categorizations of women's sexual orientation reveal unique health outcomes in a nationally representative U.S. sample. Wom Health Issues Jan-Feb 2023;33(1):87–96.
65. Shokoohi M, Kinitz DJ, Pinto D, et al. Disparities in alcohol use and heavy episodic drinking among bisexual people: A systematic review, meta-analysis, and meta-regression. Drug Alcohol Depend 2022;235:109433.
66. Mereish EH, Lee JH, Gamarel KE, et al. Sexual orientation disparities in psychiatric and drug use disorders among a nationally representative sample of women with alcohol use disorders. Addict Behav 2015;47:80–5.
67. Wheldon CW, Kaufman AR, Kasza KA, et al. Tobacco use among adults by sexual orientation: Findings from the Population Assessment of Tobacco and Health Study. LGBT Health 2018;5(1):33–44.
68. Schuler MS, Dick AW, Stein BD. Sexual minority disparities in opioid misuse, perceived heroin risk and heroin access among a national sample of US adults. Drug Alcohol Depend 2019;201:78–84.
69. Duncan DT, Zweig S, Hambrick HR, et al. Sexual orientation disparities in prescription opioid misuse among U.S. adults. Am J Prev Med 2019;56(1):17–26.
70. Boyd CJ, Veliz PT, McCabe SE. Severity of DSM-5 cannabis use disorders in a nationally representative sample of sexual minorities. Subst Abus 2020;41(2): 191–5.
71. Kerridge BT, Pickering RP, Saha TD, et al. Prevalence, sociodemographic correlates and DSM-5 substance use disorders and other psychiatric disorders among sexual minorities in the United States. Drug Alcohol Depend 2017;170:82–92.
72. Schuler MS, Stein BD, Collins RL. Differences in substance use disparities across age groups in a national cross-sectional survey of lesbian, gay, and bisexual adults. LGBT Health 2019;6(2):68–76.
73. Cotaina M, Peraire M, Bosca M, et al. Substance use in the transgender population: A meta-analysis. Brain Sci 2022;12(3). https://doi.org/10.3390/brainsci12030366.
74. Scheidell JD, Kapadia F, Turpin RE, et al. Incarceration, social support networks, and health among black sexual minority men and transgender women: Evidence from the HPTN 061 study. Int J Environ Res Public Health 2022;19(19). https://doi.org/10.3390/ijerph191912064.
75. Hughto JMW, Reisner SL, Kershaw TS, et al. A multisite, longitudinal study of risk factors for incarceration and impact on mental health and substance use among young transgender women in the USA. J Public Health 2019;41(1):100–9.
76. Moleiro C, Pinto N. Sexual orientation and gender identity: review of concepts, controversies and their relation to psychopathology classification systems. Front Psychol 2015;6:1511.
77. Li CC, Matthews AK, Aranda F, et al. Predictors and consequences of negative patient-provider interactions among a sample of African American sexual minority women. LGBT Health 2015;2(2):140–6.
78. Ayhan CHB, Bilgin H, Uluman OT, et al. A systematic review of the discrimination against sexual and gender minority in health care settings. Int J Health Serv 2020; 50(1):44–61.
79. Bass B, Nagy H. Cultural competence in the care of LGBTQ patients. StatPearls Publishing; 2022 [updated 2022 Oct 3]. StatPearls [Internet]. https://www.ncbi.nlm.nih.gov/books/NBK563176/.

80. Arthur S, Jamieson A, Cross H, et al. Medical students' awareness of health issues, attitudes, and confidence about caring for lesbian, gay, bisexual and transgender patients: a cross-sectional survey. BMC Med Educ 2021;21(1):56.
81. Bosworth A, Turrini G, Pyda S, et al. Health insurance coverage and access to care for LGBTQ+ individuals (Issue Brief No. HP-2021-14). Office of the Assistant Secretary for Planning and Evaluation, U.S. Department of Health and Human Services; 2021.
82. American Psychiatric Association. Diagnostic and statistical Manual of mental disorders, . Text Revision (DSM-5-TR). 5th edition. Arlington, VA: American Psychiatric Publishing; 2022.
83. Independent Forensic Expert Group. Statement on conversion therapy. J Forensic Leg Med 2020;72:101930.

Working with Survivors of Sex Trafficking

Mental Health Implications

Abigail H. Conley, PhD[a],*, Kellie E. Carlyle, PhD, MPH[b],
Gary Cuddeback, PhD, MSW, MPH[c], Susan G. Kornstein, MD[d]

KEYWORDS

- Sex trafficking • Sexual violence • Risk factors • Prevalence, and screening
- Mental health sequalae

KEY POINTS

- Sex trafficking is the most common form of human trafficking, and it involves the use of force, coercion, or fraud to compel an adult to engage in a commercial sex act.
- Any commercial sex act with a minor is sex trafficking.
- Survivors of sex trafficking experience significant physical, emotional, and sexual trauma that places them at increased risk of poorer health outcomes.

BACKGROUND

Globally, human trafficking is a multibillion-dollar industry and persistent public health problem. Human trafficking involves the enslavement and commoditization of persons using force, fraud, or coercion. The Trafficking Victims Protection Act (TVPA)[1] defines sex trafficking as "the recruitment, harboring, transportation, provision, obtaining, patronizing, or soliciting of a person for the purpose of a commercial sex act." Additionally, any commercial sexual activity with a minor is considered sex trafficking. The most common forms of sex trafficking include escort services, pornography, illicit massage, residential-based commercial sex, personal sexual servitude, outdoor solicitation, strip clubs, and other emerging types.[2]

[a] Department of Counseling and Special Education, Virginia Commonwealth University, 1015 West Main Street, Richmond, VA 23284, USA; [b] Department of Social and Behavioral Health, Virginia Commonwealth University, One Capitol Square, 830 East Main Street, 4th Floor, Room 4-120, Richmond, VA 23219, USA; [c] School of Social Work, Virginia Commonwealth University, Academic Learning Commons, 1000 Floyd Avenue, Box 842027, Richmond, VA 23284, USA; [d] Department of Psychiatry and Institute for Women's Health, Virginia Commonwealth University School of Medicine, PO Box 980319, Richmond, VA 23298, USA
* Corresponding author. VCU School of Education, Box 842020, 1015 West Main Street, Richmond, VA 23284-2020.
E-mail address: ahconley@vcu.edu

Psychiatr Clin N Am 46 (2023) 597–606
https://doi.org/10.1016/j.psc.2023.04.013
0193-953X/23/Published by Elsevier Inc.
psych.theclinics.com

In 2020, the National Human Trafficking Hotline and BeFree Textline identified 16,658 survivors of human trafficking who sought emergency housing, transportation, trauma counselors, and local law enforcement services.[3] The majority of hotline callers reported being age 15 to 17 at the time the trafficking exploitation began. Of those identified, the majority experienced sex trafficking (65%) followed by labor trafficking (22%), sex and labor trafficking (4%), and other or not specified (10%). As with many other forms of interpersonal violence, preventing human trafficking requires a shift from the reactive, criminal justice perspective, to a proactive public health approach. This article describes the prevalence and health consequences of trafficking with a particular focus on sex trafficking. We highlight specific populations at high risk for trafficking, including women, girls, sexual and gender minorities, and sex workers, and conclude with specific considerations for mental health treatment and clinical care.

PREVALENCE AND RISK FACTORS

In the fourth edition of the *Global Report on Trafficking in Persons* compiled by the United Nations Office on Drugs and Crime (UNODC),[4] almost 25,000 trafficking victims were reported across the 142 countries surveyed. Of the trafficking victims reported to the UNODC, 59% were sex trafficked. However, this is considered a gross underestimate as it is believed that only a small number of victims of trafficking are actually detected. For example, according to a Dutch research brief referenced by UNODC, a Multiple Systems Estimation (MSE) estimated that there were four to five times more victims of human trafficking than detected. UNODC also reported regional overviews of trafficking. Of the 10 regions, North America had the third highest number of trafficking victims detected at about 1.5 victims per 100,000 people. Sex trafficking was the most commonly reported form of trafficking in North America, occurring in 71% of reported cases.[4]

Risk factors for human trafficking included recent migration, substance use, homelessness, mental health challenges, and foster care involvement.[2] Perpetrators of human trafficking target individuals who are disproportionately unemployed, belong to impoverished communities, have lower educational attainment, are vulnerable, and who are searching for a better life.[5] Stigma, limited access to resources, and lack of coordinated care contribute to underreporting of human trafficking among those representing marginalize communities most at-risk for becoming victims.[6–8] Victims of human trafficking are often detained in jails, runaway shelters, and group homes that do not adequately meet their needs.[7]

Physical and mental consequences of human trafficking are serious and include infectious diseases such as HIV/AIDS and STIs; exacerbations of chronic diseases such as asthma, heart disease, and diabetes; and mental health disorders.[9–11] Survivors of human trafficking experience significant physical, emotional, and sexual trauma that places them at increased risk of poorer health outcomes including substance abuse, exposure to communicable diseases, reproductive health issues, and mental health challenges.[6,12]

High Risk Populations

From a public health perspective, it is important not only to help individuals improve the quality of life as well as increase years of healthy life, but it is also important to work toward eliminating health disparities among different segments of the population. Women, minors—especially minor females—LGBTQI + identifying youth, and college age sex workers are all at elevated risk for sex trafficking.

According to the UNODC 2018 global report, trafficking for sexual exploitation accounts for 58% of all trafficking cases detected globally. Of these, 71% of victims of sex trafficking were adult and 29% were minors, with women and girls accounting for the majority of cases.[4] The Federal Human Trafficking Report stated that 65.8% of the active sex trafficking cases involved only minors, 17.6% involved only adults, and 15.4% included both minors and adults.[13] Overall, in 2016, the International Labor Organization (ILO) estimated that 3.8 million adults and 1 million minors were victims of sex trafficking. However, providing estimates for trafficking prevalence is exceptionally difficult, and the ILO suggests that all estimates be considered conservative.

The most common form of trafficking is commercial sexual exploitation of children and includes child pornography, prostitution of children, child marriage, use of children in live sex shows, and the exchange of sex with adolescents for gifts.[14] Children of any sociocultural or socioeconomic status can become sex trafficked, but children who have been abused, have an unstable living environment, and have caregivers battling addiction are at the highest risk.[15] Children and adolescents are much more likely to be trafficked by people they know, including family. And, while the majority of victims are women and girls, men and boys are also impacted. Most child sex traffickers recruit victims by building trust then manipulating them into sexual exploitation. Importantly, in the United States, anyone involved in commercial sex work and is under 18 is a victim of sex trafficking.[16]

Among youth, homeless LGBTQIA + identifying youth are at the highest risk for sex trafficking and sexual exploitation, are less likely to report their victimization to local authorities and have decreased the utilization of health and support services.[6,8] An estimated 20 to 40% of homeless youth who are LGBTQIA + identifying are vulnerable to coerced prostitution due to familial estrangement. [7] Additionally, LGBTQIA + identifying youth are increased risk of contracting HIV and other sexually transmitted diseases. [6]

Lastly, there is also a growing body of research that examines the presence of sex work among college students.[17,18] Sex work is defined as receiving some form of compensation for sex or intimacy-related activities.[18] Although willing sex work is not the same as human trafficking (the former suggests the individual involved has agency whereas the latter involves force, fraud or coercion), both dynamics involve conditions of vulnerability that are conducive to exploitation. College students experience intense economic challenges (eg, increasing tuition rates, student loans, housing) and are vulnerable to pursuing sex trade as a form of income.[19]

Indeed, in Sagar and colleagues's[18] landmark study, 4.8% of college students surveyed reported engaging in sex work to some capacity. Supporting academic pursuits was a major contributing factor to participants' motivation to do sex work. About 57% of the students used income from sex work to pay for higher education, while 45% and 39% did so to avoid or reduce debt respectively. Additionally, about 56% reported that the flexible schedule of sex work fit with their studies. Of the participants who reported engaging in sex work, 14% responded that they felt forced to work in the sex industry and were more likely to report fear of violence, not feeling safe during their work, and diminished self-esteem. College students who reported receiving compensation for sexual acts were more likely to also report mental health concerns, such as symptoms of PTSD, anxiety, low self-esteem, substance use disorders, gambling disorder, and impulsivity. Physical health concerns included a reported history of sexually transmitted infections (STIs) and exploitation of substance abuse was factor in sex work, as half the students who did sex work reported doing so in exchange for drugs.[17]

Mental Health Sequelae

Physical and mental health consequences of sex trafficking are numerous and serious and include infectious diseases, exacerbations of chronic diseases, and mental health disorders such as depression, post-traumatic stress disorder, and suicidality.[9–11] Sex trafficking survivors are exposed to constant physical abuse and sexual violence, often resulting in untreated wounds and bruises on their bodies including to their sexual organs. Individuals may present with complex physical health problems that may include dermatological, neurological, musculoskeletal, gastrointestinal, and/or gynecological issues in addition to their psychiatric needs.[20]

In addition to treating the physical effects of trauma, treatment of sex trafficking victims should be focused on possible post-traumatic stress disorder (PTSD) The emotional effects of trauma can be persistent and debilitating. Sex trafficking survivors often report intrusive and recurrent thoughts and memories of their abuse, difficulty sleeping, hyperarousal, social isolation, exaggerated startle response and hyper vigilance, and suicidal ideation.[21] Because of the repeated trauma associated with trafficking, especially in the case of child sex trafficking, the consequences of the prolonged trauma experienced by victims are better explained by complex post-traumatic stress disorder (CPTSD).[22] Although not included in DSM-5 or DSM-5-TR, CPTSD was incorporated into the 11th edition of the *International Classification of Diseases* (ICD-11); CPTSD is diagnosed when individuals meet the criteria for PTSD and experience affect dysregulation, negative self-concept, and interpersonal disturbances and sensitivity.[23]

Trafficking survivors often present with co-occurring disorders and experience significant pathology in multiple domains including cognitive, behavioral, somatic, affective, and relational. Survivors may experience depression, anxiety, panic disorder, dissociation, antisocial behaviors, substance use disorders, and eating disorders.[24,25] Research has yielded mixed results when examining the impact of comorbidities such as depression, dissociation, and shame on treatment outcomes (eg,[26,27]) Additionally, there is a lack of consensus among researchers regarding which PTSD interventions are optimal for which patients.[28] Experts generally agree on using a multi-phase or sequenced treatment tailored to specific symptoms, yet there is no consensus on the expected course of symptom improvement or duration of treatment.[29]

Treatment Considerations

Despite the fact that it is widely understood that human trafficking remains a serious problem, evidence-based prevention and treatment guidelines remain sparse. Survivors of sex trafficking often report childhood sexual, emotional, and physical abuse, as well as periods of homelessness, family instability, and other forms of maltreatment.[30] Treatment should include a biopsychosocial assessment across the lifespan to conceptualize how childhood trauma and related risk factors intersect with forced sexual exploitation.[31] It is important to note that the experience of prolonged trauma is a risk factor for PTSD and CPTSD, not a requirement. Therefore, it is important to gain a comprehensive and nuanced understanding of current symptoms and impairment alongside trauma history. Trauma complexity is associated with symptom complexity,[28] therefore, treatment should tailor interventions to the identification of symptoms that are clinically significant and associated with functional impairment. Trauma-informed treatment centers on the survivor's experience; therefore, clinicians should empower survivors to direct treatment to what they consider to be their most distressing experiences and symptoms. For example, it is not uncommon for sex trafficking victims to experience trauma bonding with their trafficker or fellow trafficking victims.[32] For some survivors, adjusting to life without their perceived intimate relationship with their trafficker could be more traumatic than the forced sexual exploitation itself.[31]

Public Health Framework

One of the factors contributing to the lack of evidence-based strategies for sex trafficking prevention is the overwhelming reactive, criminal justice approach to the issue, as opposed to a proactive, public health approach. Basile[33] argues that it is appropriate to consider violence as a public health issue for several reasons. First, the sheer magnitude of the problem should make it a public health consideration. Second, many of its effects are related to health. Moreover, the CDC states that interpersonal violence can also affect future health behaviors, including an increased engagement in risky sexual behaviors, substance use, and unhealthy eating behaviors. Lastly, Basile[31] asserts that violence should be considered a public health issue because it is amenable to prevention: "implicit in the public health focus are the ideas that public health problems are preventable, and that more emphasis should be placed on the front end before a problem begins or becomes widespread" (P. 447). Basile argues that by approaching violence as a disease affecting the public's health, the public health model will not only be appropriate to address this issue, but also be a more effective strategy than a criminal justice focus alone.

Using the public health model to prevent violence in the areas of child abuse and neglect, sexual violence, and intimate partner violence has been effective.[34] Although the CDC recognizes sex trafficking under the same umbrella as these other violence issues, the evidence base for sex trafficking prevention is in its infancy. As such, lack of evidence about how to best prevent trafficking and reduce the associated adverse health outcomes among trafficking victims is a critical barrier to progress. Although primary prevention is always ideal, we know that there are currently innumerable trafficking victims who need to be identified and connected to resources. Healthcare providers can create these "exit ramps" for trafficking victims by successfully screening for, and intervening with trafficking victims, and connecting them with community resources.

Screening

In the general population, healthcare providers are often the only ones in a position to encounter human trafficking victims while they are still being controlled.[11] As such, screening for trafficking by healthcare providers represents an important secondary prevention strategy that has the potential to reduce the long-term health consequences associated with trafficking. However, victims may not feel comfortable disclosing their situation, and often healthcare providers are unfamiliar with the warning signs for human trafficking as well as common barriers for disclosure.[35,36] **Box 1** presents human trafficking warning signs for healthcare providers from Physician's Weekly.

Healthcare providers express concern with how screening and potential disclosures could affect the patient-provider relationship, the patients' safety in the home with their partner, and could be emotionally upsetting for patients.[37] Despite these challenges, there is evidence to support the positive effects of training on health providers' abilities to screen for violence and improve the standard of care.[37,38] Even simple trainings can have a significant impact on healthcare professionals' ability to recognize signs of human trafficking and care for victims.[39,40]

To best meet the needs of sexual violence survivors, providers should prompt for disclosures, recognize the signs, use a patient-centered and culturally competent approach, and create a safe environment.[41] Research evidence supports the idea

Box 1
Human trafficking warning signs

Healthcare providers should be on the look for.

- Bruising, scars, burns, cuts, especially those in non-apparent places
- Multiple STD or pregnancy tests
- Fearful, anxious or depressed mood
- Cash payments, no insurance
- Malnourished
- A third party may speak for the patient and not allow them to speak
- Substance addiction or the appearance of withdrawal symptoms
- Lying about age
- Patient transient or no address (or the patient doesn't know what city they are in)
- Tattoo of a name or strange symbol

that effective screening goes beyond asking probing questions and should integrate empathy and a trauma-informed approach into screening practices to promote trust, safety, and support disclosures.[37,38] **Fig. 1** displays the Substance Abuse and Mental Health Services Administration's (SAMHSA) six key principles to a trauma-informed approach and **Fig. 2** lists the six elements of trauma-informed services.

After the initial crisis phase and after safety has been secured, treatment should be person-centered and trauma-informed aimed at restoring both the physical and mental health of the trafficking victim. A recent meta-analysis[43] highlighted the key services during this recovery phase: (1) legal aid, (2) medical care, (3) psychosocial care, (4) accommodation (**Box 2**).

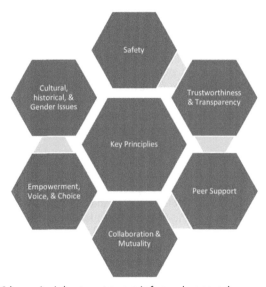

Fig. 1. SAMHSA's 6 key principles to a trauma-informed approach.

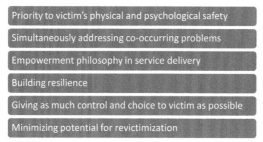

Fig. 2. Elements of trauma-informed services.[42]

Box 2
Clinics care points

1. Legal aid

   Trauma-informed legal aid includes providing clear, understandable, and developmentally appropriate information on the victim's rights that validate their status as a victim of exploitation rather than a criminal or an accomplice.[4] The victim should not be pressured into pressing charges and the offer of legal aid should not be contingent upon their cooperation to prosecute. Legal aid is most often needed to help navigate immigration status, prosecute against the trafficker, and claim compensation.[44]

2. Accommodation

   Safe and secure accommodation is an important component of aftercare for trafficking survivors. Service providers should maintain up to date resources and referrals for safe and secure accommodations, including emergency shelters, transit homes, rehabilitation centers, long-term shelters, and foster care if working with minors. Accommodations should not further traumatize survivors, or violate their rights to privacy, freedom of movement, and/or access to family and/or the community. Accommodations should honor and support culture, religion, age, gender, and dietary needs.

3. Medical care

   Trafficking survivors often have complex medical needs and need access to both general practitioners and medical and dental specialists. Trauma-informed medical care should include age-appropriate, literacy-sensitive language provided in a cultural- and gender-sensitive manner. Medical care should be patient-centered and coordinated wherever possible.

4. Psychosocial care

   Psychosocial care should begin as soon as possible and follow an individualized treatment plan. Trafficking survivors should be empowered to give input to their treatment plan and be continuously reevaluated collaboratively. Treatment teams will likely include individual and group counseling if the victim is staying in a shelter or group home, addiction specialists, psychotherapy and psychiatric care. All members of the treatment team (including interpreters) should be trained in trauma-informed, and developmentally appropriate care.

While healthcare providers cannot singlehandedly solve the crisis of sex trafficking, they do play an important role in approaching prevention from a public health framework. We encourage all providers to be aware of the warning signs among patients, engage in routine screening, and have the knowledge to connect at-risk patients to resources in the community. Together, we can make an impact.

FUNDING SOURCES AND CONFLICTS OF INTEREST

The authors have nothing to disclose.

REFERENCES

1. Grassley C. Trafficking Victims Protection Act of 2017. https://www.congress.gov/bill/115th-congress/senate-bill/1312.
2. Typology of Modern Slavery. https://polarisproject.org/wp-content/uploads/2019/09/Polaris-Typology-of-Modern-Slavery-1.pdf.
3. Analysis of 2020 national human trafficking hotline data - polaris. Published January 6, 2022. https://polarisproject.org/2020-us-national-human-trafficking-hotline-statistics/. Accessed 2 December, 2022.
4. Global report on trafficking in persons. United Nations Office on Drugs and Crime; 2018.
5. Trafficking in persons report. United States Department of State; 2010. Available at: https://www.state.gov/j/tip/rls/tiprpt/2010/index.htm.
6. Martinez O, Kelle G. Sex trafficking of lgbt individuals: a call for service provision, research, and action. Int Law News 2013;42(4).
7. Orme J, Ross-Sheriff F. Sex trafficking: policies, programs, and services. Soc Work 2015;60(4):287–94.
8. Robertson MA, Sgoutas A. Thinking beyond the category of sexual identity: at the intersection of sexuality and human-trafficking policy. Pol & Gen 2012;8(03):421–9.
9. Lederer LJ, Wetzel CA. The Health Consequences of Sex Trafficking and Their Implications for Identifying Victims in Healthcare Facilities. Ann Health Law 2014;23(1):61–91.
10. Oram S, Stöckl H, Busza J, et al. Prevalence and risk of violence and the physical, mental, and sexual health problems associated with human trafficking: systematic review. In: Jewkes R, editor. PLoS Med 2012;9(5):e1001224.
11. Stoklosa H, Grace A, Littenberg N. Medical education on human trafficking. AMA Journal of Ethics 2015;17(10):914–21.
12. Rothman EF, Stoklosa H, Baldwin SB, et al. Public health research priorities to address us human trafficking. Am J Public Health 2017;107(7):1045–7.
13. Currier A, Feehs K. Federal human trafficking report. Human Trafficking Institute; 2018.
14. The state of the world's children. UNICEF; 2012.
15. Fedina L, Williamson C, Perdue T. Risk factors for domestic child sex trafficking in the united states. J Interpers Violence 2019;34(13):2653–73. https://doi.org/10.1177/0886260516662306.
16. Sex trafficking|sexual violence|violence prevention|injury center|cdc. Published February 4, 2022. https://www.cdc.gov/violenceprevention/sexualviolence/trafficking.html. Accessed 2 December, 2022.
17. Blum AW, Lust K, Christenson G, et al. Transactional sexual activity among university students: Prevalence and clinical correlates. Int J Sex Health 2018;30(3):271–80.

18. Sagar T, Jones D, Symons K, et al. Student involvement in the UK sex industry: motivations and experiences: Student involvement in the UK sex industry. Br J Sociol 2016;67(4):697–718.

19. Roberts R, Jones A, Sanders T. Students and sex work in the UK: providers and purchasers. Sex Educ 2013;13(3):349–63.

20. Oram S, Ostrovschi NV, Gorceag VI, et al. Physical health symptoms reported by trafficked women receiving post-trafficking support in Moldova: prevalence, severity and associated factors. BMC Wom Health 2012;12(1):20.

21. Pascual-Leone A, Kim J, Morrison OP. Working with victims of human trafficking. J Contemp Psychother 2017;47(1):51–9.

22. Herman JL. Complex PTSD: A syndrome in survivors of prolonged and repeated trauma. J Traum Stress 1992;5(3):377–91.

23. World Health Organization (2018). International Classification of Diseases for Mortality and Morbidity Statistics (11th Revision). Https://Icd.Who.Int/En.

24. Cole J, Sprang G, Lee R, et al. The trauma of commercial sexual exploitation of youth: a comparison of cse victims to sexual abuse victims in a clinical sample. J Interpers Violence 2016;31(1):122–46.

25. Miller-Perrin C, Wurtele SK. Sex trafficking and the commercial sexual exploitation of children. Women Ther 2017;40(1–2):123–51.

26. Hagenaars MA, van Minnen A, Hoogduin KAL. The impact of dissociation and depression on the efficacy of prolonged exposure treatment for PTSD. Behav Res Ther 2010;48(1):19–27.

27. van Minnen A, Arntz A, Keijsers GPJ. Prolonged exposure in patients with chronic PTSD: predictors of treatment outcome and dropout. Behav Res Ther 2002;40(4): 439–57.

28. Cloitre M. The "one size fits all" approach to trauma treatment: should we be satisfied? Eur J Psychotraumatol 2015;6(1):27344.

29. Cloitre M, Courtois CA, Charuvastra A, et al. Treatment of complex PTSD: Results of the ISTSS expert clinician survey on best practices: Treatment of Complex PTSD. J Traum Stress 2011;24(6):615–27.

30. Franchino-Olsen H. Vulnerabilities relevant for commercial sexual exploitation of children/domestic minor sex trafficking: a systematic review of risk factors. Trauma Violence Abuse 2021;22(1):99–111.

31. Litam SDA, Neal S. Trauma-informed interventions for counselling sex trafficking survivors. Int J Adv Counselling 2022;44(2):243–62.

32. Casassa K, Knight L, Mengo C. Trauma bonding perspectives from service providers and survivors of sex trafficking: a scoping review. Trauma Violence Abuse 2022;23(3):969–84.

33. Basile KC. Implications of public health for policy on sexual violence. Ann N Y Acad Sci 2006;989(1):446–63.

34. The public health approach to violence prevention |violence prevention|injury center|cdc. Published July 5, 2022. https://www.cdc.gov/violenceprevention/about/publichealthapproach.html. Accessed 2 December, 2022.

35. Beck ME, Lineer MM, Melzer-Lange M, et al. Medical providers' understanding of sex trafficking and their experience with at-risk patients. Pediatrics 2015;135(4): e895–902.

36. Tracy EE, Konstantopoulos WM. Human trafficking: a call for heightened awareness and advocacy by obstetrician–gynecologists. Obstet Gynecol 2012;119(5): 1045–7.

37. Dyer AM, Abildso CG. Impact of an intimate partner violence training on home visitors' perceived knowledge, skills, and abilities to address intimate partner violence experienced by their clients. Health Educ Behav 2019;46(1):72–8.

38. Burton CW, Carlyle KE. Screening and intervening: evaluating a training program on intimate partner violence and reproductive coercion for family planning and home visiting providers. Fam Community Health 2015;38(3):227–39.

39. Chisolm-Straker M, Richardson LD, Cossio T. Combating slavery in the 21st century: the role of emergency medicine. J Health Care Poor Underserved 2012;23(3):980–7.

40. Grace AM, Lippert S, Collins K, et al. Educating health care professionals on human trafficking. Pediatr Emerg Care 2014;30(12):856–61.

41. Lanthier S, Du Mont J, Mason R. Responding to delayed disclosure of sexual assault in health settings: a systematic review. Trauma Violence Abuse 2018;19(3):251–65.

42. Macy RJ, Johns N. Aftercare services for international sex trafficking survivors: informing u. S. Service and program development in an emerging practice area. Trauma Violence Abuse 2011;12(2):87–98.

43. Muraya DN, Fry D. Aftercare services for child victims of sex trafficking: a systematic review of policy and practice. Trauma Violence Abuse 2016;17(2):204–20.

44. Blue BlindFold. Services for victims of child trafficking. Department of Justice and Equality; 2012.

Reproductive Rights and Women's Mental Health

Nada Logan Stotland, MD, MPH

KEYWORDS

- Reproductive rights • Abortion • Women's health • Reproductive health care
- Access

KEY POINTS

- Attempts to manage their reproductive lives have been universal and crucial to women throughout history.
- Reproductive rights are essential to the recognition and treatment of women as human beings. Barriers to comprehensive reproductive health care pose a grave danger to women's well-being and to that of society.
- There is a solid body of evidence demonstrating that abortion does not cause mental illness.
- Barriers, misinformation, intrusion, and coercion affecting sex education, contraception, abortion, and perinatal care are an ongoing and serious danger to women's mental and physical health and to the well-being of their families.
- Mental health professionals need to know the facts and laws affecting reproductive health care, to communicate them clearly to patients, the public, and policy makers. The latest Supreme Court decision, and some resulting state laws, require care providers to weigh their obedience to the law against their professional ethics.

INTRODUCTION

On June 24, 2022, the US Supreme Court, in an unprecedented and poorly argued decision, deprived not only women, but all Americans, of a fundamental human right: the right to abortion.[1] The decision ignores the realities of women's lives, the history of reproductive health care, and the profound dangers to health when care is denied or coerced.[2] Women care deeply about having children when they have the capacity to care for them. The notion that, from the fertilized egg onward, the products of conception are entitled to the full rights of citizenship is implicit or explicit in some state laws. It justifies not only abortion bans but also counterproductive, inequitable, punishments of pregnant women and coerced interventions on them.[3] It negates the

The author has no relationship with any commercial entity related to the subject of this article. The author is a past Board member of Physicians for Reproductive Choice and Health.
5511 South Kenwood Avenue, Chicago, IL 60637-1713, USA
E-mail address: nada.stotland@gmail.com

Psychiatr Clin N Am 46 (2023) 607–619
https://doi.org/10.1016/j.psc.2023.04.014
0193-953X/23/© 2023 Elsevier Inc. All rights reserved.

personhood of women who are or may become pregnant, reducing them to environments for the unborn. We have been left with not only our reactions and those of our patients but also a morass of Draconian, ambiguous, and conflicting state laws, which will lead to years of debate and legal appeals—which will ultimately be decided by the same Supreme Court. This article reviews the history of reproductive rights and behavior; the impact of religion; the widespread misinformation and misunderstanding about sex education, contraception, abortion, and perinatal care; the status of access to and barriers to them; the evidence that abortion is psychologically and physically safe; current laws; and the role of psychiatrists.

DEFINITIONS: LANGUAGE

People with female anatomy and physiology can become pregnant whether identifying as male or female. However, because it is female anatomy and physiology that are concerned with reproductive rights, female nouns and pronouns are used in this article.

The common terms for people opposed to and in favor of abortion are "pro-life" and "pro-choice." These terms convey deleterious and inaccurate messages. The term "pro-life" implies that proponents of abortion access are anti-life, when in fact they are deeply concerned about human life. The antiabortion movement is completely silent about other protection for human life: from the death penalty, from want of basic necessities, from violence. On the other side, "pro-choice" diminishes the nature of advocacy for abortion care. People "choose" what brand of toothpaste to buy. Women make decisions after considering the realities of their circumstances—their capacities to assume responsibility for a baby, while continuing to fulfill other ongoing obligations, when they find themselves pregnant under problematic circumstances.

The one positive result of the Dobbs decision is the emergence of the word "abortion" from the stigmatized shadows into open public discourse.

The unacknowledged negative connotations of abortion were manifested in a remarkable announcement by Chrissy Teigen, a much-admired model and celebrity married to a major popular singer, John Legend. The couple had joyfully announced that Chrissy was pregnant with their third child, and then, sadly, that Chrissy had had a miscarriage. Only recently did Chrissy realize, she reported, that she had had an abortion, not a miscarriage. Terminating her much-wanted pregnancy because of serious maternal or fetal complications had not seemed to her to be an abortion until, in response to the Dobbs decision, women and obstetricians on television talked about the importance of abortion in cases like hers. She had not thought that an intervention performed for a serious complication, one that left her feeling sad, could be an abortion. This perspective brings to light the assumption that women who have abortions do not take pregnancy seriously, happily getting rid of an inconvenient conception.

BACKGROUND

The World Health Organization declares reproductive rights to be essential human rights and has issued many statements and guidelines for the implementation of those rights.[4]

The medical community of the United States has also taken a strong stand.[5] The American Psychiatric Association has adopted a series of policies—beginning before the passage of Roe v Wade in 1973—recognizing reproductive rights and advocating against barriers to their fulfillment.[6,7] The American College of Obstetricians and Gynecologists (ACOG) has issued positions and guidelines unequivocally recognizing the rights of women to make autonomous decisions about pregnancy.[8] It is striking, and important, that there are no other circumstances in American law that allow forced bodily intrusion on competent human beings. It is not legal to take one drop of blood from an unwilling individual, even when that drop could save a life.

These positions remind us that reproductive rights extend far beyond the right to safe and legal abortion. Women have a right to contraception and sterilization. They have a right, as long as they are legally competent to consent, to refuse sterilization: the right to bear children, regardless of someone else's feelings that she ought not. They have a right to quality perinatal care, regardless of their race, gender identity, or ability to pay. The United States' maternal mortality greatly exceeds that of other developed countries. The rate is particularly high for black women and in states with the fewest or no abortion services.[9]

ABORTION DEMOGRAPHICS

The Guttmacher Institute offers definitive, up-to-date data on abortion, contraception, HIV, sexually transmitted diseases, pregnancy demographics worldwide as well as interactive information about state abortion laws and studies on the impact of anti-abortion legislation on various populations. Representative statistics are addressed in later discussion.

In the United States, approximately half of pregnancies are unintended. Of those, about one-third end in abortion.

As of May 2016, in the United States,

75% of abortion patients were poor or low income
49% were at or below the legal poverty level
62% identified a religious affiliation:
  24% Catholic
  17% mainline Protestant
  13% Evangelical Protestant
  8% other
59% had existing children
60% were in their 20s
12% were teens, of whom 4% were minors. The proportion of abortion patients who are teenagers has been declining.
39% were white; 28% black, 25% Hispanic, 6% Asian or Pacific Islander, and 3% other.

The cost was paid out-of-pocket by 53% and by Medicaid for 24%. Only 31% had private health insurance.

HISTORY

The concept of reproductive rights is relatively new—although the practice of abortion is not. Throughout history, there have been penalties for women who become pregnant outside of marriage: some formal, others cultural or interpersonal. Children conceived or born outside of marriage were officially called "bastards" and did not enjoy the rights of children born within marriage. These social mores and practices made unmarried women desperate to terminate pregnancies.

Although effective contraception and safe abortion became available only in mid-twentieth century, historical and anthropological studies reveal that contraception and abortion were attempted or practiced in a wide variety of times and places. Abortion techniques are described in Egyptian medical papyruses dating from 1700 BC. The

Hippocratic Oath, traditionally taken by graduating medical students, contains language forbidding a particular abortion technique. Paradoxically, this language in the Hippocratic Oath is evidence that abortion was practiced in fifth century BC Greece. Several ancient medical or gynecologic texts describe abortifacient drugs, and ancient tools used for surgical abortions have been discovered.[10] Anthropological studies indicate that abortion occurs in every society.[11]

All this prevailed while abortion was fraught with a high risk of physical pain, morbidity, and mortality until the advent of sterile technique and anesthesia.

The fact is that neither civil laws, religious prohibitions, pain, nor the very real fear of death prevents millions of women from attempting abortions. It is estimated that 56.3 million women worldwide per year have abortions and that well over 20,000 women per year who must resort to illegal, unsafe abortions die from them--leaving thousands of their existing children, for whose benefit many of these abortions are undertaken, motherless. This is testimony to the intensity, the desperation, with which women regard control of their procreative functions. Women take motherhood very, very seriously.

ABORTION METHODS AND SAFETY

Abortion can be accomplished medically, on an outpatient/at-home basis, using oral mifepristone to block the progesterone essential to the maintenance of the uterine lining, followed by misoprostol to induce contractions and empty the uterus. Years of experience with medical abortion, now the most widely used method in North America, have led experts to lessen the recommended dose, to widen the window of effectiveness, and to relax standards for observation. Prompted by the COVID-19 pandemic, we learned that the whole process can be successfully completed by patients, at home, without the patient ever seeing a medical practitioner.[12] The process causes cramping and bleeding but does not require anesthesia. In an outpatient clinic, an early pregnancy can be terminated via suction or dilatation and evacuation (D and E), using local anesthesia. The advantage of surgical abortion is that the process is complete when the patient leaves the clinic.

So-called Plan B, the use of doses of contraceptives to prevent pregnancy for 1 to 2 days after unprotected sexual intercourse, is regarded by some antiabortion activists as abortion. The medical definition of pregnancy requires that the fertilized egg be implanted in the uterine lining. Plan B prevents implantation. Many fertilized eggs, in the normal course of events, never implant and dissolve or are washed away by menstruation. The women inside whom those eggs are fertilized are never considered to be pregnant.

Abortion in the second and third trimester requires the induction of labor, or cervical dilation, followed by expulsion of the fetus or its removal. Third-trimester abortion is very rare and almost always performed because of a fetal abnormality incompatible with extrauterine life. ACOG has determined that the safest method for the mother begins with the emergence from the birth canal of a body part of the fetus. This method has been dubbed "partial birth abortion" by the antiabortion lobby, which leads people to believe that it is used at earlier stages of pregnancy as well. Despite ACOG's recommendation, some states forbid the technique safest for the mother.

The data on the physical risks are clear and impressive. Despite allegations leading to a major commission finding that abortion does not raise the risk of breast cancer, some states require that patients be told that it does, and that it causes infertility, difficulty bonding with future children, and/or alcoholism and suicide—also without evidence. Induced abortion is among the safest interventions in medicine. Childbirth, the only alternative for the pregnant woman, carries orders of magnitude greater risk of psychological and physical morbidity, including mortality.[13]

RELIGION AND REPRODUCTIVE RIGHTS

Many Americans may mistakenly believe that abortion is completely forbidden by all major religions. A blanket prohibition on abortion is not part of the ancient JudeoChristian tradition. Traditional Judaism allowed for abortion at early stages of pregnancy, at least under some circumstances, including danger to the mother's health. Similar latitude exists in the Islamic tradition. The early Roman Catholic Church regarded abortion as acceptable until the fetus was believed to have a soul, as evidenced by the mother's ability to feel fetal movements: "quickening." Note that, like the Hippocratic Oath, proscriptions against abortion in doctrine demonstrate that a significant number of abortions were being performed. Current Church doctrine, although forbidding abortion regardless of the circumstances, states that there is disagreement among theologians as to when the embryo becomes a person and is thus entitled to the protections due a person. Many non-Evangelical Protestant denominations, as well as reform and conservative Jewish scholars, support latitude in abortion decisions. In fact, some have argued that abortion prohibitions violate their practitioners' religious beliefs.[14] Although traditional Taoism, Buddhism, and Hinduism forbid abortion, abortion is widely practiced in China, India, and other countries where these faiths are prominent.[15]

Religion in the United States has been used to justify other barriers to reproductive health services. Some state laws allow anyone potentially involved in the abortion process to refuse their services. The clerk registering patients for inpatient or outpatient services may refuse to register a patient presenting for abortion, sterilization, or contraception. The anesthesiologist may refuse to provide anesthesia.[16] Recently, the federal government intervened to order that pharmacists dispense prescribed medications, including contraceptives and Plan B, regardless of the pharmacist's religious beliefs. Nevertheless, it is not clear what a woman with a prescription for medication can do when refused the medication. She is not likely to be in a geographic location where the local law enforcement officials will enforce the order. Last, pregnant women with fatal medical conditions or injuries have been kept artificially alive, despite their expressed wishes and those of their family, until the fetus is mature enough to survive outside the womb.[17]

In practice, women of various religion affiliations obtain abortions in the same ratio as in the general population.

BASIC REPRODUCTIVE KNOWLEDGE

The right to know is central to reproductive health and health care. Many women cannot draw a substantially accurate representation of their reproductive organs. They do not know when, during their menstrual cycles, they are most likely to conceive. Misinformation about conception and contraception is rife.[18]

Unfortunately, much sex education—where there is sex education—in the United States is predicated on the false belief that the provision of information about sex encourages sexual activity. The US government funds "abstinence-only" sex education. To encourage abstinence, the effectiveness of contraception is downplayed, and the risks are exaggerated. The students are given no realistic approaches to their own sexuality, and those who do have intercourse are less likely to use contraceptives.[19] Young women are not given the information they need about exerting their right to make their own decisions about sexual activity.

REASONS FOR ABORTION

There is no evidence that women forego contraception, using abortion instead.[20] Some women become pregnant by coercion, because they do not have access to contraceptives, because their partners refuse to use condoms, or because contraceptives fail. Some women simply do not want to have children. Many abortions happen because of poverty, abuse, ongoing responsibilities, including existing children, and the lack of social supports for parenthood. A woman's hope for support from her sexual partner may vanish in the context of pregnancy. Interpersonal violence increases during pregnancy.[21] There are strong links between domestic violence and abortion; abusers may coerce women into unprotected intercourse, refuse or forbid the use of contraception, and, of course, make the domestic situation dangerous for both mother and an anticipated child.[22]

Women with serious mental illnesses may choose abortion for several reasons. Women with depression may be unable to assert themselves against unwanted sex. Women with mania may conceive during a promiscuous episode. Women may be concerned about the effects of their psychotropic medications on a fetus. It should not be assumed that women with psychotic symptoms are unable to make autonomous, informed decisions about pregnancy, or that anyone else, including a health professional, should be allowed to make those decisions for them. However, any kind of illness, mental or physical, may make a woman feel that she could not be an adequate mother to the embryo or fetus she is carrying.[23]

MENTAL HEALTH OUTCOMES OF ABORTION

Purported mental health risks have been used as an excuse to limit abortions. There is a solid body of evidence that abortion does not cause mental illness. Thorough literature reviews have been published by the American Psychological Association[24] and the Royal College of Physicians.[25] There is, in contrast, a string of methodologically unacceptable papers alleging adverse psychiatric sequelae. Poorly done studies, for example, compare the mental well-being of women who have abortions with that of women who decide to give birth or with the general population. They fail to recognize that the circumstances of women who have abortions are not comparable with either. They do not provide baseline data about the mental health of the woman before the abortion. They do not take the circumstances that occasioned the decision for abortion into account. The reasons women decide to abort, just discussed, are all mental health risk factors: poverty, lack of social supports, domestic violence, rape, incest, overwhelming responsibilities, lack of education—and preexisting mental illness. The strongest predictor of a woman's mental health after an abortion is her mental health before the abortion. Abortion may be associated with alcoholism, substance abuse, suicidality, depression, and anxiety, but it does not cause them. Difficulty obtaining an abortion for whatever reason increases a woman's stress, as does exposure to antiabortion clinic demonstrators. To address the methodologic challenges posed by outcome studies, researchers at the University of California, San Francisco, compared the women seeking abortions whose pregnancies were very close to the legal limit for gestational age and those whose pregnancies were just over the limit and therefore denied abortion. The patients who had abortions fared better, psychologically and socially, than those turned away.[26,27]

The publication of the poorly performed studies claiming to demonstrate negative mental health effects of abortion has led to consternation in the scientific community and the publication of reanalyses pointing out the gross methodologic errors that invalidate the conclusions, ultimately resulting in the disavowal of one paper by the editors of the journal that published it.[28] A similar effort is underway regarding another such paper.

Nevertheless, misinformation is rampant.[29] A Google search on abortion led to a Web site called TeenBreak, which states that abortion causes depression, suicide, and other dire mental health outcomes. Many of the resources listed at the top of such searches are "pregnancy crisis centers," funded by the government, which advertise help for pregnant women, but exist solely to deter women from having abortions. There are more than twice the number of these centers than there are abortion clinics. The "crisis centers" provide misinformation and antiabortion persuasion. Some offer free ultrasound imaging—by untrained staff—and deliberately delay conveying the results until the pregnancy has progressed beyond the legal limit for abortion. They lead women to believe that the state will successfully force the fathers to support them. The centers themselves have a policy of not providing any support beyond a token package of diapers.

The decision to terminate a pregnancy may be easy or difficult, depending on a woman's circumstances and beliefs. After abortion, women experience a wide variety of feelings, including guilt and sadness; the most common is relief.[30,31] Negative feelings must not be confused with psychiatric disorders. Like all feelings, they evolve over time, depending on ensuing experiences. There is no evidence that abortion leads to more regret than any other life decision; often women who report regret realize that it was the best option under the circumstances.

PSYCHOSOCIAL UNDERPINNINGS OF ANTIABORTION FERVOR

Strong feelings about mothers in general, and one's own mother, are core elements of human psychology. Anxiety about one's own wantedness may give rise to objections to abortion. Disability advocates voice concern that the abortions of fetuses diagnosed as abnormal mean that their own existence is not worthwhile. For some, abortion symbolizes the rejection of women's submissive, maternal role, threatening male dominance and women who feel that motherhood is their reason for being.

Unplanned pregnancy in a sexual partner can arouse a wide variety of psychological reactions in a man. He may be proud of his virility. He may be gratified at the prospect of having a child. On the other hand, he may feel tricked and trapped into a lifetime of responsibility and ties to the pregnant woman. He may feel guilty for impregnating his partner. If his partner opts to terminate the pregnancy, he may feel helpless to protect, and deprived of, his potential child.

Attitudes toward women's sexuality color beliefs and attitudes toward contraception and abortion. Women have been, and continue to be, held accountable for male sexual aggression. It was Eve who ate the forbidden apple and sexually seduced Adam. Orthodox Judaism, Hinduism, and Islam require women to cover their bodies and limit their activities. The unspoken rule is that men cannot control, and therefore cannot be held accountable for, sexual attacks on women. Rape is blamed on lapses in women's adherence to social rules, such as how to dress and where to go. Women's sexual desires are stigmatized. If a woman voluntarily engages in sexual activity and becomes pregnant, continuing the pregnancy, as reflected in laws and public opinion, becomes a responsibility—a punishment, rather than a blessing.

A significant number of women oppose abortion in theory but terminate pregnancies they experience as untenable. Physicians who work in abortion facilities report that some antiabortion demonstrators request abortions to be performed outside regular hours so that the other demonstrators do not see them. After their own abortions, they resume demonstrating. Some have told the physicians who performed the requested abortion that, "You are still a murderer"; some look down on the other abortion patients. It is hard to consider these paradoxic behaviors with equanimity. Nevertheless, it is possible to consider some behavior, such as murder, as sinful, but to accept the possibility that it is essential or even positive under some circumstances, such as an attack on civilians. Perhaps that is an explanation for the discordance between the frequency with which women terminate pregnancies and the attitudes they express to family, in public, in opinion polls—and in casting votes for government office. Approximately one-third of women in the United States have an abortion.

Thus, public attitudes toward abortion, as reported in polls, are probably misleading. It is essential to know precisely what questions were asked, and in what context. Most polls offer stark alternatives, sometimes skewed in favor of prohibitions: should abortions be available simply on demand? Or should abortion be banned? Most people are uncomfortable with the idea of unlimited abortion, but also uncomfortable with the notion that government should intrude on an intimate decision, the reasons for which are only known to the pregnant woman. Most people endorse the idea that abortion should be allowed in cases of rape or incest—again, because the sex was involuntary. Polls may be important not only for policy/legislative decisions but also because people contemplating abortion for themselves or someone close to them may be influenced by what they understand public opinion to be.[32]

The Dobbs decision has had an unanticipated and powerful effect on public opinion and public discourse. It seems that the brutal reality of state abortion bans has jarred people out of their comfort zones. The legislature of Kansas decided to hold a referendum as evidence of state support for the abolition of abortion. The result was that only a minority favored that policy. In general, the word "abortion" has traditionally been avoided in public statements. Since Dobbs, electoral campaign ads feature physicians and members of the public using the word abortion. Hearing and reading this word will impact public opinion.[33]

ABORTION AND YOUTH

The policy of abortion providers is to encourage young patients to involve their parents and to help them prepare to do so.[34] They also recognize that there are circumstances in which that is not a good idea. Some girls are pregnant by family members or close friends. That revelation may cause a family cataclysm. Some parents will refuse to believe their pregnant daughter; others may be inspired to violence against the perpetrator. There are also parents who are abusive or likely to throw the girl out of the house or punish her severely. No one knows those possibilities better than the girl herself.

States that mandate parental involvement allow a "judicial bypass." The girl can go to court; if she can convince the judge she is at risk and that she is mature enough to make the decision, the judge may allow the abortion to proceed. The likelihood of obtaining permission varies widely. Relying on the judicial exception assumes that every pregnant girl in a risky situation is aware that the process exists, can identify the appropriate court, can get there during court hours, and has no reason to fear that someone in the community or the courthouse will learn what she is doing. If a girl gets to an abortion clinic, the staff there can assist her. If not, she is on her own.

There is a powerful paradox in this. The decision to have a baby or an abortion is not a cognitively complicated one. The procedure is straightforward. Abortion poses far less physical and emotional risk than childbirth. The girl who wants an abortion but is deemed too immature to make the decision will, in a few short months, go through childbirth and become the mother of a newborn—for which she will be responsible and have full legal authority. That will take a quantity of maturity that most adults only strive to fulfill.[35] Abortion poses no greater psychiatric risk for the young than for older patients.[36]

THE RIGHT TO NOT BECOME PREGNANT

Most Planned Parenthood and many other abortion clinics provide contraceptive and general medical care. The closing of these clinics in states that outlaw abortion leaves hundreds of thousands of women without contraceptive care, not to mention screening for breast and uterine malignancies. Most people with private health insurance get it through their jobs. Recent Supreme Court decisions allow employers to refuse to include contraceptive care in the health plans they offer, if the employer has a religious objection to contraception.[37]

FETAL PERSONHOOD

Fetal personhood has ominous significance for women's rights and women's health. The moment a fetus is legally a person, the pregnant person becomes legally less than a person. Many women in the United States have been arrested, prosecuted, and imprisoned on charges that they damaged a fetus in some way. One way was imprisonment for having attempted suicide while pregnant. Almost universally, the accusations and prosecutions were based on flawed medical grounds, often that the use of an illegal substance had damaged the fetus. One woman spent 2 years in jail, separated from her children, awaiting sentencing because, after she experienced a stillbirth, investigators had found inquiries about medical abortion on her computer. There was no evidence that she had even attempted to obtain, much less use, abortifacients. There have also been forced fetal surgeries and surgical deliveries,[38] against the explicit wishes of the pregnant woman and against ACOG policy.[39] In the states that prosecute women for alleged fetal damage, women are less likely to seek prenatal care. These prosecutions happen almost exclusively to poor and minority women.[40]

STATE LAWS: THE IMPACT OF BARRIERS AND DENIALS

The US Supreme Court 1973 *Roe v Wade* decision permitted states to mandate limitations so long as they did not constitute "undue burdens" on women seeking abortion. Subsequent Court decisions allowed state laws that did and do pose undue burdens, especially on the poor women and mothers who constitute many of the women who have abortions. These include the provision of negative and/or incorrect information about abortion—never with parallel, essential information about the alternative—childbirth—required in consent procedures for other treatments. Some states mandate medically unnecessary ultrasound tests. Many mandate waiting periods, often necessitating 2 separate visits, although many women have to travel a considerable distance to an abortion provider. States have ratcheted down the gestational age beyond which abortion is forbidden. Restrictions in Catholic health systems are total, even when the mother's life is at stake.[41]

What is relatively new under Dobbs are laws designating abortion as murder and abortion providers and/or patients as murderers. The Dobbs decision has resulted in a patchwork of frequently changing laws and court challenges to those laws. At least 3 major issues will result in years of uncertainty and misery. States banning abortion will try to criminalize leaving the state, or helping someone leave the state, to obtain an abortion in a state where abortion is permitted. States will try to ban the mailing or other provision of abortion medications to residents of their states. Last, gynecologists in some states are terrified, afraid to care for patients having spontaneous miscarriages because those are impossible to differentiate from abortions. Similarly, no one knows where abortions are allowed only to save the woman's life or health, just how sick a patient must be before aborting a fetus deemed to be alive, even when it has a condition incompatible with extrauterine life. Mental health is explicitly excluded. Undoubtedly some obstetricians/gynecologists will leave states where they have to practice under these conditions, and some medical students will choose not to train there.[42] Many of these states were already poorly staffed with obstetrician/gynecologist care, especially for the poor.

It is not clear, if embryos are legal persons, what is to be done with frozen embryos in fertility clinics. Fertility specialists do not know whether they will be allowed to destroy embryos with genetic defects or whether they will have to put all the embryos from a woman into that woman, risking multiple pregnancies, whether they will be allowed to reduce the number of fetuses when that number threatens the outcome of the pregnancy. Reportedly, some are shipping embryos out of states with bans.[43] Reportedly, there is a significant uptick in the number of men seeking vasectomies. There are also laws requiring that clinics and hospitals send the names and contact information of every patient who has an abortion. This is dangerous in light of the growing tendency of individuals to publicly threaten or enact violence against people whose behavior they dislike. The states allowing abortion care are already inundated with requests for abortion from patients traveling from states with bans. There are waiting lists, and this is a very time-sensitive procedure.

GUIDANCE FOR THE PSYCHIATRIST

First of all, each of us will have to know the current state of the law in the state or states in which we practice.

Generic mental health treatment recommendations have not changed. When a patient is actively considering whether to terminate a pregnancy, it is helpful to review, with her, her experiences and expectations with regard to both abortion and childbearing, and her beliefs and attitudes. Misconceptions can be addressed; for example, patients need to know whether their psychotropic medication can be continued during pregnancy. Next is a realistic review of her current circumstances and expectations for them. Then, the patient can be asked to imagine her state of mind and her circumstances a week after, a year after, and 5 years after having either an abortion or a baby.[44] It is perfectly normal, although not universal, to be ambivalent. It is only paralyzing ambivalence that calls for targeted psychiatric referral. Some laws impose criminal sanctions on anyone who helps a woman obtain an abortion. This puts not only clinicians, but everyone a patient might want to talk to, at legal risk.[45]

The Dobbs decision raises additional issues for patients. Some patients do not believe that they or any loved one will ever need an abortion, or are pleased with the overturning of Roe v Wade. Most women are very upset about the decision, not only with regard to abortions they or their loved ones may need, but also because the decision reflects a dire misunderstanding of and concern for the lives of women, portending more attacks on women's rights. We can and should sympathize. Some psychiatrists practice in places where they are forbidden to discuss abortion with patients. In states where it is illegal to help a woman obtain an abortion, each of us has to decide whether to follow medical ethics requiring us to do whatever is in a patient's interest—or the law.[46] It is painful to contemplate caring for a patient desperate to obtain an abortion and unable to get one. Are we to advise her of helpful resources? Our professional organizations all have voiced strong objections to the law.

Consequently, we are faced with decisions about civil disobedience. We do have prescribing privileges. No one knows just how long the medications in an abortion "kit" will be effective, but we might consider prescribing one of those, and one of Plan B, to every patient, right now. They can put them away safely in a drawer; they may well prove useful, not to say lifesaving, for themselves or someone they know. These are hard times for women's rights and mental health and for those of us who care for them.

REFERENCES

1. Alito S. Thomas E. Dobbs, State Health Officer of the Mississippi Department of Health, et al v Jackson Women's Health Organization, et al. Supreme Court of the United States, 2022.
2. Arey W, Lerma K, Beasley A, et al. A preview of the dangerous future of abortion bans—Texas Senate Bill 8. NEJM 2022;387(5):388–90.
3. Paltrow LM, Flavin J. Arrests of and forced interventions on pregnant women in the United States, 1973-2005: implications for women's legal status and public health. J Health Polit Policy Law 2013;38:299–343.
4. World Health Organization. Reproductive, maternal, newborn and child health and human rights: a toolbox for examining laws, regulations, and policies. World Health Organization; 2014. p. 106.
5. American College of Obstetricians and Gynecologists. More than 75 health care organizations release joint statement in opposition to legislative interference with abortion care. 2022. Available at: https://www.acog.org/en/news/news-releases/2022/07/more-than-75-health-care-organizations-release-joint-statement-in-opposition-to-legislative-interference. Accessed September 6, 2022.
6. American Psychiatric Association. Position on family planning. Washington DC. Am J Psychiatry 1973;131(4):498. Reaffirmed, 2007.
7. American Psychiatric Association. Abortion and women's reproductive health care rights. Am J Psychiatry 2010;167(6). reaffirmed 2014.
8. American College of Obstetricians and Gynecologists. Opposition to criminalization of individuals during pregnancy and the postpartum period. Available at: https://www.acog.org/clinical-information/policy-and-position-statements/statements-of-policy/2020/opposition-criminalization-of-individuals-pregnancy-and-postpartum-period. Accessed May 23, 2022.
9. Stevenson AJ. The pregnancy-related mortality impact of a total abortion ban in the United States: a research note on increased deaths due to remaining pregnant. Demography 2021;58(6):2019–28.
10. Riddle JM. Contraception and abortion from the ancient world to the renaissance. Cambridge(MA): Harvard University Press; 1992.
11. Devereux G. A Study of Abortion in Primitive Societies: a typological, distributional, and dynamic analysis of the prevention of birth in 400 preindustrial societies. NY: International Universities Press, Inc.; 1976.
12. Aiken ARA, Romanova EP, Morber JR, et al. Safety and effectiveness of self-managed medication abortion provided using online telemedicine in the United States: a population-based study. Lancet Regional Health-Americas 2022. https://doi.org/10.1016/j.lana.2022.100200.
13. Raymond EG, Grimes DA. The comparative safety of legal induced abortion and childbirth in the United States. Obstet Gynecol 2012;119(2pt 1):215–9. https://doi.org/10.1097/AOG.0b013e31823fe923.

14. Pew Research Center. Religion and public life. Religious groups' official positions on abortion. 2013. Available at: http://pewforum.org/2013/01/16/religiousgroups-official-positions-on-abortion/.
15. Damian CI. Abortion from the perspective of Eastern religions: Hinduism and Buddhism. Rom J Bioeth 2010;8(1). http://www.bioetica.ro/index. 149/227.
16. American College of Obstetricians and Gynecologists. Committee Opinion no.385: the limits of conscientious refusal in reproductive medicine. Obstet Gynecol 2007; 110(5):1203–8. http://www.acog.org/Resources-and-Publications/Committee-Op inions/Committee-on-Ethics/The-Limits-of-Conscientious-Refusal-in-Reproducti ve-Medicine.
17. Sonfield A. Learning from experience: where religious liberty meets reproductive rights. Guttmacher Policy Rev 2016;19(1):1.
18. Lundberg LS, Pal L, Gariepy AM, et al. Knowledge, attitudes, and practices regarding conception and fertility: a population-based survey among reproductive-age United States women. Fertil Steril 2014;101(3):767–74.
19. Ott MA, Santelli JS. Abstinence and abstinence-only education. Curr Opin Obstet Gynecol 2007;19(5):446–52.
20. Moore AM, Singh S, Bankole A. Do women and men consider abortion as an alternative to contraception in the United States: an exploratory study. Glob Public Health 2011;6(suppl 1):S25–37.
21. Silverman JG, Decker MR, Reed E, et al. Intimate partner violence victimization prior to and during pregnancy among women living in 26 U.S. states: associations with maternal and neonatal health. Am J Obstet Gynecol 2006;195(1): 140–8.
22. Miller E, Jordan B, Levenson R, et al. Reproductive Coercion: connecting the dots between partner violence and unintended pregnancy. Contraception 2010;81(6): 457–9.
23. Finer LB, Frohwirth LF, Dauphinee LA, et al. Reasons U.S. women have abortions: quantitative and qualitative perspectives. Perspect Sex Reprod Health 2005; 37(3):110–8. https://search.datasite.org/works/10.1363/3711005.
24. Major B, Appelbaum M, Dutton MA, et al. Report of the American Psychological Association Task Force on Mental Health and Abortion. Washington DC: APA; 2008. Available at: http://www.apa.org/pi/wpo/mental-health-abortion-report.pdf.
25. Royal College of Physicians. Induced abortion and mental health: a systematic review of the mental health impact of induced abortion. London: RCP; 2011.
26. Foster DG. The Turnaway study: the cost of denying women access to abortion. Simon and Schuster; 2020.
27. Foster DG, Biggs MA, Ralph L, et al. Socioeconomic outcomes of women who receive and women who are denied abortions in the United States. Am J Public Health 2018;108(3):407–13. https://doi.org/10.2105/AJPH.2017.304247.
28. Steinberg JR, Finer LB. Coleman, Coyle, Shuping and Rue make false statements and draw erroneous conclusions in analyses of abortion and mental health using the National Comorbidity Survey. J Psychiatr Res 2012;46:407–9.
29. Rowlands S. Misinformation on abortion. Eur J Contracept Reprod Health Care 2011;16(4):233–40.
30. Adler NE, David HP, Major BN, et al. Psychological responses after abortion. Science 1990;248:41–4.
31. Munk-Olsen T, Laursen TM, Pedersen CB, et al. Induced first-trimester abortion and risk of mental disorder. NEJM 2011;364:332–9.
32. Lipka M. Pew Research Center online. 6/27/2016. Population attitudes towards abortion.

33. Simon MA. The A Word-Our Collective Scarlet Letter. JAMA Surg 2022. https://doi.org/10.1001/jamasurg.2022.6638.
34. Henshaw SK, Kost K. Parental involvement in minors' abortion decisions. Fam Plann Perspect 1992;24(5):196–207, 213.
35. Steinberg L, Cauffman E, Woolard J, et al. Are adolescents less mature than adults? Am Psychol 2009;64(7):583–94.
36. Leppalahti S, Heikinheimo O, Kalliala I, et al. Is underage abortions associated with adverse outcomes in early adulthood? A longitudinal birth cohort study up to 25 years of age. Hum Reprod 2016;31:2141–9.
37. Rovner J. High court allows employers to opt out of ACA's mandate on birth control coverage. LNP;2020. Available at: httpss://search-proquest-com.proxy.cc-c.uic.edu/docview/242114268877.
38. Stewart K. Overturning Roe Isn't Just About Abortion. NYT 2/27/22,p7.
39. American College of Obstetricians and Gynecologists. Available at: https://www.acog.org/clinical-information/policy-and-position-statements/statements-of-policy/2018/global-womens-health-and-rights.
40. Davis D. Reproductive injustice: racism, pregnancy, and premature birth. Soc Forces 2020. https://doi.org/10.1093/sf/soaa067.
41. Kaye J, Amiri B, Melling L, et al. Health care denied: patients and physicians speak out about catholic hospitals and the threat to women's health and lives. American Civil Liberties Union; 2016.
42. Vinekar K, Karlapudi A, Nathan L, et al. Projected implications of overturning Roe v Wade on abortion training in U.S. obstetrics and gynecology residency programs. Obstet Gynecol 2022. https://doi.org/10.1097/AOG.0000000000004832.
43. US Centers for Disease Control and Prevention. 2019 assisted reproductive technology: fertility clinic and national summary report. Available at: https://www.cdc.gov/art/reports/2019/pdf/2019-Report-ART-Fertility-Clinic-National-Summary-h.pdf. Accessed 20 May 2022.
44. Stotland NL. Abortion: facts and feelings. Washington DC: American Psychiatric Press; 1998.
45. Cohen IG, Mello MM. Big data, big tech, and protecting patient privacy. JAMA 2019;322(12):1141–2. https://doi.org/10.1001/jama.2019.11365.
46. Sawicki NN. Protections from Civil Liability in State Abortion Conscience Laws. 2019. https://jamanetwork.com/journals/fullarticle/2755604?gue...mpaign=article_alert-jama&utn_content=etoc&utm_term=111919.

Psychiatric Issues in Women Veterans

Elizabeth Alpert, PhD[a,b],*, Allison L. Baier, PhD[a,b],
Tara E. Galovski, PhD[a,b]

KEYWORDS

- Women veterans • Trauma • Military sexual trauma • PTSD • Depression
- Substance use disorders • Eating disorders • Suicide

KEY POINTS

- Many women veterans thrive during and after military service, yet they are at disproportionate risk for negative mental health outcomes compared to civilian women.
- Women veterans face increased risk for certain stressors and traumatic events before, during, and after military service and are uniquely impacted by military sexual trauma, combat trauma, and reintegration stress.
- Depression, anxiety, eating disorders, and suicide attempts are more prevalent among women veterans than both civilian women and veteran men; posttraumatic stress disorder and substance use disorders are additionally more prevalent among women veterans than civilian women.
- Mental health symptoms contribute to functional impairment across important life domains, which, in turn, predicts worse mental health symptoms.
- Evidence-based treatments are available, but barriers to care (including providers' lack of military cultural competence and paucity of providers trained in these treatments) remain. Providers can ask about military history and related stressors, engage in training on military cultural competence, and provide evidence-based interventions to women veteran patients.

INTRODUCTION/HISTORY/DEFINITIONS/BACKGROUND
Nature of the Problem

While still very much a minority in the military population, women veterans are the fastest-growing segment of the veteran population and are a particularly diverse group

Author Note: The views expressed in this article are those of the authors and do not necessarily reflect the position or policy of the Department of Veterans Affairs or the United States government.
[a] National Center for PTSD Women's Health Sciences Division at VA Boston Healthcare System, 150 South Huntington Avenue (116B-3), Boston, MA 02130, USA; [b] Boston University Chobanian & Avedisian School of Medicine, Boston, MA, USA
* Corresponding author.
E-mail address: Elizabeth.Alpert@va.gov

Psychiatr Clin N Am 46 (2023) 621–633
https://doi.org/10.1016/j.psc.2023.04.015
0193-953X/23/Published by Elsevier Inc.

in terms of race and ethnicity.[1,2] While many of the women who have entered military service enjoy personal and professional growth,[3,4] many also return from service to face significant challenges, including mental health problems and related functional impairment. Differences in life experiences between men and women in service as well as between women who enter military service and civilian women may contribute to the unique challenges faced by women veterans. For example, women have historically been prohibited from having the same military jobs as men and often experience marginalization while in service, frequently with the added stressor of an intersecting marginalized identity.[5,6] These and other circumstances may contribute to women veterans' elevated rates of exposure to trauma as compared to their male veteran counterparts and to civilian women.[5,7–9] Unique predisposing risk factors, military experiences, and elevated risk for exposure to traumatic events contribute to risk for mental health problems and functional impairments that, in turn, mutually influence each other and can have a long-lasting impact (**Fig. 1**).

Increasing awareness of women veterans' unique life experiences and mental health needs is essential for providing them optimal care. This review is not intended to be comprehensive, but instead, we summarize the mental health needs of the women veteran population, evidence related to mental healthcare in this population, and considerations and recommendations for healthcare and future research.

Exposure to Trauma Among Women Veterans

Trauma exposure is a key factor differentiating women veterans from other populations and can have lasting impacts on mental health. More than half of women veterans report experiencing trauma (eg, physical or sexual violence) before joining the military. Indeed, many report joining the military to escape traumatic environments.[9,10] Women veterans report higher rates of premilitary trauma compared to veteran men[7] and report more exposures to childhood trauma and adverse childhood experiences than both veteran men[5] and civilian women.[8] In total, 81% to 93% of women veterans report at least one traumatic event in their lifetime, which is higher than the rate of trauma exposure among civilian women.[9,11]

Once women enter the military, the nature of their work confers trauma risk that is unique to service, including exposure to combat and military sexual trauma (MST). MST is defined as any sexual assault or harassment experienced at any time during military service.[12] A recent meta-analytic study including active duty and veteran samples found that 38% of women (compared to 4% of men) endorsed MST when both harassment and sexual assault were assessed. For studies in which only sexual assault was assessed, 24% of women endorsed MST (compared to 2% of men).[13] Additionally,

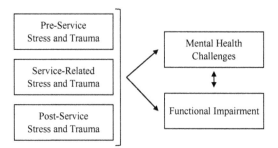

Fig. 1. Guiding model of relationships among pre-service, service-related, and post-service stress and trauma and subsequent mental health problems and functional impairment.

one in 4 women seeking VA care in a national sample reported experiencing MST.[14] Women service members are more likely than their male counterparts to experience sexual assault, sexual harassment, gender-related discrimination, and nonsexual harassment during military service.[5] People who have experienced MST often report feeling betrayed by the military institution and describe barriers to reporting these crimes including consequences such as demotions, unwanted assignments, ostracism, loss of support, disruption in unit cohesion, and risk of additional violence.[15] Service members who have experienced MST often must continue to work and live with perpetrators and even depend on perpetrators in potentially life-threatening situations, contributing to MST-related distress and serving as a risk factor for mental health difficulties.[15] The experience of MST is associated with a higher likelihood of being diagnosed with a mental health disorder,[16] including posttraumatic stress disorder (PTSD), depression, anxiety, and substance use disorder (SUD),[9] as well as higher risk of suicidal ideation and attempts.[17] Indeed, MST confers greater risk of mental health problems and functional impairment than other types of traumatic experiences.[18]

Combat exposure is a unique military experience shared by both men and women. While rates of combat trauma are higher among men than women veterans,[5,19] women service members have increasingly experienced combat and combat-related trauma over the course of military history, particularly as bans on women in combat have been lifted.[5,6] Combat exposure contributes to the already high trauma burden born by many women veterans. Combat-related stress in women veterans contributes to symptoms of PTSD, depression, and SUD.[19]

Intimate partner violence (IPV) is another experience that is unfortunately prevalent among women veterans. Approximately a third of women veterans endorse a history of intimate partner violence (IPV), which could have occurred before, during, or after military service. Some studies suggest higher rates of IPV among women veterans compared to their civilian counterparts.[20] A recent meta-analysis found that self-reported rates of lifetime IPV victimization among women veterans range from 25% to 86%, and past-year IPV victimization ranges from 12% to 25%.[21] Childhood sexual trauma and MST histories, both prevalent among women veterans, are associated with higher risk of IPV after service.[22] Experiencing IPV is also associated with poorer mental health outcomes.[20]

Challenges of Reintegration

Women veterans' unique experiences continue after separation from service. Reintegration into civilian communities after leaving military service is a challenging process with unique impacts on women veterans.[23] During this time, women must contend with reintegration stress and, in some cases, exposure to additional trauma and stressors. Indeed, women veterans report more stressors and trauma after military service than men.[7] While strong social support and reintegration services can be protective against reintegration difficulties for women veterans, postservice stressors and barriers to reintegration can include lack of access to high-quality reintegration and mental health services, difficulty trusting others, lack of social support, loneliness and isolation, and lack of recognition of women's service.[23] Such stressors predict poor mental and physical health outcomes in this population,[24] and well-being can decline in the first few years after separation, particularly among women veterans.[25]

MENTAL HEALTH PROBLEMS AMONG WOMEN VETERANS

Next, we review the prevalence of the most common mental health conditions among women veterans and describe relationships between women veterans' life experiences and mental health challenges after service. Notably, women veterans are more likely than veteran men to meet criteria for a mental health disorder in the first year after separating from service,[26] and this discrepancy increases over time.[25] Women veterans are also more likely than civilian women to meet criteria for at least one mental health disorder[3] and to attempt or complete suicide.[27,28]

Posttraumatic Stress Disorder

Posttraumatic stress disorder prevalence rates are elevated among women veterans, likely due to their high risk of trauma exposure. Findings from a nationally-representative sample found that lifetime PTSD is more prevalent among women veterans (13.4%) compared to both civilian women (8.0%) and veteran men (7.7%).[29] When comparing men and women veterans who have experienced combat, studies have largely found similar PTSD prevalence among men and women.[5] PTSD is the most common service-connected disability among women veterans[6] and is the most prevalent disorder to develop secondary to experiences of MST.[16] In fact, experiencing MST may contribute to PTSD symptoms among women more so than men, suggesting a unique impact of MST on mental health among women veterans.[30] Risk factors such as pre-deployment interpersonal victimization and combat-related stressors during deployment may also be more strongly related to post-deployment PTSD among women than men.[31] This symptom picture is further complicated by high rates of comorbidity with PTSD; women veterans with PTSD and a history of MST are more likely than their male counterparts to have comorbid depression, anxiety, and eating disorders.[32]

Mood Disorders

Major depressive disorder (MDD) is the second most common service-connected disability among women veterans[6] and is highly comorbid with PTSD.[33–35] In contrast to the PTSD literature noted above, research consistently shows depression prevalence is greater for women veterans than men.[25,34] In a sample of over 10,000 veterans engaged in VA primary care, 20% of women compared with 12% of men met screening criteria for probable current MDD.[36] Women veterans are more likely than men to meet criteria for depression in the first year after separating from service,[26] and this gap increases over the first few years after separation.[25] Furthermore, lifetime MDD is higher for women veterans (46.5%)[35] than both men veterans (36.3%)[35] and women in the general population (22.1%),[37] suggesting that both military service and female gender may confer risk for depression.

Anxiety Disorders

Anxiety disorders are also prevalent among women veterans. A nationwide survey found that women veterans self-reported a lifetime anxiety disorder prevalence of 19.5%, compared with 16.3% among their civilian counterparts.[38] As with depression, women veterans are also more likely than men to meet criteria for an anxiety disorder in the first year after separating from service,[26] and this gap increases over the first few years after separation.[25] Anxiety disorders are more common for women veterans with a history of MST, comorbid PTSD,[32] and comorbid MDD.[35]

Substance Use Disorders

SUD prevalence is greater among women veterans than civilian women,[39] but women veterans are less likely to be diagnosed with SUD than veteran men.[7,34,40] SUD is highly comorbid with depression[35] and PTSD[32] and is associated with childhood adversity,[39] trauma exposure,[7] and suicidal ideation and suicide.[41] Research further suggests that women veterans may use substances to cope with depressive symptoms more so than with PTSD symptoms.[42] SUD is also a strong risk factor for homelessness[43] and contributes to a "downward spiral" of economic, legal, medical, and interpersonal challenges for women veterans.[44]

Eating Disorders

Eating disorders in women veterans are more prevalent as compared to veteran men and civilian women, with rates among women veterans ranging from 2.8% to 4.6%.[35,45,46] Women with a history of MST are more likely to be diagnosed with an eating disorder,[32] as are women veterans with another mental health diagnosis, including PTSD, depression, anxiety, and SUD.[35,47,48] It is hypothesized that the military culture of fitness and body composition testing may influence the onset of eating disorders.[49]

Suicidality

Longitudinal national data show the completed suicide rate is nearly three times higher for women veterans than civilian women (9.8 vs 3.4 per 100,000) and that women veterans are more likely to use firearms than their civilian counterparts.[28] Lifetime suicidal ideation and attempts are higher for women veterans than veteran men, and lifetime suicide attempts, but not ideation, are higher for women veterans than civilian women.[27] Gender-specific risk factors for suicide attempts and death among women include younger age, being unmarried, mental health symptoms, history of IPV, and history of childhood trauma [50]; as reviewed above, many of these risk factors disproportionately affect women veterans. Of mental health disorders, SUD confers the highest suicide risk for women veterans relative to other psychiatric disorders.[51] Suicide risk is also elevated among those with personality disorders, with a particularly high risk for veterans diagnosed borderline personality disorder (BPD). This risk associated with BPD is compounded by the high rates of comorbidity of BPD with other mental health conditions that confer additional risk for suicide (eg, PTSD, depression, SUD) in this clinically complex population.[52]

RELATED FUNCTIONAL IMPAIRMENT AMONG WOMEN VETERANS

Experiencing mental health symptoms, among other types of stressors, translates to difficulties in functioning across important life domains. These relationships are bidirectional, with functioning challenges contributing to mental health problems as well. Regarding physical health and functioning, PTSD is associated with worse physical functioning among women veterans [53]: in a national sample of over 90,000 post-9/11 veterans accessing care through VA, women with PTSD had twice the number of medical conditions as women without PTSD.[54] MST[15] and depression[53] are also associated with worse physical health outcomes among women veterans. PTSD and post-deployment stress are specifically associated with worse reproductive health outcomes among women veterans such as pregnancy complications and adverse pregnancy outcomes.[55] Worse physical health functioning in turn predicts later PTSD and depression severity.[53]

Relationships between traumatic experiences, mental health difficulties, and relationship functioning are also well-established: MST, combat exposure, PTSD, depression, and suicidal ideation can contribute to worse sexual,[15,56–58] intimate relationship,[15,59–61] family,[60,62] and social functioning.[11] Difficulties with intimate relationship functioning in turn predict later increases in PTSD and depression symptoms[63] and suicidal ideation.[61] PTSD, depression, substance use, and postdeployment stress predict impairment in parental functioning among women veterans,[59,60] and these relationships are stronger for women than men veterans.[59] Likewise, impairment in work functioning is also associated with PTSD symptoms[62,63] and depression [63]; difficulties in work functioning, in turn, predict more severe PTSD and depression.[63] Finally, PTSD,[11] depression,[64] and anxiety[65] are related to worse overall well-being and quality of life among women veterans.

THERAPEUTIC OPTIONS, CLINICAL OUTCOMES, AND CLINICAL CONSIDERATIONS

Fortunately, robust evidence-based treatments are increasingly available. Evidence-based treatments shown to improve mental health and functioning include individual and group therapies such as those for PTSD,[66] MST,[15] anxiety disorders,[67] mood disorders,[68] eating disorders,[69] and substance use disorders [70]; couples therapy [71]; and family therapy.[72] Complementary, integrative, and alternative treatments including trauma-informed yoga,[73] mindfulness,[74] and skills training[75] also show promise in reducing the mental health symptoms and improving functioning among women veterans. In VA, mental health services for women veterans are increasingly offered in specialty gender-specific clinics (eg, women's primary care clinics, specialized women's trauma clinics) designed to better meet women veterans' needs and preferences.[76–78]

Despite the availability of evidence-based therapies, only half of women veterans in need of care seek services.[79] Veterans face numerous barriers to care, including stigma, logistical barriers (eg, distance from clinic, childcare coverage), and socioeconomic factors (eg, health insurance coverage, financial hardship).[80] Women veterans are more likely to experience difficulties finding childcare,[79] and among women veterans with PTSD, being a parent is associated with lower psychotherapy retention.[81] The delivery of evidence-based interventions via telehealth may increase access and address some of these barriers to care.[82] Furthermore, massed care—the delivery of an intervention daily over the course of 1 to 2 weeks—may also increase access when the logistics of weekly sessions present barriers to care.[83] Emerging research also suggests some veterans may prefer and benefit from mobile application ("app") and internet-based approaches.[84]

Linking women veterans to the plethora of available veteran resources can be challenging because many veteran services and events are generally geared toward men. Women veterans accessing these resources may find that they are the only woman in attendance and unfortunately often report that their service was unrecognized or, worse, questioned.[85] In recognition of this problem and need, the VA Center for Women Veterans (https://www.va.gov/womenvet/) offers information about healthcare, benefits, services, and programs for women veterans and may be a helpful resource for both patients and providers. Peer-support initiatives (eg, the Women Veterans Network[86]) also bolster connectedness and support among women veterans and reduce risk factors for negative mental health outcomes such as isolation and loneliness.

RECOMMENDATIONS FOR PROVIDERS

Understanding women veterans' unique experiences and elevated risk factors for mental health challenges is an important first step in optimizing clinical care to address these needs. More than half of mental health and primary care providers report they do not regularly ask patients about military history.[87] Given the unique life experiences and challenges faced by the veteran population, it is critical for community healthcare providers to query military service for both men and women patients[88] and to screen for military-related experiences such as combat, MST, and reintegration stress.[15] Furthermore, it is important for providers to familiarize themselves with evidence-based treatments and resources available to veterans, both to better serve this population and, if needed, to make referrals to appropriate care.[89] Providers in both public and private sectors may consider enrolling in any number of military cultural competence trainings in order to increase their knowledge about the experiences of the veteran population, including the unique challenges women veterans face. Licensed providers may benefit from participating in free, online, accredited continuing education webinars such as through the Center for Deployment Psychology (https://deploymentpsych.org/psychological-training) or the Home Base Training Institute (https://homebase.org/resources/training-institute/). Furthermore, a thorough assessment of mental health symptoms, functioning, and the roles of military service and reintegration into civilian life in current clinical presentations will help providers formulate optimal treatment plans. Relying on clinical practice guidelines published by the VA and Department of Defense (DoD)[90] among other organizations and implementing the recommended evidence-based therapies will optimize outcomes for veterans.

DISCUSSION

Understanding women veterans' unique life experiences and mental health needs is critical for providing optimal care and improving patient outcomes. Women veterans are more likely than their civilian counterparts to experience a range of pre-service stressors including childhood adversity and trauma. Women veterans may be at greater risk for experiencing MST and deployment-related stressors while serving and may face greater challenges with reintegration after military service. These stressors combined put women veterans at elevated risk for mental health problems and associated functional impairment. Further, emerging evidence shows that historically marginalized groups (eg, racial/ethnic minorities, sexual/gender minorities) within the women veteran population may be at particularly high risk for poorer mental health and functioning.[91] Efforts to increase access to evidence-based interventions, remove barriers to care, and improve provider competency working with this population are critical to optimize outcomes.

SUMMARY

Many women veterans thrive during and after military service, yet the disproportionate risks for negative mental health outcomes cannot be denied. As the number of women veterans grows, so will the need for effective, culturally competent clinical care. Future research might seek to better understand the unique challenges faced by women veterans and develop and enhance interventions designed to meet their needs.

CLINICS CARE POINTS

- In light of women veterans' unique life experiences and mental health needs, it is critical for providers to ask about military history and screen for experiences of combat trauma, military sexual trauma, intimate partner violence, and reintegration stress to inform case conceptualization and treatment planning.

- Evidence-based treatments that can improve mental health and functioning are available and should be offered to women veterans. Women veterans may also benefit from complementary, integrative, and alternative treatments, as well as peer-support programs.

- Barriers to care include stigma, logistical barriers, and socioeconomic factors. Telehealth, massed treatment delivery, and app-based care may help improve access.
- Resources are available for clinicians to improve military cultural competency and learn more about care in this population, including free accredited online training.

DISCLOSURE

The authors have no conflicts of interest to disclose.

REFERENCES

1. Department of Veterans Affairs. Women Veterans in Focus. Department of Veterans Affairs; 2022. https://www.womenshealth.va.gov/WOMENSHEALTH/docs/VHA-WomensHealth-Focus-Infographic-2022-v02.pdf.
2. U.S. Department of Veterans Affairs. Profile of Women Veterans: 2015.; 2016. https://www.va.gov/vetdata/docs/specialreports/women_veterans_profile_12_22_2016.pdf.
3. Vogt D, Borowski S, Maguen S, et al. Strengths and vulnerabilities: Comparing post-9/11 U.S. veterans' and non-veterans' perceptions of health and broader well-being. SSM - Popul Health 2022;19:101201.
4. Vogt D, Smith BN, Fox AB, et al. Consequences of PTSD for the work and family quality of life of female and male U.S. Afghanistan and Iraq War veterans. Soc Psychiatry Psychiatr Epidemiol 2017;52(3):341–52.
5. Street AE, Vogt D, Dutra L. A new generation of women veterans: Stressors faced by women deployed to Iraq and Afghanistan. Clin Psychol Rev 2009;29(8):685–94.
6. Department of Veterans Affairs, *National Center for Veterans Analysis and Statistics. Women Veterans Report: The Past, Present and Future of Women Veterans*, 2017. Available at: https://www.va.gov/vetdata/docs/specialreports/women_veterans_2015_final.pdf. Accessed May 15, 2023.
7. Kelley ML, Brancu M, Robbins AT, et al. Drug use and childhood-, military- and post-military trauma exposure among women and men veterans. Drug Alcohol Depend 2015;152:201–8.
8. Blosnich JR, Garfin DR, Maguen S, et al. Differences in childhood adversity, suicidal ideation, and suicide attempt among veterans and nonveterans. Am Psychol 2021;76(2):284–99.
9. Zinzow HM, Grubaugh AL, Monnier J, et al. Trauma among female veterans: A critical review. Trauma Violence Abuse 2007;8(4):384–400.
10. Sadler AG, Booth BM, Mengeling MA, et al. Life span and repeated violence against women during military service: Effects on health status and outpatient utilization. J Womens Health 2004;13:799–811.
11. Kelly UA, Skelton K, Patel M, et al. More than military sexual trauma: Interpersonal violence, PTSD, and mental health in women veterans. Res Nurs Health 2011;34(6):457–67.
12. United States Government. Counseling and Treatment for Sexual Trauma, 38 U.S. Code § 1720D.
13. Wilson LC. The prevalence of military sexual trauma: A meta-analysis. Trauma Violence Abuse 2018;19(5):584–97.

14. Skinner KM, Kressin N, Frayne S, et al. The prevalence of military sexual assault among female Veterans' Administration outpatients. J Interpers Violence 2000; 15(3):291–310.
15. Galovski TE, Street AE, Creech S, et al. State of the knowledge of VA military sexual trauma research. J Gen Intern Med 2022. https://doi.org/10.1007/s11606-022-07580-8.
16. Kimerling R, Street AE, Pavao J, et al. Military-related sexual trauma among Veterans Health Administration patients returning from Afghanistan and Iraq. Am J Publ Health 2010;100(8):1409–12.
17. Monteith LL, Holliday R, Schneider AL, et al. Identifying factors associated with suicidal ideation and suicide attempts following military sexual trauma. J Affect Disord 2019;252:300–9.
18. Surís A, Lind L, Kashner TM, et al. Mental health, quality of life, and health functioning in women veterans: Differential outcomes associated with military and civilian sexual assault. J Interpers Violence 2007;22(2):179–97.
19. Vogt D, Vaughn R, Glickman ME, et al. Gender differences in combat-related stressors and their association with postdeployment mental health in a nationally representative sample of U.S. OEF/OIF veterans. J Abnorm Psychol 2011;120(4): 797–806.
20. Gerber MR, Iverson KM, Dichter ME, et al. Women Veterans and Intimate Partner Violence: Current State of Knowledge and Future Directions. J Womens Health 2014;23(4):302–9.
21. Sparrow K, Dickson H, Kwan J, et al. Prevalence of self-reported intimate partner violence victimization among military personnel: A systematic review and meta-analysis. Trauma Violence Abuse 2020;21(3):586–609.
22. Iverson KM, Mercado R, Carpenter SL, et al. Intimate partner violence among women veterans: Previous interpersonal violence as a risk factor. J Trauma Stress 2013;26(6):767–71.
23. Hawkins BL, Crowe BM. Contextual facilitators and barriers of community reintegration among injured female military veterans: A qualitative study. Arch Phys Med Rehabil 2018;99(2):S65–71.
24. Demers AL. From death to life: Female veterans, identity negotiation, and reintegration into society. J Humanist Psychol 2013;53(4):489–515.
25. Vogt D, Borowski SC, Godier-McBard LR, et al. Changes in the health and broader well-being of U.S. veterans in the first three years after leaving military service: Overall trends and group differences. Soc Sci Med 2022;294:114702.
26. Vogt DS, Tyrell FA, Bramande EA, et al. U.S. military veterans' health and well-being in the first year after service. Am J Prev Med 2020;58(3):352–60.
27. Hoffmire CA, Monteith LL, Forster JE, et al. Gender differences in lifetime prevalence and onset timing of suicidal ideation and suicide attempt among post-9/11 veterans and nonveterans. Med Care 2021;59:S84–91.
28. Kaplan MS, McFarland BH, Huguet N. Firearm suicide among veterans in the general population: Findings from the National Violent Death Reporting System. J Trauma Inj Infect Crit Care 2009;67(3):503–7.
29. Lehavot K, Katon JG, Chen JA, et al. Post-traumatic stress disorder by gender and veteran status. Am J Prev Med 2018;54(1):e1–9.
30. Tannahill HS, Livingston WS, Fargo JD, et al. Gender moderates the association of military sexual trauma and risk for psychological distress among VA-enrolled veterans. J Affect Disord 2020;268:215–20.
31. Polusny MA, Kumpula MJ, Meis LA, et al. Gender differences in the effects of deployment-related stressors and pre-deployment risk factors on the

development of PTSD symptoms in National Guard Soldiers deployed to Iraq and Afghanistan. J Psychiatr Res 2014;49:1–9.

32. Maguen S, Cohen B, Ren L, et al. Gender differences in military sexual trauma and mental health diagnoses among Iraq and Afghanistan veterans with post-traumatic stress disorder. Wom Health Issues 2012;22(1):e61–6.

33. Smith TC, Ryan MAK, Wingard DL, et al. New onset and persistent symptoms of post-traumatic stress disorder self reported after deployment and combat exposures: Prospective population based US military cohort study. BMJ 2008; 336(7640):366–71.

34. Maguen S, Ren L, Bosch JO, et al. Gender differences in mental health diagnoses among Iraq and Afghanistan veterans enrolled in Veterans Affairs health care. Am J Publ Health 2010;100(12):2450–6.

35. Curry JF, Aubuchon-Endsley N, Brancu M, et al. Lifetime major depression and comorbid disorders among current-era women veterans. J Affect Disord 2014; 152-154:434–40.

36. Davis TD, Campbell DG, Bonner LM, et al. Women veterans with depression in Veterans Health Administration primary care: An assessment of needs and preferences. Wom Health Issues 2016;26(6):656–66.

37. Kessler RC, Petukhova M, Sampson NA, et al. Twelve-month and lifetime prevalence and lifetime morbid risk of anxiety and mood disorders in the United States: Anxiety and mood disorders in the United States. Int J Methods Psychiatr Res 2012;21(3):169–84.

38. Lehavot K, Hoerster KD, Nelson KM, et al. Health indicators for military, veteran, and civilian women. Am J Prev Med 2012;42(5):473–80.

39. Evans EA, Upchurch DM, Simpson T, et al. Differences by Veteran/civilian status and gender in associations between childhood adversity and alcohol and drug use disorders. Soc Psychiatry Psychiatr Epidemiol 2018;53(4):421–35.

40. Iverson KM, Hendricks AM, Kimerling R, et al. Psychiatric diagnoses and neurobehavioral symptom severity among OEF/OIF VA patients with deployment-related traumatic brain injury: a gender comparison. Wom Health Issues 2011; 21(4):S210–7.

41. Chapman SLC, Wu LT. Suicide and substance use among female veterans: A need for research. Drug Alcohol Depend 2014;136:1–10.

42. Kelley ML, Runnals J, Pearson MR, et al. Alcohol use and trauma exposure among male and female veterans before, during, and after military service. Drug Alcohol Depend 2013;133(2):615–24.

43. Tsai J, Rosenheck RA. Risk factors for homelessness among US veterans. Epidemiol Rev 2015;37(1):177–95.

44. Hamilton AB, Poza I, Washington DL. Homelessness and trauma go hand-in-hand": Pathways to homelessness among women veterans. Wom Health Issues 2011;21(4):S203–9.

45. Forman-Hoffman VL, Mengeling M, Booth BM, et al. Eating disorders, post-traumatic stress, and sexual trauma in women veterans. Mil Med 2012;177(10): 1161–8.

46. Mitchell KS, Rasmusson A, Bartlett B, et al. Eating disorders and associated mental health comorbidities in female veterans. Psychiatr Res 2014;219(3): 589–91.

47. Buchholz LJ, King PR, Wray LO. Rates and correlates of disordered eating among women veterans in primary care. Eat Behav 2018;30:28–34.

48. Mitchell KS, Wolf EJ. PTSD, food addiction, and disordered eating in a sample of primarily older veterans: The mediating role of emotion regulation. Psychiatr Res 2016;243:23–9.

49. Gaviria D, Ammerman A. Eating disorders and disordered eating in servicemen and women: A narrative review. J Clin Psychol 2022. https://doi.org/10.1002/jclp.23424. jclp.23424.

50. Stacy M, Kremer M, Schulkin J. Suicide among women and the role of women's health care providers. Obstet Gynecol Surv 2022;77(5):293–301.

51. Ilgen MA, Bohnert ASB, Ignacio RV, et al. Psychiatric diagnoses and risk of suicide in veterans. Arch Gen Psychiatr 2010;67(11):1152.

52. Nelson SM, Griffin CA, Hein TC, et al. Personality disorder and suicide risk among patients in the veterans affairs health system. Personal Disord Theory Res Treat 2022;13(6):563–71.

53. Serier KN, Vogt D, Pandey S, et al. Analysis of the bidirectional relationships between posttraumatic stress and depression symptoms with physical health functioning in post-9/11 veteran men and women deployed to a war zone. J Psychosom Res 2022;162:111034.

54. Frayne SM, Chiu VY, Iqbal S, et al. Medical care needs of returning veterans with PTSD: Their other burden. J Gen Intern Med 2011;26(1):33–9.

55. Gawron L, Mohanty A, Kaiser J, et al. Impact of deployment on reproductive health in U.S. active-duty servicewomen and veterans. Semin Reprod Med 2018;36(06):361–70.

56. Schnurr PP, Lunney CA, Forshay E, et al. Sexual function outcomes in women treated for posttraumatic stress disorder. J Womens Health 2009;18(10):1549–57.

57. Pulverman CS, Christy AY, Kelly UA. Military sexual trauma and sexual health in women veterans: A systematic review. Sex Med Rev 2019;7(3):393–407.

58. Rosebrock L, Carroll R. Sexual function in female veterans: A review. J Sex Marital Ther 2017;43(3):228–45.

59. Zelkowitz RL, Archibald EA, Gradus JL, et al. Postdeployment mental health concerns and family functioning in veteran men and women. Psychol Trauma Theory Res Pract Policy 2022;15(4):705–14.

60. Creech SK, Swift R, Zlotnick C, et al. Combat exposure, mental health, and relationship functioning among women veterans of the Afghanistan and Iraq wars. J Fam Psychol 2016;30(1):43–51.

61. Lawrence KA, Vogt D, Nigam S, et al. Temporal sequencing of mental health symptom severity and suicidal ideation in post-9/11 men and women veterans who recently separated from the military. Chronic Stress 2021;5. https://doi.org/10.1177/24705470211061347. 247054702110613.

62. Smith BN, Taverna EC, Fox AB, et al. The role of PTSD, depression, and alcohol misuse symptom severity in linking deployment stressor exposure and post-military work and family outcomes in male and female veterans. Clin Psychol Sci 2017;5(4):664–82.

63. Lawrence KA, Vogt D, Dugan AJ, et al. Mental health and psychosocial functioning in recently separated U.S. women veterans: Trajectories and bidirectional relationships. Int J Environ Res Publ Health 2021;18(3):935.

64. Vogt D, King MW, Borowski S, et al. Identifying factors that contribute to military veterans' post-military well-being. Appl Psychol Health Well-Being 2021;13(2):341–56.

65. Mendlowicz MV, Stein MB. Quality of life in individuals with anxiety disorders. Am J Psychiatry 2000;157(5):669–82.

66. Galovski TE, McLean CP, Davis CA, et al. Psychosocial treatments for PTSD. In: Friedman MJ, Keane TM, Schnurr PP, editors. Handbook of PTSD: science & practice. 3rd edition. New York, NY: Guilford Press; 2021. p. 330–59.

67. Todd G, Branch R, editors. Evidence-based treatment for anxiety disorders and depression: a cognitive behavioral therapy compendium. 1st edition. Cambridge University Press; 2022.

68. Hollon SD, Dimidjian S. Cognitive and behavioral treatment of depression. In: Gotlib IH, Hammen CL, editors. Handbook of depression. New York, NY: Guilford Press; 2014. p. 513–31.

69. Cuthbert K, Hardin S, Zelkowitz R, et al. Eating disorders and overweight/obesity in veterans: Prevalence, risk factors, and treatment considerations. Curr Obes Rep 2020;9(2):98–108.

70. Department of Veterans Affairs, Department of Defense. VA/DoD clinical practice guideline for the management of substance use disorders, 2021, 187. Available at: https://www.va.gov/vetdata/docs/specialreports/women_veterans_2015_final.pdf. Accessed May 15, 2023.

71. Snyder DK, Halford WK. Evidence-based couple therapy: current status and future directions: Evidence-based couple therapy. J Fam Ther 2012;34(3):229–49.

72. Meis LA, Griffin JM, Greer N, et al. Couple and family involvement in adult mental health treatment: A systematic review. Clin Psychol Rev 2013;33(2):275–86.

73. Kelly U, Haywood T, Segell E, et al. Trauma-sensitive yoga for post-traumatic stress disorder in women veterans who experienced military sexual trauma: Interim results from a randomized controlled trial. J Altern Complement Med 2021;27(S1). https://doi.org/10.1089/acm.2020.0417. S-45-S-59.

74. Niles BL, Mori DL, Polizzi C, et al. A systematic review of randomized trials of mind-body interventions for PTSD. J Clin Psychol 2018;74(9):1485–508.

75. Cloitre M, Koenen KC, Cohen LR, et al. Skills training in affective and interpersonal regulation followed by exposure: A phase-based treatment for PTSD related to childhood abuse. J Consult Clin Psychol 2002;70(5):1067–74.

76. Kimerling R, Bastian LA, Bean-Mayberry BA, et al. Patient-centered mental health care for female veterans. Psychiatr Serv 2015;66(2):155–62.

77. Runnals JJ, Garovoy N, McCutcheon SJ, et al. Systematic review of women veterans' mental health. Wom Health Issues 2014;24(5):485–502.

78. Yano EM, Haskell S, Hayes P. Delivery of gender-sensitive comprehensive primary care to women veterans: Implications for VA patient aligned care teams. J Gen Intern Med 2014;29(S2):703–7.

79. Department of Veterans Affairs. Study of Barriers for Women Veterans to VA Health Care.; 2015. https://www.womenshealth.va.gov/docs/Womens%20Health%20Services_Barriers%20to%20Care%20Final%20Report_April2015.pdf.

80. Tsai J, Mota NP, Pietrzak RHUS. female veterans who do and do not rely on VA health care: Needs and barriers to mental health treatment. Psychiatr Serv 2015;66(11):1200–6.

81. Farmer CC, Rossi FS, Michael EM, et al. Psychotherapy utilization, preferences, and retention among women veterans with post-traumatic stress disorder. Wom Health Issues 2020;30(5):366–73.

82. Chen CK, Palfrey A, Shreck E, et al. Implementation of Telemental Health (TMH) psychological services for rural veterans at the VA New York Harbor Healthcare System. Psychol Serv 2021;18(1):1–10.

83. Wright EC, Wachen JS, Yamokoski CA, et al. Clinical and administrative insights from delivering massed trauma-focused therapy to service members and veterans. Cogn Behav Pract. Published online, in press.

84. Gutner CA, Pedersen ER, Drummond SPA. Going direct to the consumer: Examining treatment preferences for veterans with insomnia, PTSD, and depression. Psychiatr Res 2018;263:108–14.

85. Goldstein AN. Women are the most visible servicemembers, and the most invisible veterans. Center for a new American security. 2018. https://www.cnas.org/publications/reports/women-are-the-most-visible-soldiers-and-the-most-invisible-veterans. Accessed October 28, 2022.

86. Galovski TE, Street AE, McCaughey VK, et al. WoVeN, the Women Veterans Network: an innovative peer support program for women veterans. J Gen Intern Med 2022;37(S3):842–7.

87. Kilpatrick DG, Best CL, Smith DW, Kudler H, Cornelison-Grant V. Serving Those Who Have Served: Educational Needs of Health Care Providers Working with Military Members, Veterans, and Their Families.; 2011. https://www.mirecc.va.gov/docs/visn6/serving_those_who_have_served.pdf.

88. Burgo-Black AL, Brown JL, Boyce RM, et al. The importance of taking a military history. Public Health Rep 2016;131(5):711–3.

89. Richards LK, Bui E, Charney M, et al. Treating veterans and military families: Evidence based practices and training needs among community clinicians. Community Ment Health J 2017;53(2):215–23.

90. U.S. Department of Veterans Affairs. VA/DoD clinical practice guidelines. Published 2022. https://www.healthquality.va.gov/index.asp. Accessed October 28, 2022.

91. Lehavot K, Beckman KL, Chen JA, et al. Race/ethnicity and sexual orientation disparities in mental health, sexism, and social support among women veterans. Psychol Sex Orientat Gend Divers 2019;6(3):347–58.

Moving?

Make sure your subscription moves with you!

To notify us of your new address, find your **Clinics Account Number** (located on your mailing label above your name), and contact customer service at:

Email: journalscustomerservice-usa@elsevier.com

800-654-2452 (subscribers in the U.S. & Canada)
314-447-8871 (subscribers outside of the U.S. & Canada)

Fax number: 314-447-8029

Elsevier Health Sciences Division
Subscription Customer Service
3251 Riverport Lane
Maryland Heights, MO 63043

*To ensure uninterrupted delivery of your subscription, please notify us at least 4 weeks in advance of move.

Printed and bound by CPI Group (UK) Ltd, Croydon, CR0 4YY

03/10/2024

01040468-0009